ADOLESCENT PSYCHIATRY

DEVELOPMENTAL AND CLINICAL STUDIES

VOLUME X

Annals of the American Society for Adolescent Psychiatry

ADOLESCENT PSYCHIATRY

DEVELOPMENTAL AND CLINICAL STUDIES

VOLUME X

Edited by
SHERMAN C. FEINSTEIN
JOHN G. LOONEY
ALLAN Z. SCHWARTZBERG
ARTHUR D. SOROSKY

The University of Chicago Press
Chicago and London

The University of Chicago Press, Chicago 60637
The University of Chicago Press, Ltd., London

© 1982 by The University of Chicago
All rights reserved. Published 1982
Printed in the United States of America

International Standard Book Number: 0-226-24056-8
Library of Congress Catalog Card Number: 70-147017

CONTENTS

PART III. PSYCHOPATHOLOGICAL ASPECTS OF
ADOLESCENT DEVELOPMENT

AFFECTIVE DISORDERS IN CHILDREN AND ADOLESCENTS
CLARICE J. KESTENBAUM, Special Editor

PART IV. THE ADOLESCENT, THE FAMILY, AND THE
HOSPITAL

EDWARD R. SHAPIRO, Special Editor

PART V. PSYCHOTHERAPEUTIC ISSUES IN ADOLESCENT
PSYCHIATRY

IN MEMORIAM
Selma H. Fraiberg
1918–1981

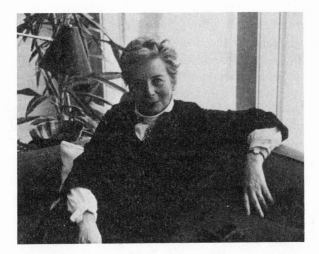

Selma Fraiberg was a gifted psychotherapist, teacher, researcher, writer, and humanist. Originally trained in social work, she refined her clinical skills with psychoanalytic training and developed a special interest in early childhood development. She first achieved national acclaim with the publication of *The Magic Years* (1959), in which she not only displayed a unique capacity to enter the inner world of the child but also revealed the rare gift of being able to communicate the essence of psychoanalytic developmental theory in a clear yet scientifically accurate fashion. Her later major works included *Insights from the Blind* (1977), *Every Child's Birthright: In Defense of Mothering* (1977), and *The First Year of Life* (1980).

Born in Detroit, Michigan, in 1918, she was from July 1979 professor of child psychoanalysis at the University of California, San Francisco, after previously serving at the University of Michigan and Tulane University. At the University of Michigan she was director of the Child Development Project, supervisor of child psychoanalysis at the Michigan Psychoanalytic Institute, and became professor emeritus of child psychoanalysis in 1980. Professor Fraiberg died in December 1981, after a brief illness, from metastatic cancer.

Those who were privileged to hear her William A. Schonfeld Distinguished Service Award lecture on "The Adolescent Mother and Her Infant" at the annual meeting of the American Society for Adolescent Psychiatry, May 1981, were deeply impressed, not only with the clarity and quality of her presentation, the accuracy of her research design, but also with the deep sense of caring, commitment, and patience that she brought to her work with very deprived and depressed adolescent mothers, struggling for their own sense of autonomy. She emphasized the need for adequate support and education for these teenaged mothers before the therapist could deal with earlier developmental conflicts associated with problems of attachment and detachment.

Selma Fraiberg's death was untimely and a great loss to the whole field of child and adolescent psychiatry. This volume is dedicated to her memory.

PREFACE

With the completion of ten volumes of *Adolescent Psychiatry,* a summing up is in order. The coordinating editor will retire with this issue,
an act of generativity according to Erik Erikson, an act which should
encourage productivity and creativity.

On looking back, the original editors (Sherman C. Feinstein, Peter L.
Giovacchini, and Arthur A. Miller) noted that there was increasing
psychiatric interest in adolescence as a stage of life stemming from
several sources: the need for the utilization of specialized therapeutic
techniques, the further understanding of growth and development, and
the impact of adolescents on the world. These ideas have proved to be
critical interest areas, and an examination of the contents of the *Annals
of the American Society for Adolescent Psychiatry* shows the impact of
youth on all levels of our culture and the diversity of the authors who
have written about adolescence (the greatest reward).

For the future, it is comforting to know that Max Sugar will assume the editorship assisted by an editorial group of the highest devotion. What form the publication will take is speculative but certainly
the emergence of increasing research in adolescent development, psy-
chophysiology, and psychopharmacology will be influential.

Many friends have contributed to my editorship over the years, and I
am immeasurably indebted to them for their support and criticisms. A
few names must be mentioned: Arthur Rosenthal, Roy R. Grinker, Sr.,
Daniel Offer, Serge Lebovici, E. James Anthony, Mary Staples, and
Deborah Spector.

SHERMAN C. FEINSTEIN

PART I

ADOLESCENCE:
GENERAL
CONSIDERATIONS

EDITORS' INTRODUCTION

A crucial developmental task for all adolescents is the achievement of healthy separation-individuation leading to establishment of a stable ego identity. Identity formation is significantly affected not only by early identifications but also by multiple social, vocational, and sexual factors along with basic ego endowment and ego adaptive capacity. The chapters in this part range from the developmental conflicts resulting in early adolescent pregnancy and parenthood to the vicissitudes of adolescents coping with adaptation to work as well as the devastating effect of loss of employment. Specialized problems are explored in a large group of adolescents who experienced great stress in having to hide a felt sense of homosexual identity as well as a much smaller and unique group of adolescents who struggle and identify with Holocaust survivor parents presenting with unresolved issues of grief, guilt, separation, and loss.

Selma Fraiberg in her William A. Schonfeld Distinguished Service Award lecture describes some clinical observations of a group of young mothers struggling with formidable developmental conflicts of adolescence along with their new and uncertain identity as mother to an infant. The girls and their families were locked together in morbid conflict, and the attachment and detachment problems of the mother were mirrored in the disorders of attachment seen in the babies. Another dimension of conflict was maternal depression which manifested as rejection, neglect, or abuse. Professor Fraiberg presents an example of the treatment approach to such adolescent mothers and concludes that therapeutic work with adolescent mothers and their babies must accommodate objectives for the treatment of both the mother and child.

3

Saul V. Levine reviews the psychological and social effects of youth unemployment and focuses on the repetitive patterns of emotional reactions experienced by this group. He delineates stages in the reaction to loss of job as optimism, ambiguity, and despair, and discusses the boredom, identity diffusion, self-esteem problems, guilt and shame, anxiety and fear, anger, depression, demoralization, and alienation of unemployed young people. Levine proposes an action strategy to deal with this major dilemma in young people in order to give them meaning and a sense of participation.

Lois T. Flaherty examines the complex changes in the quality of female participation in the work force and its impact on psychological developments during adolescence. Material from the psychotherapy of adolescent girls is analyzed to give further insight into the development of attitudes toward future work. Flaherty concludes that the older female adolescent's anxiety related to work may be overlooked or considered to be of less significance than other issues. The importance of work as a means of gaining autonomy is stressed.

A. Damien Martin discusses how the gay person in general and the gay adolescent in particular are stigmatized within our society. He contends that negativism toward homosexuals is primarily a result of prejudicial attitudes (homophobia) that reduce gay people to members of a minority group, cause homosexuals to hide their sexual identity, and deprive the gay adolescent of suitable role models. He explains how the homosexually oriented person is denied social identities, is often forced to hide rather than accept a gay identity, and avoids being discredited by becoming discreditable, with resultant intrapsychic distortion and isolation. Martin believes that negative sensitization can be changed only if young people are exposed to alternatives to prevent stigmatization. He exhorts professionals to work against discriminatory practices.

Rudolph G. Roden and Michelle M. Roden write about the unique aspects of Holocaust survivors and their children—the common bond, the mourning, the impetus toward life as well as death, and their struggle with self-image. The children possess, as their own, the emotions that grew out of their parents' uprooting, persecution, and near extermination. They are burdened by their spoken and unspoken communication that they must provide meaning for their parents' perceived empty life.

The chapters by Levon D. Tashjian and Jon A. Shaw demonstrate the reciprocal contributions of psychoanalytical developmental theory and the study of lives. They provide a framework for the examination and understanding of autobiographic reflections, while the self-revelations represent a useful body of data through which developmental theories can be refined.

Levon D. Tashjian examines the problem of how an adolescent—with a reasonable constitution, environment, and development—arrives at self-definition. He studied James Joyce's *Portrait of the Artist as a Young Man,* a literal transcript of the first twenty years of Joyce's life, and describes the surge toward identity formation in terms of the separation-individuation process. He also explores those critical nodal points necessary for any adolescent to integrate diverse experiences into an inner psychic vision in terms of epiphany, a galvanizing force that illuminates and enlightens.

Jon A. Shaw, using autobiographical material of John Stuart Mill, explores a profound postadolescent crisis in terms of intrinsic conflicts of adolescence and those particular tasks whose resolution is required for the consolidation of mature character formation. Specifically, he discusses Mill's struggles to loosen his infantile ties, to consolidate a sexual identity, to establish an enduring sense of identity, and to master an infantile trauma.

Aaron H. Esman discusses Levon D. Tashjian's and Jon A. Shaw's chapters and emphasizes the creativity and productivity of their subjects, whose characters were both shaped by a relationship with a powerful father. He explores the occurrence of moments of revelation which serve as crucial self-organizers during adolescence. Esman concludes that most young people must settle for a gradual reshaping of the ego ideal, reorganization of identification systems, and adaptation of early superego rigidities to the demands of life in the real world.

Hyman L. Muslin examines the tragedy of *Romeo and Juliet* from a self-psychology perspective. He sees Shakespeare's play as illustrating the fatal results of unempathic self-absorption by the lovers' parents. The adolescents, Romeo and Juliet, are viewed as instances of a self/selfobject unit in formation. Muslin discusses the reluctance and ambivalence around confronting self/selfobject ties and achieving selfhood as a fundamental part of adolescent development.

1 THE ADOLESCENT MOTHER AND HER INFANT

SELMA FRAIBERG

In this chapter I will describe our work with adolescent mothers and their infants in an infant psychiatry program. I have gathered together some of our clinical observations of a group of young mothers struggling with formidable developmental conflicts of adolescence and their new and uncertain identity as mother to an infant. Later I will describe our treatment of one sixteen-year-old, severely depressed mother and her failure-to-thrive infant.

As the basis for this presentation I have chosen a group of ten babies and their eight adolescent mothers who constituted a subgroup in our intensive treatment case load in our University of Michigan program during the period from November 1972 to October 1978. The ten babies represented 20 percent of our intensive treatment case load of fifty. Since the only criteria for entering our intensive treatment program were our assessment of need for this form of treatment and the practical limitations of a small staff, it is important to note that teenage mothers constituted a substantial number of those we had identified as severely impaired in critical areas of functioning.

Characteristics of the Group

The ages of the mothers at the time of delivery ranged from sixteen to eighteen. Five were unmarried girls. Of the three mothers who were married, one was separated from her husband. The five fathers in the

William A. Schonfeld Distinguished Service Award Address presented at the annual meeting of the American Society for Adolescent Psychiatry, New Orleans, May 1981.

never-married group are unknown to us and, in fact, broke connections with the girls soon after pregnancy was confirmed. They appear in our records as nameless, faceless partners in casual encounters.

Seven of the ten babies were firstborn. All of the babies were full term with birth weights within the normal range. Congenital defects were later identified in three of the children. All of the mothers were living in poverty. The five unmarried mothers were supported by welfare services. In nearly all cases the young mother was living apart from her family of origin, and encounters with the extended family were caught up in conflict and turmoil. There was no psychological support for mother and baby nor were there traditions of child rearing to guide a young girl who was unready for motherhood.

The five unmarried mothers were attending school or were enrolled in job training. Their babies were being cared for in day-care centers or family day care. Mainly, the day-care arrangements, which we ourselves could assess through visiting, were poor and offered little more than custodial care. In three cases there was outright neglect of infants. As we came to know the babies and their families, we were sobered by the fact that the child, endangered by the considerable pathology in the mother and already showing signs of a severe attachment disorder, was further endangered by the circumstances in which he received indifferent or neglectful substitute-mother care. The baby who needed an optimal day-care program was receiving substitute care of the poorest quality.

The babies and their mothers had been referred to us by physicians, nurses, and social workers in Washtenaw County (population approximately 300,000). The babies of teenage mothers were, as a group, among the most severely impaired children in our case load. A primary attachment disorder was present at the time of referral in each case. Four of the babies had been hospitalized for failure to thrive. The teenage mothers, as a group, showed grave impairment in psychological functioning and were virtually incapacitated in mothering a baby. Although they had been labeled by their community as "neglectful" and "rejecting," none of them had been evaluated by a psychiatric team before coming into our program. Ideally, we would like to see a psychosocial assessment of the teenage mother in every case at the point where the pregnancy is first identified by the health-care provider. After our own diagnostic study, six of the eight mothers were seen by us as severely depressed. Depression in each of these cases had been present for many months and even years before the baby was conceived. In fact, as I shall later discuss, depression and the unsatisfied psychological hungers which were entwined with depression had found their way into longing for a baby.

Developmental Conflicts of Adolescent Motherhood

When I speak of the interlocking developmental conflicts of adolescence and motherhood that we saw in this group of young girls, I should preface these remarks with some caution. Clearly, the severely disordered teenage mothers in our case load do not represent the larger population of teenage mothers, in which we can find a fair amount of adequate or excellent mothering. The adolescent and mothering conflicts which we encountered are not typical but are exaggerated and heightened conflicts in which universal problems of adolescent maturation become distorted by disorder in the adolescent personality and the inability of the primary family of the girl to provide the vital pathways to resolution of conflict. The girls and their families, in our cases, were locked together in a morbid conflict.

The diagnostic study and treatment of this group of young mothers and their infants brought into focus the interlocking conflicts of adolescent development and mother-infant relationships. Each of these mothers had become pregnant at a point in psychological development when attachment and detachment from the primary family figures had produced conflicts of considerable magnitude. The unresolved conflicts of adolescence became the focus of new conflicts which embraced the child. The attachment and detachment problems of the mother were mirrored in the disorders of attachment that we saw in the baby.

The baby was caught up in the morbid past and uncertain present of his mother. But he was also, most poignantly, the symbol of hope and self-renewal in his mother. Each of the unmarried girls had examined the alternatives of abortion and adoption and had chosen to keep the baby. They wanted their babies and kept them against the wishes of their own parents. In each case, the baby, when we met him, was manifestly neglected and showed impoverishment in all areas of human attachment. The contradiction between the adolescent mother's daydreams for the baby and the actual state of the baby needed to be understood.

As we came to know these adolescent mothers, we saw how many of the typical conflicts of adolescence had become intensified and magnified for each of these girls before they became pregnant. Their own mothers were at the center of these conflicts. By the time we came to know them, these conflicts appeared to consume the life energies of each. In normal adolescence we may see the love-hate conflicts of the girl surface in daily life, but after the storm the beloved aspects of the mother can be reclaimed. What is preserved and eventually consolidated in the course of adolescence becomes available for positive identification and integration of personality in late adolescence. But among the young girls in our group, the mother as enemy and betrayer dominated the theater of conflict. There appeared to be no aspect of this mother that could serve maturation and identification. It also seemed to us that the mothers of these girls had become the unwitting collaborators in this tense family drama, transforming themselves into the enemy, so that the fantasy mother and the real mother sometimes merged.

Side by side with these consuming struggles with the mother was dependency in the girl and a longing for nurturance from the mother, which was explicitly brought to us in their stories and reenacted in transference with the therapist. Often, when the therapist was visiting the young mother and her baby in the home, there were two crying children in that living room.

The unresolved maternal conflicts of the girl became impediments to mothering and to the attachment of the girl to her baby. A girl who is fighting against her tie to her mother, who sees her mother as an enemy without redeeming features, has nothing good or solid to hold onto when she seeks a model for herself as a mother. And a girl who is still longing for a mother, who wants a mother to hold her close and nourish her, is not ready to become a mother herself.

Much of the important work that we accomplished in our treatment of these teenage mothers grew out of our exploration of the mother conflicts which were paralyzing the girl in her own psychological development. We examined the love-hate relationships to the mother, as they were described to us and as they were reenacted in transference to the therapist. We provided, through our treatment, a form of psychological nurturance for hungry girls. We offered a relationship in which independence could grow out of dependency. Affection and trust for the therapist could provide the conditions for new identifications with an adult figure and alternative models for mothering. The listening and understanding which the therapist gave the young mother could be transformed into listening to and understanding a baby. Again and again, in our records, the therapist is in a room with a crying mother and a neglected and crying baby. The therapist offers words of comfort to the mother and the mother turns to the crying baby as if she has heard him for the first time.

The adolescent girl's father, as he was described to us and revealed through the eyes of the girl, was also at the center of love-hate conflicts. We expect that in the normal adolescent process the girl's attachment to her father is gradually modified, that the oedipal wishes and fantasies are transformed, and that resolution paves the way to the discovery of new partners in love. Among the adolescent mothers in our group, the childhood daydream of father love had been preserved and was reenacted with male partners who appeared as transient lovers—if, indeed, the word "lovers" should be used.

Since the attachment to the father was still primary, there was no possibility of forming an enduring bond with another male partner. Typically, among our girls, sexual activity had begun at the age of thirteen or fourteen. The sexual partners were distantly remembered and seemed to have no more substantiality than figures in a fantasy. And, in fact, the sexual experiences resembled fantasies in which each partner was interchangeable with the other, like the masturbation fantasies of early adolescence. What was acted out in these transient sexual episodes was the fantasy of forbidden and dangerous love, a transparent oedipal fantasy. When pregnancy occurred, the unconscious childhood fantasy of having a baby with the father added another psychological dimension to a crisis, and the baby, when he arrived, became the embodiment of a shameful secret, a "child of sin," in the old-fashioned phrase.

The baby was also the child of a profound disappointment, the result of a promise that was not kept by whoever it is in our society who makes promises to the young. In the hyped-up sexual climate of our times, it is easy for the young to believe that puberty carries a passport into sexual bliss. But not one of the young girls in our group had experienced sexual pleasure of any kind in her many encounters. In fact, the serial encounters were motivated by the search for sexual joy. "It'll be different with the next fellow." But it never was. These girls were, in fact, unready for sexual fulfillment, like the majority of adolescents in their early and mid teens. But clearly, for the girl who is still pursuing a childhood fantasy love with her father, there is no place yet for a new partner and uninhibited sexual joy. The father love becomes the inhibitor.

The father love also becomes an impediment to motherhood. A girl

11

who is still playing out an unconscious childhood fantasy of make-believe love and make-believe union with her father is likely to continue this fantasy as a make-believe mother with a make-believe baby. And this, in fact, is what we saw when we first met the mothers and babies in our group. Motherhood was somehow unreal; the baby was not quite real.

In our infant-focused psychotherapy, we listened to the tangled stories of fathers and lovers and helped the adolescent mother to find new solutions to old griefs and old longings. As we watched the mother and her baby together in session after session, we were attentive to those aspects of the baby and of mothering which were caught up in the old daydream. Where the baby was somehow unreal, and motherhood was unreal, we could make them real. This was not a fantasy baby to us; he was a person with all the unique qualities of his own personality. She was not a pretend mother to us; she was a real mother with real concerns for her baby and real problems. We played with this real baby and revealed his marvelous attributes to his mother. We talked to the real mother and most respectfully gave her the authority and prestige of mother. She was not a child to us, innocent and blundering, but a mother trying very hard to be a mother in the midst of terrible hardship.

The unresolved conflicts of childhood embraced every aspect of the childhood family. Repeatedly, in our work with adolescent mothers, we saw intense sibling conflicts reenacted with the baby. Jealousy toward the baby, competition with the baby, anger toward the baby, and the feeling of being robbed of something precious by the baby were recurring themes which we could trace back in treatment to a sibling who had been a rival in childhood. Normally in adolescence, the sibling conflicts of childhood undergo resolution along with other early and intensive love-hate relationships of the family. When the adolescent process has not been completed through maturation, the old jealousies and hostilities stand ready for transference to other objects. Tragically, in the case of teenage motherhood the new baby may come to represent the old rivals in the family of childhood.

In our work with the adolescent mother, we examined those ways in which the baby was caught up in old memories and the conflicts of the childhood family of the mother. We helped the mother to disentangle her baby from the figures of childhood and free the baby from the ghosts in the maternal past.

The inventory of unresolved adolescent conflicts in motherhood should include conflicts between self-love and love of others. Adolescence is normally a period in which self-love appears in heightened forms. The egocentricity and narcissism of the adolescent are, under all normal circumstances, only headaches that parents and teachers need to live with for a while. But when the adolescent becomes a parent, the self-love and self-centered goals come into conflict with the needs of a baby and the requirements of parenthood. A mother needs to put the child's needs before her own needs and is able to do this when psychological maturation has given her the possibility of subjugating self-interest and self-love in the interest of a child. The adolescent girl who has not completed this maturational step finds herself strained, or actually incapable, at times, of ministering to the ordinary needs of a helpless baby.

It is this colossal narcissism in the young that evokes anger in the parent generation. When the adolescent is also a mother, the self-centeredness of the mother united with neglect of her infant evokes anger in those who are called upon to help her. By the time we met our young mothers, they had been scolded by public health nurses, doctors, and social workers and grimly prepared themselves for a scolding from us. They seemed surprised, but certainly relieved, when no scolding awaited them.

Narcissism in parenthood, it strikes us, has two faces. There is the self-love that can endanger the child, and there is the self-love that can embrace the child. There is a large measure of healthy narcissism that goes into the parenting of many good and normal people. The baby is the most remarkable baby in the world. He's a genius, if we have to say it ourselves. Every achievement, even his first tooth, is somehow a credit to us, as parents. All this, the healthy narcissism, is available to the teenage parent, too. We began to see it happen in our work. As the baby began to thrive and reward his mother for her efforts, he became, for his young mother, a marvel, a precocious child, destined for a brilliant future.

From this brief summary, we can see how the intense unresolved conflicts of adolescence become psychological obstacles to the nurturance of a child and may, in fact, provide a theater in which the baby is caught up in the reevoked childhood griefs and disappointments of the mother. In our group, however, there was still another dimension of conflict which exerted its morbid influence upon the baby, and this was maternal depression.

Six of the eight adolescent mothers were suffering from severe and incapacitating depression. If these girls had not been mothers, they would have required intensive psychotherapy and, in two cases, might have required hospitalization for depression-related anorexia. While these young mothers had been labeled by their communities as rejecting, neglectful, or abusive toward their children, our clinical inquiry led us to understand that these were young girls who were barely able to function. In each case, the depression had antedated pregnancy and the birth of the child by many months and even years. Since each of these girls had considered the alternatives of abortion and adoption, the decision of these depressed young girls to keep their babies needed to be understood. What did the baby represent? In the course of our work we began to understand. In the hopelessness of depression the baby represented hope and renewal, the chance to live another life through the baby of fantasy. The hunger for love in the adolescent and the unsatisfied hungers seen in depression found the dream of a baby's love. And not only love, we saw, as we began to unravel the complex meanings of the baby. Periodically, in the course of treatment, the depressed young girl would speak of feelings of emptiness and a yearning for something to fill the emptiness. And, as we moved back into the historical events that had led to pregnancy and the decision to keep the baby, we began to understand. The yearnings for a baby seemed linked to an imperative need to fill the emptiness.

The baby, being a baby, could not fill the emptiness for needy and hungry girl-mothers. The baby, in fact, was a disappointment. Neither did the baby bring self-renewal or the fulfillment of old dreams. More likely, the bad dreams of childhood were reevoked by him. The baby had become the center of morbid conflicts by the time we met him.

The Babies: Disorders of Attachment

It is time to talk about the babies. In each of these cases the baby had come to us because of severe disorders of attachment. Here, I am not generalizing to the larger population of infants of teenage mothers. We must remember that, as a psychiatric clinic, we were preselected by referring agencies for our expertise in the area of attachment disorders. The babies, as a group, were among the most severely impaired children in our case load. They were joyless, listless babies, who showed virtually none of the age-appropriate signs of attachment to the mothers, or who had a limited repertoire of attachment behaviors along with a constricted range of affect. Four of the ten babies were referred to us following diagnosis of failure to thrive.

As we follow the links between the adolescent conflicts of the mothers in our group and the disorders of attachment we identified in their babies, we can see how every component of the unresolved adolescent conflicts became an impediment to the attachment of mother to baby and baby to mother. Where resolution of childhood conflicts paves the way for parenthood and identification with one's own parents, nonresolution brings unreadiness, disappointment, and a turning away from the baby or the investment of the baby with the love-hate conflicts of the mother's own childhood. Where self-love is still dominant in adolescent psychology, there cannot be the selfless love of a parent. And when we add to this inventory of adolescent afflictions the severe depressions we encountered among the mothers in our group, it appears as if everything in the parental personality is negating the possibility of attachment.

Yet this is by no means a hopeless picture for therapy. Remarkably, when we consider the psychopathology we saw in mothers and babies, we found that we were able to engage each of these mothers in work on behalf of their babies and themselves, and the therapeutic gains were substantial in all but one case.

CLINICAL ILLUSTRATION

The case of sixteen-year-old Karen and her baby, Nina, illustrates many of the interlocking disturbances of mother and baby.[1] It also illustrates our methods of diagnostic study and the formulation of treatment alternatives which grow out of the initial assessment.

No case can stand by itself in illustrating the clinical picture that we saw in our case load of teenage mothers and their babies. However, the case of Karen and Nina demonstrates many of the characteristics of our larger group. Nina, the seven-month-old baby, is referred to us following hospital diagnosis of "nonorganic failure to thrive due to maternal deprivation."

At birth, Nina had been a full-term healthy baby, birth weight six pounds one ounce (tenth percentile) and height twenty inches (seventy-fifth percentile). At the time of hospitalization for failure to thrive, Nina's weight had dropped to below the third percentile and height had fallen to below the twenty-fifth percentile. Medical study revealed no organic cause for failure to thrive, and the referring pediatrician and nurses concluded that growth failure was caused by severe maternal deprivation.

Her sixteen-year-old mother is unmarried and attending high

school. The mother is described as neglectful and unable to cooperate with physicians and nurses who have offered their help. When
we meet the mother and baby, we see a young mother who is
suffering with a severe depression and a depression-related
anorexia which has antedated the birth of the baby by several years.
Karen, the mother, weighs approximately eighty-five pounds. Food
is repulsive to her, she tells us, and she eats barely enough for
sustenance. She knows the doctors are concerned about Nina, but
she is not sure why. Nina looks chubby to her, she says.

Karen and Nina are supported by welfare services. They are
living in the home of the maternal grandparents in the midst of
domestic chaos. There are violent quarrels between Karen's
mother and father with periodic separations. Karen and Nina are
given grudging shelter in this home. Nina is unwanted. Karen is
taunted daily by her parents for bringing a baby into this home. No
help is offered Karen. Karen would like to find another place to live,
but she is afraid to live alone. She is a child herself, of course. The
grandparents themselves are hostile to the treatment offered Karen
and Nina. They will not permit us to visit the home. If Karen wants
our help she will have to see us at our office. With all these constraints we will need to provide treatment for this endangered baby
and her mother.

In the course of the initial evaluation period, we are asking
ourselves many questions. The developmental testing of Nina will
give us a fair assessment of the motor and cognitive development of
Nina and the areas of deficit. But the test will not help us to discern
the qualities of infant-mother relationship. In our observations, we
want to look for the age-appropriate indicators of human attachment in the baby, the ability of the mother to respond to the range of
signs and signals which a baby can send to the mother, and the
ability of the mother to initiate and exchange social and affectionate
signs with her baby.

In our initial observations we see a severely depressed young
mother and her child who is suffering from growth failure and a
severe attachment disorder. The depression of the mother is mirrored in the baby's face. The baby is silent, stares off into space,
uninvested in her surroundings. She rarely turns to her mother for a
social exchange or for comfort. In our broader observations, we see
a limited number of attachment indicators. There is discrimination
of her mother from others, there is preference for her mother. Nina

has a limited repertoire of attachment behaviors, but they are muted and joyless. Similarly, Karen shows some signs of affection for her baby, but she sinks back into depression and solitude after each exertion.

As we look at the depressed and anorectic mother, we also look at our own therapeutic dilemma. Karen cannot read the signs of hunger and satiation in herself; how can she read the signs of hunger and satiation in her baby? In fact, in every observation during this assessment period of seven sessions, Karen seems unable to read hunger in Nina, or she misreads the signs.

Ideally, we would want our therapy to focus on the interlocking aspects of Karen's depression and her baby's attachment disorder. But soon after treatment begins, we find ourselves facing a formidable therapeutic problem. If the therapist begins to speak about feelings with Karen, to speak of sadness or anger, to touch ever so gently on the defenses against affect, Karen's depression deepens and her symptoms are exacerbated.

Clearly, we cannot yet deal with Karen's internal and objective conflicts without precipitating a grave conflict in personality and worsening the situation for Karen and Nina. We decide, then, that we will work with Karen and Nina, for the indefinite future, within the context of supportive treatment and developmental guidance. This treatment brings about very substantial changes for Karen and Nina.

Our treatment focused on both the nutritional and psychological aspects of Nina's and Karen's interlocking conflicts. But both aspects of this treatment were solidly embedded in the context of human attachments. On the nutritional side, we worked with Karen and the nursery in providing an optimal diet for Nina. Karen and the nursery staff were helped to see how a baby's pleasure in eating was intimately related to pleasure in the arms of a partner, most particularly the mother. Karen was encouraged to take over the lunch feedings in the nursery as often as possible. One or, at most, two aides at the nursery were assigned as Nina's special caregivers.

In our own sessions, with Karen and Nina and the therapist together in our playroom, the therapy focused on the relationship between Nina and Karen, emphasizing in every way possible how Karen was the most important person in the world to her baby, how no one, not even the therapist, could get the special smiles or comfort Nina in distress as well as her mother could. Karen, who had never in her life believed she was important or special to anyone, was deeply touched as she learned to recognize these signs of preference and love in her baby. And Nina, like all babies, gave generous rewards to her mother. Within four months of work, Nina made tremendous progress toward nutritional and psychological adequacy.

Karen, watching the therapist talk to Nina, was initially puzzled. After all, Nina could not understand English. Karen had no traditions in her family for talking to a baby, or, indeed, for conferring personality on a baby. As Karen watched her therapist, she saw that Nina began to make responsive sounds, and it was easy for the therapist to begin to speak about how babies learn to talk. Within a short time, mother-baby dialogues appeared in all of our sessions, and the quiet baby who never uttered a sound became positively garrulous.

Karen's conflicts with her own parents gave her no models for parenting. Her own mother did not like babies and considered a baby who cried as "just plain spoiled." Her own mother did not believe that a baby of Nina's age cared who took care of her. Mothers were not important. Karen's therapist listened to Karen and Nina with most respectful attention to each. To understand why Nina cried or what Nina was trying to tell us became central to every session. To understand Karen's sadness, inarticulate cries, and griefs was equally central to the sessions. Karen was profoundly touched by her therapist's concern for her, her listening, her sympathy, her praise, and her confidence in Karen. No one had ever cared for her in this way. Later she told the therapist how much this caring had meant to her. Karen, whose own griefs were listened to, then became a mother who could listen, in every sense of the word, to her child's cries and the everyday griefs of a small girl. She began to understand Nina's pain at separation from her each day at the door of the nursery. She had no alternatives in care for Nina, but she could now find words of sympathy and understanding for Nina which made the pain bearable. In short, what Karen received in emotional sustenance from her therapist, she could now give to her own baby.

At fourteen months of age Nina had reached weight adequacy. She also achieved adequacy in our affective-social evaluation and made substantial gains in cognitive motor development. Our health evaluation showed that Nina had gained weight steadily in these seven months. Her weight was now nineteen pounds, which placed her between the tenth and twenty-fifth percentiles. She was bright-eyed, animated, strong, active, and had good color and muscle tone. (She sustained these gains in later years.)

In the affective-social areas which had been seriously affected by the time we first met her at seven months, Nina was now age adequate. She had a good range of affective expression. She had strong and stable ties to her mother, with strong preference for and valuation of her mother (as we saw in social situations as well as need states). Her pleasure in being with her mother was manifest through warm and special smiles for her, animated "conversations" with her mother, and seeking her mother to share special moments and to touch base with her. She showed age-appropriate reactions to the daily separations from her mother at the nursery. She protested but then settled down (with resignation) to the less than ideal circumstances provided by this substitute care.

There were advances in cognitive motor development. At fourteen months she scored an MDI on the Bayley of 133. Her first testing at seven months had actually placed her within normal range (110), but now we could see that Nina's potential in mental development was higher than average. The gains reflected to some measure the tremendous progress in language development which was one result of our work.

During this period we saw Karen develop into a responsible and affectionate mother. It is important, however, to keep in mind that Karen was still a seriously depressed girl and was still anorectic. We had already discovered that our treatment of Karen had to be modified because of her inability to tolerate exploration of her profound conflicts (mainly internalized rage). She could not tolerate even the gentlest therapeutic probing of her feelings toward her mother and father, yet found comfort in the understanding and sympathy which the therapist expressed as she listened to the reports of fights between the maternal grandparents, their constant blame of Karen for bringing a baby into this home, and their depreciation of Karen as mother.

Thus our work with Karen was mainly supportive, and the supportive work was united with observations of Nina and developmental guidance. All of this brought significant developmental

19

progress for Nina, as we have seen. And for Karen, too, there was brightening of mood, enhancement of self-image, and new confidence in herself as a mother. But the anorexia remained. Karen could now feed her baby, but she could not feed herself.

In describing the therapeutic approach to Karen, I should say that I am not generalizing about work with adolescents or work with adolescent parents. In nearly every other case we have worked with we were able to deal therapeutically with the inner conflicts of our adolescent parents and to do this fairly early in treatment. Only in Karen's case was such an approach contraindicated.

Actually, we had to wait two more years before Karen's love-hate conflicts toward her parents could be dealt with therapeutically (and, I believe, with great benefit to her). But what we learn from this work is that long before the clinical picture of a mother's disorder can change, there are large possibilities for change in the capacity to mother which can be brought about through supportive treatment and guidance.

Between Nina at age fourteen months and twenty-two months, we continued to work with mother and baby. For Nina, all gains in health and affective and cognitive development were sustained.

At twenty-two months, Nina was a healthy, enthusiastic, buoyant, outgoing child. In nursery school (a new school) she was regarded by her teachers as intelligent, creative, and socially mature for her age. She was well liked by her teachers and her peers. In doll play in our observation sessions we saw Nina as a tender and solicitous mother. She loved feeding and cooking for her dolls. We could not see residues of early oral conflicts.

Karen, herself, was a proud mother. Through guidance she had become a very sensitive and empathic reader of signs and needs in her child. She enjoyed Nina. She was proud of her spunkiness and assertiveness (a vicarious pleasure for a young woman now eighteen years old, who could not yet assert herself with her own parents, except in defending Nina). Some measure of Karen's self-confidence was brought to improved schoolwork and a decision to enroll in a community college after high school graduation.

It was not until the final year of treatment, when Nina was three years old, that Karen's profound conflicts, which centered on the relationship to her own parents, could be dealt with. At last she felt strong enough as a person to allow herself to feel rage and disappointment toward her own parents and to speak of the heartbreaks, the childhood sense of worthlessness, and the fear of parental explosions. The depression lifted. The last vestiges of anorexia disappeared.

Karen's joy in her child had been sustained through our work. But now there was the beginning of pleasure for herself. Karen, at last, was ready to move out of her parental home. She made good plans for herself and Nina and entered a community college technical training program. With the liberation from parental love-hate bonds, Karen fell in love with a stable young man who became devoted to her and to Nina. Within a year after termination of treatment they were married.

Discussion

A single case of an adolescent mother and her baby cannot, of course, illustrate all of the factors which I have identified as characteristics of the unresolved conflicts of adolescence which impinge on motherhood.

What we can see in the case of Karen and Nina are the effects of profound inner conflicts in adolescence on the capacity to mother a baby. Karen, when we met her, was a child herself, caught in a morbid love-hate conflict with her own parents. Her depression and anorexia spoke for intense internalized rage toward her own parents. The unsatisfied longings and hungers of adolescence had led her to early sexual experience with boys in casual encounters. She became pregnant. And she wanted to keep her baby. When we first met Karen and Nina we saw a starving mother and baby living in the home in which Karen's family gave grudging shelter and neither affection nor support to their child or their grandchild. If we give clinical attention only to Karen's own adolescent conflicts, the therapeutic task appears a formidable one: the anorexia is severe enough to warrant hospitalization. Depression has depleted Karen's resources. She is barely able to function in school. Failures in love have marked her life from childhood to adolescence, now marked again by the failures in seeking love from boys. There are unresolved oedipal problems in the pursuit of "forbidden love" through transient boys.

But this adolescent, with some ordinary and many extraordinary developmental problems, was a mother. And her baby was in great danger.

Anorexia has distorted Karen's ability to read her own signs of

21

hunger and satiation. Anorexia has blotted out her recognition of hunger and satiation in her infant. Depression, which makes her psychologically absent in all social relationships, has made her psychologically absent to a baby who is in need of mother nurture.

The baby, herself, seems not quite real to Karen when we first meet her. She is uncertainly a mother. She still needs a mother herself. Her own longings for nurture collide at times with the baby's needs for nurture. And the fantasy baby, who would satisfy longings to be loved and the yearning for self-renewal which are universal in adolescence, is after all only a baby with imperative demands and no promise of bringing self-renewal. The baby of fantasy who would fill the emptiness only enlarges the sense of emptiness. At best, if Karen summons all of her meager resources, she can give mechanical care to Nina since Karen has no models for mothering. Her own mother's failure to mother leaves Karen bereft of knowledge and tradition.

We can sketch the treatment for Karen if Karen were not a mother. Many months of intensive work would be required. Hospitalization of Karen might be desirable. But Nina, the baby, is our patient, too. She cannot wait for her mother's depression to lift or for resolution of the complex problems that are bound together in anorexia.

Our work with Karen and Nina focused on the needs of both the baby and the mother. It was a delicate balance to sustain, for Karen, like many adolescent mothers we know, was desperately needy herself. Most sessions were held with both mother and baby in the room. When necessary, private sessions for Karen, herself, were arranged.

Psychotherapy is a form of undoing of the past. And so it was for Karen, too, even though our access to the emotionally laden memories of the past was limited by Karen's own defenses against powerful affects. Where rejection by parents had led to Karen's feelings of worthlessness, the relationship to the therapist could give to Karen a sense of worth as an adolescent and as a mother. Where unsatisfied longings for mother love had led to morbid symptoms, therapy could provide a form of psychological nurturance which sustained the adolescent girl and had the effect of undoing some part of the injuries of the past. Where failures in understanding had marked the relationship with parents, understanding and profound sympathy from a therapist had the effect of healing the old wounds. Where the baby was somehow "a child of sin" with echoes from an unremembered past and censorship from the maternal parents, the baby was given, through our work, the rights of every baby to be cherished and to bear no shameful stigma.

Where the baby was a fantasy baby who belonged to an oedipal romance, we helped to make her a real baby, a real person, which had the effect of detaching the baby from childhood conflicts even though we were unable to deal with those fantasies directly. And long before we were able to deal with the inner conflicts of Karen in our treatment, Nina, herself, began to fulfill her mother's adolescent dream of renewal of self, a rebirth through giving birth to a child. Nina, through our work, became a loving, intelligent, social person who gave her mother huge rewards for motherhood. The mother who could not love herself or value herself when we first met her could know love and valuation from her child. Some measure of self-love could now grow in Karen—which means, of course, that for Karen, as well as all parents, a loving and rewarding child brought enhancement of self-love, the healthy narcissism that is the privilege of all parents.

Nina's progress in treatment was far in advance of her mother's during the first two years. Nina was brought to adequacy on all measures of personality development by the time she was fourteen months old. But in this work we had two patients, a mother and a baby. As long as Karen's depression remained, Nina was regarded by us as at risk and her mother's psychological state was regarded as precarious. When treatment was terminated at Nina's age three and a half, we were satisfied that Karen's internal conflicts had found resolutions and that Nina was progressing sturdily in her own development.

Conclusions

Therapeutic work with adolescent mothers and their babies needs to accommodate objectives for the treatment of two patients, each of whom may be suffering from a developmental disorder. This therapy has the aim of bringing optimal development for an adolescent who is also an adolescent mother and for a baby whose development is endangered.

NOTE

1. A full clinical report of this case and three other cases of adolescent mothers are included in Fraiberg (1980).

REFERENCE

Fraiberg, S., ed. 1980. *Clinical Studies in Infant Mental Health: The First Year of Life*. New York: Basic.

2 THE PSYCHOLOGICAL AND SOCIAL EFFECTS OF YOUTH UNEMPLOYMENT

SAUL V. LEVINE

For at least the last century there have been myriad analyses of the effect of work or the lack of it on individuals and communities. These reports differ greatly because the work ethic varies considerably from time to time, from society to society, or from subgroup to subgroup. Over the generations, the meaning of work has ranged widely, from punishment to divine inspiration, duty to society, basic psychological need, constitutional right, and crass means to an end (Burstein, Tienhaara, Hewson, and Marrander 1975; Harris 1972; Inglis 1971; Tilgher 1958; and Unemployment Insurance Commission of Canada 1978). Similarly, unemployment, the fact of not working, has meant different things to different people. It is clear, however, that nonworkers who are physically and mentally able to be part of the labor force are viewed with disdain by a large number of their working fellow citizens. The former are perceived as lazy, exploitative "ne'er-do-wells who rip off the system" and steal middle-class taxes, people who could work if only they wanted to—the implicit corollary being that there are large numbers of jobs available.

Most of the earlier studies in this area were done on employed and unemployed individuals who were adult members of families, usually fathers, heads of households, or mothers (Ginsburg 1942; Jahoda, Lazarsfeld, and Zeisal 1971). The focus was on the terrible effects of the Depression in 1929 and the early 1930s on many North American families (Eisenberg and Lazarsfeld 1938; Pieroni 1978; Pilgrim Trust 1968). We have experienced in the mid and late 1970s a situation that the Western world has seen before, that of youth unemployment. But the extent and chronicity of the problem is a relatively new phenomenon. An economic downturn disproportionately affects employable young people. In addition to being unemployed per se, they are the last hired, the first laid off, and are given the least rewarding jobs, financially and meaningfully. Advanced technology has made the youngest workers the most expendable. Perhaps this is understandable in terms of seniority and experience, but this issue is a growing problem for society. While there are innumerable economic and statistical indices to measure the extent of youth unemployment, there are very few data, in human terms, on the effects on the young people who cannot find work. Because they are young, with relatively few responsibilities, it has been assumed that no great harm can come to them. There is even less examination of the implications for a society which espouses individuality, achievement, competition, and materialism and yet cannot provide meaningful work for many of its young adult citizens.

The Facts of Youth Unemployment

There is no one culture of youth, any more than there is one culture of poverty or one youth personality profile. There is no one work ethic or one education ethic among youth. There is, however, rhetoric, bias, and polarization. And there is a mélange of facts, prejudices, and mythologies that have served to muddy the waters of an already turbulent stream (Levine 1975).

We shall explore the reactions of young people to a situation that is affecting the contemporary Western world—large-scale youth unemployment. In the process of debunking some mythologies, let us look at some of the facts.

1. First and foremost, the vast majority of young people, from all social strata, want to work (Burstein et al. 1975; Goodwin 1972; Yankelovich 1978). Many young people see work instrumentally as a means to an end (money, leisure, acquisition, and power), many others perceive work as part of their identity, and a growing number want to derive some intrinsic satisfaction from their work itself. In all, however, there is a desire to work. Gainful, meaningful (if possible) work is a common goal.

2. In Canada and the United States, the youth (ages sixteen to twenty-four) unemployment rate, the relative number of young people looking for work compared with that age group in the work force, currently runs between 14 percent and 70 percent, depending on the specific area of the population one is studying. This accounts, again

with some variation, for almost half the unemployment currently in both countries. That is, the unemployment rate for youth is approximately double what it is for the rest of the population (Citizens' Policy Center 1977; Social Planning Council of Metropolitan Toronto 1978; Statistics Canada 1978; U.S. Department of Labor, Manpower Administration 1974).

3. There is no evidence that youth en masse abuse the unemployment insurance program. In fact, young people consistently underuse that system. Less than half the eligible recipients of benefits are actually claimants of that compensation. The majority of young people who are on unemployment insurance benefits have lost their jobs or have been laid off—relatively fewer youths than older workers quit of their own volition (Social Planning Council of Metropolitan Toronto 1978; Unemployment Insurance Commission of Canada 1978).

4. The vast majority of unemployed youth would rather work than accept government compensation in the form of welfare or insurance (Larter and Eason 1978; National Council of Welfare of Canada 1975; Yankelovich 1978).

5. There is no doubt that the majority of unemployed youth are from low-socioeconomic-level backgrounds (Citizens' Policy Center 1977; National Council of Welfare of Canada 1975), but youth unemployment is spreading to affect the middle class as well (Coleman 1973; Conger 1977).

6. Level of education is a strong indicator of potential unemployment. The earlier the departure from school, the greater the chances of unemployment. However, education itself is a poor guarantee of entry into the labor force. Unemployed youth most often have poor school histories and speak of their unhappiness at school. Many feel glad to be out of school, although they realize the consequences.

We have a paradoxical situation. Those who quit school early are ill prepared for jobs requiring even a modicum of skill. Those who complete school at a secondary or even higher level find that they, too, do not have the necessary skills to fill available jobs. And both groups discover readily that there simply are not enough jobs available for those looking for work (Social Planning Council of Metropolitan Toronto 1978). The school system effectively removes young people from contact with adults, falsely raises expectations early on, stratifies youth socioeconomically and racially, and usually succeeds only in preparing some students for more schooling, nothing else. Schools by and large are not set up to deal with the large numbers of young people who do not "fit in" to "standard operating procedures" (Mihalka 1974).

School is thus seen as irrelevant to a large number of young people, and this is reflected in the increasing dropout statistics from many urban high schools (Bachman, Green, and Wirtanen 1971; Peebles 1973; Social Planning Council of Metropolitan Toronto 1978). If schools are in the business of developing responsible, competent citizens, surely that goal is being thwarted by these realities (Coleman 1973; Evans 1968).

Effects of Youth Unemployment

What happens to young people who are unemployed? There have been numerous studies and reports which indicate that the cost to society in social and economic terms is immeasurable (Aiken, Forman, and Shappared 1968; Report of the Special Task Force to the Secretary of Health, Education, and Welfare 1972). There are suggestions that every 1 percent rise in unemployment leads to an exponential increase in such indices as mental hospital admissions, homicide, suicide, and arrests (Brenner 1979). There is clinical evidence that the high school dropout rate and youth unemployment are closely tied to crimes of violence, vandalism, delinquency, suicide, and heavy drug abuse (Campbell 1978; Guttentag 1968; Lester 1970; Pitman 1977; Ross 1977; Wenk 1974). These phenomena can and have been translated into actual losses of millions of dollars to society each year. When reading about the social problems and the attendant economic losses, one is appalled at the phenomenal waste, the overwhelming loss of potential funds for needy individuals and projects, the cost to society as a whole. But what is obscured are the personal and human effects on these young people. The statistics actually represent various skewed samples of young people. Obviously relatively few of the unemployed youth will kill themselves or end up in jail. But what about the thousands of young people who are unemployed and do not end up in these statistics? What are their views of themselves and their society? Anyone who has worked with young people in trouble recognizes that the difficulties they have are either causally related or at least aggravated by their being out of school or unemployed. In working with unemployed youth, I have been struck by repetitive patterns of emotional reactions experienced by these young people. This report does not imply, in any way, scientific rigor; rather, it reflects extensive clinical experience of

27

professionals and others working with innumerable youth over the past few years.

Stages

Studies have shown that older individuals who are out of work or who lose jobs go through a series of stages (Coelho, Hamburg, and Adams 1974; Coleman 1974; Moos 1976) not unlike the progression of emotional and cognitive states in any type of crisis (Bakke 1969; Jahoda et al. 1971; Pieroni 1978; Report of the Special Task Force to the Secretary of Health, Education, and Welfare 1972; Wilcock and Ranko 1963; Zawadski and Lazarsfeld 1935). Similarly, a young person recently out of school enters a sequence of states. Certainly there are glaring exceptions, but the following progression of reactions of the young employed has been seen with considerable regularity. The sequence is tempered by varying circumstances. That is, a young person who has quit school recently is in a different situation from one who has lost a series of jobs. Similarly, social class differences play a major role. With the disadvantage of generalization, let us look at a lower-middle-class youth who has dropped out of high school or has recently lost his first job.

STAGE I: OPTIMISM

At first there may be a feeling almost akin to "release from bondage." The individual feels free, optimistic, and relaxed. Youthful optimism is apparent; there is less concern for long-term consequences, there are few responsibilities, and gratification can be almost immediate. There is no initial stage of shock, disbelief, or denial, unlike early responses to other crises. His hours are his own, nobody is looking over his shoulder, he enjoys his leisure. He is hopeful of finding work; he has few illusions regarding himself and even fewer expectations about his long-term future. Similarly, these feelings may pertain to someone who has recently lost one of his first jobs. There is that same initial sense of relief. During this period, he is looking for work with the full anticipation of finding it.

STAGE II: AMBIGUITY

If this period becomes prolonged (more than a few months), new feelings and experiences occur. The inactivity becomes harder to take, especially if many of the friends of the unemployed individual are in school or in jobs. Boredom predominates, but there is a new feeling of being somewhat isolated and out of the mainstream of things. Also, there is implicit and explicit pressure on the youth to get a job. "The pressure is all around you," as one young man put it. But it is especially pronounced, paradoxically, from those closest to the unemployed young person—his parents and friends. A recent study has shown that friends, more than anyone else, are opposed to a youth's quitting school (Bakke 1934)—more than parents, teachers, and counselors. Similarly, after he quits and does not have work, his mother and father are critical because he is now more financially dependent; subtle hints, empathy, and understanding soon give way to demands and ultimatums. The unemployed individual is beginning to question his own competence and self-worth (Braginsky and Braginsky 1975). A job would reverse this stage: he is still looking, but with less enthusiasm.

STAGE III: DESPAIR

Another few months of this, or of recurrent short-term employment followed by longer bouts of unemployment, a new phase is entered in which there is no confusion about feelings. The individual often becomes morose, withdrawn, and moody. He rapidly loses faith in himself and those around him. He has questions about the worth of his life and that of his society. A sense of hopelessness begins to pervade the young person's very being. He is often angry at himself, his schooling, and his parents. Depending on peer group support, or lack of it, his unhappiness might take the form of acting out via drugs, vandalism, or other antisocial activities. He may become completely apathetic and nihilistic, or he may enter into a state of despair or agitated depression. He is no longer actively looking for work.

We have, then, an individual at the potential peak of his physical health and energy, at just the time that enthusiasm and optimism should abound, at an age when ideology and commitment can be most apparent and malleable, feeling only contempt for himself, his predicament, and those responsible for this situation. There are some young people who enjoy the financial handouts from governments and the freedom from responsibility, but these are a small minority. There are others for whom work means tediousness, hassles, drudgery, yet they miss the socializing, camaraderie on the job, and especially the money that affords them the opportunity to be independent of parents (Pieroni 1978).

29

Emotional Consequences

There is a litany of negative feelings and thoughts which many out-of-work, young individuals report with regularity after a prolonged period of unemployment. Just as in our outline of the stages experienced by these young people, there are other factors aside from unemployment that determine their reactions and account for wide variability and exceptions. There are individual differences in personality types, coping styles, tolerance to stress, and personal strengths. But these notwithstanding, there are predictable emotional and cognitive consequences.

BOREDOM

The absence of things to do, the wherewithal to do them, and the people to do them with rapidly becomes of paramount importance. Day melts imperceptibly into night; sleep patterns change. The imposed structure on the day which we all bemoan is rapidly lost. But instead of the sense of relaxation, which is apparent on a working person's day off, the predominant affect and experience is boredom and some degree of confusion. There is a loss of direction of relatively clear goals. This leads to apathy and withdrawal in some young people and to agitation in others. Even on a mundane level, they lose a sense of purpose in their lives.

IDENTITY DIFFUSION

These adolescents are normally at the height of the task of coming to grips with their identity. Occupational status and role play a large part in defining a young person's sense of personal identity (Coles 1971; Eisenberg and Lazarsfeld 1938; Erikson 1968; Wilensky 1966). If the individual sees his lack of a job as being caused by external forces beyond his control, has a degree of confidence in himself, a sense of competence, and some degree of success academically or socially, his identity (and self-esteem) will not be adversely affected, at least for a while. Similarly, successful social experiences, past and present, would contribute to a successful process of identity resolution. But with any extreme prolongation of the unemployed status, even in a relatively successful individual, these mitigating circumstances would be insufficient to overcome the damage to the self-concept. Furthermore, for the majority of unemployed youth, success has not been experienced socially, academically, or vocationally. The time frame is different, but the end result in both is a sense of identity which is not resolved satisfactorily or is negatively tainted.

SELF-ESTEEM

Unemployed young individuals have lower self-esteem than those still in school or working (Braginsky and Braginsky 1975; Cohn 1978; Larter and Eason 1978). Self-esteem is a crucial variable in a young person's view of himself and his world (Rosenberg 1976). It can be a central determinant of success or failure, can serve as a powerful maturing force for different kinds of behavior, and is also inextricably tied to an individual's emotional state. It is, then, a multifaceted concept, and certainly the self as worker is only one aspect of an individual's self-definition. And yet work plays a disproportionately large role in how a young person perceives himself (Coles 1971).

Self-esteem is in part determined by one's upbringing and expectations, by his work ethic in relation to society's, and by his perception of the reactions of those around him. It also varies according to school history, type of previous job held, level of income, and prevalence of unemployment among one's peers. Low self-esteem can obviously be a lifelong problem preceding the unemployed state, but it is reinforced and aggravated by lack of work. Low self-esteem is a recurrent, predictable result of prolonged unemployment. Even those few who claim to enjoy getting unemployment insurance and not working will in confidence—and sadness—speak of their lack of respect for themselves (Pieroni 1978). It is this which pervades all thoughts, feelings, and behavior of the unemployed young person. Low self-esteem leads to demoralization (Frank 1973) and susceptibility to negative influences (Levine 1978, 1979a).

GUILT AND SHAME

Many unemployed young individuals feel humiliated by their situation. Not only do they feel that they have in part brought the situation on themselves ("I should have stayed in school"), but they feel society's censure. Face-saving is all important to many adolescents and youth. Hence, in a group situation, unemployed youth often point the finger at their peers, saying that they are lazy or irresponsible, in fact espousing the critical line directed at them. They state emphatically that they themselves cannot get jobs because of bad luck or poor connections. They are defensive and touchy. But with someone they trust, they will talk with sadness about their own failings, the guilt and the shame that they experience. These feelings may lead to obsessive ruminations, circular reasoning, and depression. The public humiliation particularly hurts them, especially if they are in a situation where the majority of their peers and elders are working (Neff 1971). If they are being hounded by their parents or others, even if they respond openly with defiance, their private guilt and shame increase. The public climate of antagonism toward them may be argued vociferously, but it is internalized and accepted.

ANXIETY AND FEAR

Young people who progress into the stage of despair express a variety of fears. Free-floating anxiety is readily apparent or reported by many, along with the usual concomitant somatic experiences (sweating, pallor, insomnia, and tremulousness). They feel psychological as well as financial insecurity. They sleep fitfully, cannot relax, and feel tense much of the time. They often look drawn and haggard. In addition they express real fear that they will never find a job, that there will be no place in society for them, that they will always have to remain dependent, or that they will feel even further rejection by their family and friends.

ANGER

A degree of resentment and anger is present in a large number of unemployed youth. The anger may be directed at single individuals, teachers, parents, employers, institutions (school, unemployment commission, government), or society in general. Sometimes the anger is directed at themselves, which relates to the guilt some experience. There are all degrees of hostility, in part dependent on the personality of the individual, as well as the particular unpleasant experiences that he or she has undergone. Usually the anger is controlled and unexpressed except verbally; at other times it evolves into rage. If the individual is involved in antisocial activities, drugs, or deviant groups, his rage at society might be expressed indiscriminately, irrationally, or destructively. Usually, however, there is general distrust which colors all relationships with prospective employers and others for the immediate future. This anger not only tends to be wasted in that there are no constructive outlets for its expression, but it is also destructive to the individual.

DEPRESSION

Many of the unemployed people who have been interviewed have a depressed affect and mood (although clinical depression is less commonly seen). The general state of dissatisfaction and sadness is related to a variety of losses—opportunities, structure to their lives, relationships, and respect from others. It is also mutually affected by low self-esteem, fears, anger at the self, and guilt and shame. While psychotherapy and medication might be helpful if a serious depression evolves, what the majority of these young people need above all is meaningful, gainful employment. Even in a despairing, crying young person, one should not too readily ascribe psychiatric labels—there is reality to this misery and it is reversible. The majority of these young people report unhappiness with their situation; they become miserable if there is any degree of persistence to the unemployed state. It is in this state most often that they cry for help. Suicide has not been shown to be more prevalent among this group.

DEMORALIZATION AND ALIENATION

All these experiences and emotions lead to individuals who are disillusioned with themselves and their society. They are demoralized—pessimism, futility, fatalism, and a low sense of personal worth characterize their consciousness (Frank 1973). They also feel alienated—feelings of powerlessness, isolation, normlessness, self-estrangement, and meaninglessness (Seaman 1959) predominate. If believing in oneself and in a cause and belonging to a highly valued, accepting group are vital psychosocial needs (Levine 1979b), as is significant self-esteem (Rosenberg 1976), then our society seems to be doing everything to obviate the possibility of attaining these goals for thousands of our young people. We espouse the desire to develop our youth into responsible, independent, competent citizens, yet the economic and social circumstances appear to be pointing to the development of individuals who have not tasted mastery and success, who may not have the skills necessary for civic competence or the mechanisms available for acquiring these skills (Bronfenbrenner 1974).

What vested interest have these young people in perpetuating the values and aspirations of a society that they feel has failed them? Alienated, demoralized young people who are, at least theoretically, at the potential peak of their physical health and power, their energy, and their idealism are being lost to themselves and, more important, to society.

There are already alienated adolescents who have been labeled by professionals and others as "deviant disturbed," "sick," or "bad." These young people will too often end up as rejects or institutionalized with significant emotional problems. But the unemployment and school dropout statistics are dominated by "normal" youth (Conger 1977). And while the unemployed young people are disproportionately from lower socioeconomic classes, middle-class youth are comprising an increasing representation in these statistics (Coleman 1974). The long-term consequences are more ominous than the immediate. There is a cumulative impact and multiplier effect on the unemployed and on their society. These young men and women will evidence signs of psychosocial disintegration (Leighton 1973) in the short run, and the delayed effects do not speak well for their future.

AN ACTION STRATEGY

A prosocial and preventive rather than repressive approach must be taken. Rather than look at dropouts and the unemployed as deviants, society can help alleviate the problem and give young people the message that they have a stake in their society. A recognition on the part of schools and government that they have a major problem on their hands would be a good start.

The secondary schools play a vital role in preparing young people for the realities and exigencies of the world outside of the educational system. This means teaching and exposing students to the meaning of work, job skills, and human-relations skills. There are many students who do not fit into traditional kinds of teaching. Schools should offer various kinds of programs, especially directed at potential dropouts and future unemployed. Students of all kinds should benefit from vocational screening and assessment to ascertain the most appropriate and rewarding path to follow (U.S. Department of Labor, Manpower Administration 1974). With the current and future surplus of teachers, we have the manpower available to provide more individually designed or at least alternative school programs. Work programs with academic credit should be present in all high schools. Job training and placement programs can be instituted in the same locales.

Vocational programs have to be upgraded and not treated as a dumping ground for second-class citizens. More student participation in developing rules and regulations—preparing them for civic competence—can and should be adopted (Neff 1971). More peer counseling in and out of school can be organized with young leaders helping their less endowed peers. The guidance and counseling programs in secondary schools should be given high priority, as high as academic subjects.

The secondary school dropout rate is a major problem. A disproportionate number of these young people become the unemployed of the immediate and long-term future. They are a population at particular risk from a social and psychological point of view, with much higher rates of delinquency and psychiatric problems than other peers. Not only do they need special academic and vocational programming, but they should be picked up early and preventive interventions instituted. These are vocational placements in the community for which academic credits are granted.

Apprenticeship systems of skill teaching should be introduced on a broad scale. Artisans, craftsmen, and skilled workers could have young people assigned to them, after careful screening, for lengthy periods. They would learn the skills necessary and receive both vocational and life guidance from their elders. This program could be subsidized by a variety of possible levels of government, as is done in Great Britain and West Germany through incentives and tax allowances.

Community economic development strategies, with short- and long-term goals, should be developed. Government, labor, and the private sector must all be involved individually and together in cooperative ventures. Make-work projects are useful only insofar as they are sustained and successful. They must be well planned, have a coherent conceptual framework, and must also be monitored and evaluated. Above all, the young people have to report the feeling that work is useful and appreciated, not just stopgap and frivolous. Job-creation programs and new business formations involving young people in the planning, learning, and working are vital, especially if these are joint ventures among public, private, nonprofit, and educational sectors of our society. Innovative, cost-effective, labor-intensive cottage industries can be established that do not compete with traditional industry yet provide jobs and training for unemployed young people. Alternative technologies, waste recovery and recycling, urban farming, and more traditional industries (new products and services) are all

35

feasible possibilities. These can be combined with an academic component to enhance the life options of dropouts.

Consciousness raising is an important part of the task. The public as well as interest groups and large bodies (government, business, labor, and schools) must be made aware of the extent of the problem, the issues involved, and the potential amelioration of the situation. This includes dissemination of information about young people in general and their place in society. Further research is necessary to look at all of the interfaces between youth and society (health care, the legal system, education, and recreation).

Conclusions

Young people who want to work and for whom there are no jobs are a vulnerable group. Many definitions of mental health cite the ability to engage in useful, satisfying work as an important facet of a positive self-concept. If society is to avoid alienation among large numbers of its young citizens, it is incumbent on it to keep youth involved, physically and spiritually, in activities that are productive to them and to their community. If this is not accomplished, the chances increase that many normal youth will deteriorate personally, engage in antisocial activities, or be attracted to socially dissonant groups which can provide them with a sense of self and a purpose in life (Levine 1978, 1979a, 1979b). Young people have to perceive that they in fact do have an important and respected role to play in a social system with a purpose.

Youth unemployment is a major problem, but it is just one aspect of the lives of young people who do not feel that they have a major role to play in their communities or country. Even if full employment is accomplished, however, we may still have to face the possibility that our current value system will not capture the imagination of many of our young. Competent, contributing citizens can best evolve in a society that is based on a meaningful raison d'être and an experience of participation in that system.

If society intends to motivate its youth to its way of life, there are a few preconditions. Adults have to believe in it themselves and show by their actions that they do. Adults have to convince young people that their society is not solely predicated on self-indulgence. We are failing at these tasks; narcissism has now supplanted altruism. The "Me Generation" must be replaced by a caring generation. If there is no demonstration that society in fact does concern itself with loftier goals than

SAUL V. LEVINE

materialism and self-aggrandizement, the problems surrounding youth unemployment will seem miniscule in comparison—and they certainly will not be solved.

REFERENCES

Aiken, M.; Forman, L. A.; and Shappared, H. L. 1968. *Economic Failure, Alienation and Extremism.* Ann Arbor: University of Michigan Press.
Bachman, J. G.; Green, J.; and Wirtanen, I. D. 1971. *Youth in Transition.* Vol. 3, *Dropping Out—Problem or Symptom?* Ann Arbor: University of Michigan Press.
Bakke, E. W. 1934. *The Unemployed Man: A Social Study.* New York: Dutton.
Bakke, E. W. 1969. *Citizens without Work.* New York: Achon.
Braginsky, D. D., and Braginsky, B. A. 1975. Surplus people: their lost faith in self and system. *Psychology Today* 3:8–72.
Brenner, H. 1979. *Estimating the Social Costs of National Economic Policy: Implications for Mental and Physical Health, and Criminal Aggression.* Washington, D.C.: Government Printing Office.
Bronfenbrenner, V. 1974. The origins of alienation. *Scientific American* 231:53–61.
Burstein, M.; Tienhaara, N.; Hewson, P.; and Marrander, B. 1975. *Canadian Work Values: Finding of a Work Ethics Survey and a Job Satisfaction Survey. Strategic Planning and Research.* Ottawa: Department of Manpower and Immigration.
Campbell, G. 1978. *Vandalism Alert.* Toronto: City of Toronto.
Citizens' Policy Center. 1977. *Open Road.* Santa Barbara: Citizens' Policy Center.
Coelho, G.; Hamburg, D.; and Adams, J. 1974. *Coping and Adaption.* New York: Basic.
Cohn, R. M. 1978. The effect of employment status change on self-attitudes. *Social Psychology* 41:81–93.
Coleman, J. C. 1973. Life stress and maladaptive behavior. *American Journal of Occupational Therapy* 27:169–180.
Coleman, J. 1974. *Youth: Transition to Adulthood.* Chicago: University of Chicago Press.
Coles, R. 1971. On the meaning of work. *Atlantic Monthly* 228:103–104.
Conger, J. J. 1977. *Adolescence and Youth: Psychological Development in a Changing World.* New York: Harper & Row.

37

Eisenberg, P., and Lazarsfeld, P. F. 1938. The psychological effects of unemployment. *Psychological Bulletin* 35:358–390.

Erikson, E. H. 1968. *Identity: Youth and Crisis*. New York: Norton.

Evans, R. N. 1968. *School for Schooling's Sake: The Current Role of the Secondary School in Occupational Preparation. The Transition from School to Work*. Princeton, N.J.: Industrial Relations Section.

Frank, J. 1973. The demoralized mind. *Psychology Today* 4:24–28.

Friendly, M.; Levine, S.; and Hagarty, L. 1979. *Child in the City: Changes and Challenges*. Vol. 2. Toronto: University of Toronto Press.

Ginsburg, S. W. 1942. What unemployment does to people: a study in adjustment to crisis. *American Journal of Psychiatry* 99:435–440.

Goodwin, L. 1972. *Do the Poor Want to Work? A Social-Psychological Study of Work Orientations*. Washington, D.C.: Brookings Institution.

Guttentag, M. 1968. The relationship of unemployment to crime and delinquency. *Journal of Social Issues* 26(1): 105–114.

Harris, J. 1972. *Unemployment and Politics: A Study in English Social Policy 1880–1914*. Oxford: Clarendon.

Inglis, B. 1971. *Poverty and the Industrial Révolution*. London: Hodder & Stoughton.

Jahoda, M.; Lazarsfeld, P. F.; and Zeisal, H. 1971. *Marientahl: The Sociography of an Unemployed Community*. New York: Aldine-Atherton.

Larter, S., and Eason, G. 1978. *"Leaving School Early" Students: Characteristics and Opinions*. Report no. 154. Toronto: Toronto Board of Education.

Leighton, A. 1973. The empirical status of the integration-disintegration hypothesis. In B. Kaplan, ed. *Psychiatric Disorder and the Urban Environment*. New York: Behavioral Publications.

Lester, D. 1970. Suicide and unemployment. *Archives of Environmental Health* 20:277–278.

Levine, S. 1975. Mythology of contemporary youth. *Canadian Medical Association Journal* 113:501–504.

Levine, S. 1978. Youth and religious cults: a societal and clinical dilemma. *Adolescent Psychiatry* 6:75–89.

Levine, S. 1979a. Adolescents, believing and belonging. *Adolescent Psychiatry* 7:41–53.

Levine, S. 1979b. Alienation as an affect in adolescents. In H. Golombek and B. D. Garfinkel, eds. *The Adolescent and Mood Disturbance*. International Universities Press, 1981.

Mihalka, J. A. 1974. *Youth and Work*. Columbus, Ohio: Merrill.

Moos, R. D. 1976. *Human Adaption: Coping with Life Crises*. Lexington, Mass.: Heath.

National Council of Welfare of Canada. 1975. *Poor Kids*. Ottawa: National Council of Welfare.

Neff, W. S. 1971. Work and human behavior. *Humanitas* 7:177–191.

Peebles, D. 1973. *Dropping Out: A Review of the Research and Literature*. Toronto: Department of Educational Research Services, Board of Education, North York.

Pieroni, R. 1978. Interviews with unemployed youth. Doctoral dissertation, University of Toronto.

Pilgrim Trust. 1968. *Men without Work*. Cambridge: Cambridge University Press.

Pitman, W. 1977. *Now Is Not Too Late*. Toronto: Government of Metro Toronto.

Report of the Special Task Force to the Secretary of Health, Education and Welfare. 1972. *Work in America*. Cambridge, Mass.: MIT Press.

Rosenberg, M. 1976. The dissonant context and the adolescent self-concept. In S. Dragastin and G. Elder, eds. *Adolescence in the Life Cycle*. New York: Wiley.

Ross, M. 1977. *Economics, Opportunity and Crime*. Montreal: Renouf.

Seaman, M. 1959. On the meaning of alienation. *American Sociolocial Review* 24(6): 783.

Social Planning Council of Metropolitan Toronto. 1978. The problem is jobs . . . not people. Toronto: Social Planning Council, October.

Statistics Canada. 1978. *The Labour Force*. Ottawa: Government Printing Office.

Tilgher, A. 1958. *Work through the Ages*. Chicago: Regnery.

Unemployment Insurance Commission of Canada. 1978. Established claims analysis. Toronto District, Unemployment Insurance Commission, February.

U.S. Department of Labor, Manpower Administration. 1974. *Manpower Report of the President*. Washington, D.C.: Government Printing Office.

Wenk, E. 1974. Schools and delinquency prevention. *Crime and Delinquency Literature* 6:236–246.

Wilcock, R. C., and Ranko, W. H. 1963. *Unwanted Workers*. London:

Free Press of Glencoe.

Wilensky, H. L. 1966. Work as a social problem. In H. A. Becker, ed. *Social Problems: A Modern Approach.* New York: Wiley.

Yankelovich, D. 1978. The new job values. *Psychology Today* 11:12–15.

Zawadski, B., and Lazarsfeld, P. 1935. Psychological consequences of unemployment. *Journal of Social Psychology* 6:224–251.

3 TO LOVE AND/OR TO WORK: THE IDEOLOGICAL DILEMMA OF YOUNG WOMEN

LOIS T. FLAHERTY

The participation of American women in labor outside the home is greater at this time than at any period in history; at the present time over half of all women over sixteen are in the labor market. Although the women's liberation movement has played a role, this rising participation is actually part of a trend which began in the early part of the twentieth century; a sharp increase occurred during World War II and did not level off as had been predicted.

Many changes in the life cycle of women have occurred. In the early 1900s the average life expectancy for women was fifty years and the average number of children per family was six. Most women who worked were young and single. Between marriage and death, women's lives centered on childbirth and child rearing. It would have been difficult to argue with Deutsch (1924) when she wrote, "The man measures and controls his ego ideal by his production through sublimation in the outside world. To the woman, on the other hand, the ego is embodied in the child, and all those tendencies to sublimation which the man utilizes in intellectual and social activity she directs to the child, which in the psychological sense represents for the woman her sublimation product."

In 1982, however, the average life expectancy of women is seventy-five years, and the average number of children per family is two. The overall "worklife" for women averages about ten years less than that of men (Kreps and Leaper 1976). These trends have been accompanied by complex changes in the quality of female participation in the work force. Upward mobility of women within organizations has been enhanced by affirmative action programs; the introduction of new, gender-free job fields, such as computer technology; and the opening up of jobs traditionally considered male (Schrank and Riley 1976). There has actually been a decline, however, in the overall job status of women relative to men and a widening of the gap between their earnings (Barrett 1976).

The impact of these social and economic trends on the psychological development of today's adolescents and young women is not altogether clear. We know that the formation of vocational and career goals, as well as the acquisition of the ability to engage in work, are key developmental tasks for adolescents. Recently there have been suggestions that young women may be opting for more traditional roles and de-emphasizing the importance of careers. The results of a *New York Times* (1980) survey, which highlighted the sense of conflict experienced by college women as they faced the future, were interpreted as indicating a trend toward rejection of committedness to career goals. Interestingly, one respondent is quoted as saying, "The fact is that we want it all." "All" in this case meant careers plus families. In fact, what the young women surveyed were rejecting was the notion that it was possible to be superwomen or do everything without having to make compromises.

Surveys and questionnaires may be misleading, however, if they force respondents into either/or choices and fail to explore fully the meaning of being forced to choose or the implications of ego ideal conflicts for women. Material from psychotherapy sessions with adolescent girls can give further insight into their experiences with respect to the development of attitudes toward future work, as themes related to work and careers often figure prominently in their ideation. Younger adolescents often strongly state preferences for careers, with little anticipation of conflict with other goals. Career choices not uncommonly include those traditionally considered male, in keeping with the preadolescent girl's bisexual trends (Harley 1971). With the onset of adolescence proper, career goals often reflect wishes for narcissistic gratification. With the increased emphasis on physical appearance, typical of this period, choices frequently include such fields as acting or modeling. The choice of such stereotypically female roles may have less to do with cultural stereotypes than with the emphasis on physical attractiveness so characteristic of this developmental stage.

During late adolescence, it becomes necessary to think more realistically about the future, and it is during this period that women commonly begin to experience conflict. The sense of omnipotentiality characteristic of late adolescence is accompanied by the realization that choice of one alternative means loss of others. For young men the choice is usually between alternative careers or life-styles. They often express a sense of intoxication with their own capabilities, which seem unlimited, and an unwillingness to limit themselves by a commitment to one goal. This has been seen as an extension of infantile omnipotence (Pumpian-Mindlin 1965).

For young women this issue is more complicated, as they often view career goals as conflicting with wishes for marriage and children. A major source of anxiety for older female adolescents has traditionally been their concern over attractiveness to males and the fear that to appear "brainy" or competitive will jeopardize their chances of finding a suitable mate. Studies done in the 1950s and the early 1960s very clearly showed this to be a paramount concern, often overtly expressed (Coleman 1963). Today, although such concerns are less likely to be stated overtly, adolescent girls are still aware that boys' preferences and ideals with regard to females' careers do not necessarily match their own.

A replication in 1974 of a study done forty years earlier dealing with college students' attitudes toward feminism and sex roles showed that boys still held less egalitarian attitudes than did girls, although in 1974 both sexes were more favorably disposed toward feminism than the students sampled in 1934 had been (Roper and Labeff 1977). An informal survey done in 1980 by a teacher in a tenth-grade class of a local private coeducational school in Baltimore indicated that while most of the girls assumed they would both work and have families, the boys tended to assume their future wives would not work outside the home. Counterbalancing this potential for conflict is the trend toward delaying marriage, which reduces the immediate anxiety over the need to find a mate; however, it is a factor which cannot be completely discounted.

Economists have suggested that many women are discouraged from pursuing careers by the perceived small payoff from a world of work in which opportunities are limited because of sexual discrimination; it simply does not seem worth the effort to them to compete with men. While it is true that women may feel less pressured to make career choices which will ensure a high income, as they do not anticipate having to support families,[1] they are apt to feel pressure to choose careers which minimize the possibility of future conflict with the anticipated demands of being a wife and mother. Thus for the older female adolescent the awareness of multiple potentials is clouded by the awareness of many limits. She fears that unless she gives up or compromises on some options she will lose out on others.

That the older adolescent experiences much conflict when forced to choose among future roles, there can be no doubt. Opinions differ, however, about the origins of this conflict. It is interesting to compare the psychoanalytic and sociological views about role conflict in women.

In early psychoanalytic thinking, a woman's wish for a career outside the home or intellectual or artistic pursuits was interpreted as a wish to compete with men in these spheres in order to compensate for her inability to compete anatomically. The term "masculine protest" was often applied to the efforts of women to pursue careers, and such efforts were attributed to the inability of such women to accept their true feminine destiny. The importance was stressed of the resolution of the conflict between masculine and feminine strivings through renunciation of the phallic need for achievement and acceptance of the feminine role of wife and mother.

Interestingly, there is a counterpart to this mode of thinking in the sociological literature, which holds to the "deviance hypothesis" to explain the fact that a relatively small number of women choose to pursue careers on the basis of their having had atypical socialization experiences (Almquist and Angist 1970).

Feminists have argued persuasively that differential sex-linked social pressures are brought to bear on children from the earliest moments of life. These result in stereotypic ideals of femininity as equivalent to passivity and subservience to males, and masculinity as equivalent to dominance and aggressiveness. The progressive deterioration in girls' goals between early and late adolescence, which has been widely documented (Matthews and Tiedman 1964; Rand and Miller 1972), is generally attributed to the impact of this differential socialization which leads them to abandon career goals in favor of love relationships as primary goals. This is not a conflict men face. For most men, any conflict between work goals and heterosexual intimacy is likely to be submerged as they are taught early to compartmentalize love and work. In the words of the poet, Lord Byron (not known for his egalitarian views of women), "Man's love is of man a thing apart/'tis a woman's whole existence."

The anxiety that college women experience when faced, not only with the prospect of making choices, but with the prospect of achievement itself, is significant. As Horner (1970) pointed out, fear of failure and fear of success often coexist simultaneously, placing women in a no-win, double-bind situation. To do well academically or in a career means risking disapproval, while not to achieve means being a failure.

Feminist literature tends to play down the inherent potential for conflict between career and family, attributing conflict, when it exists, to husbands' failure to share enough in household responsibilities, thereby placing excessive demands on wives. There is undoubtedly some validity to this view: studies seem to show less role conflict among working mothers who are heads of single-parent households than among those who are married (Laws 1978).

The older adolescent, then, begins for the first time to experience a sense of discord that may in varying degrees be experienced subjectively as an intrapsychic conflict (between conflicting ego ideals, or ego ideal and superego), a conflict between self and society in general, or a specific interpersonal conflict between self and family, self and friends, or self and boyfriend. In an attempt to resolve this conflict she may feel a need to make a decisive choice between career goals and family goals. Although she may be less likely than her mother to feel that her marketability as a wife will suffer if she pursues a career, she may decide to pursue work which would have little likelihood of conflicting with marriage or child rearing, that is, would be easily interruptible and would not involve skills which require great investments of time or energy to attain. In general, this kind of work tends to be low paying, low status, and has a low probability of advancement. As Osterman (1980) has pointed out, these work patterns are characteristic of youth who by their tentative participation in the labor force can be conceptualized as acting out their needs for a psychological moratorium. Choosing such a compromise, then, amounts to choosing to remain in a moratorium stage with respect to a work identity.

The following case history illustrates the dilemmas faced by the older female adolescent.

The patient, initially seen at age sixteen, remained in psychotherapy over a period of five years. At the initial interview, she described a generalized sense of incompetence with respect to peer relationships and school. She had, in fact, been recurrently school phobic. During the same interview, she described herself as a good student who planned to go to college and "do something in photography or graphic art." Although she experienced minor successes with her artistic ef-

45

forts, on the whole her involvement in school and social activities remained marginal.

During one summer she obtained a job as a camp counselor. A letter she wrote during this time detailed her anxiety and turmoil over being thrust into what was, for her, intense social involvement. At the same time she commented, "The job itself I'm totally satisfied with." This short-lived period of success was not maintained once she returned to her old home and school environment. She eventually dropped out of school, becoming quite isolated and regressed. Real progress was only possible when at the age of twenty she enrolled in a five-day-per-week, residential, vocational rehabilitation program, remaining there for a year and continuing psychotherapy. During this period her therapy sessions often reflected her preoccupation with working out her sense of identity with respect to male-female relationships as well as work. She was excited and pleased about being the object of male attention, and for a while she threw herself into sexual activity in an almost compulsive manner, going from one brief and intense relationship to another. At the same time she received recognition for her skill as an artist, both in her graphic illustration class and informally, as she was commissioned to do portraits by peers and staff members. Experiencing success in her work was pleasurable but anxiety provoking. She commented, "Sometimes I realize I could be a successful artist. Sometimes I don't think I've got the brain power. It means losing people, it's too risky. It means being a 'hot shot.'" Her associations to "hot shot" were her father and brother, males whose success she envied but whom she saw as egotistical and self-centered. As she thought more about her relationships with other males, she concluded that they were not really interested in her work or what was important to her, but only in what she could offer them in terms of narcissistic gratification. She wondered if it was possible to have an intimate heterosexual relationship and put energy into finding and keeping a job at the same time. "Maybe sex after marriage is the best idea after all."

It is not difficult to see that for this young woman career aspirations were associatively conceptually linked with masculinity. This was a source of anxiety and conflict; to be successful in the world of work meant being masculine and most unlike her mother, who was, in her words, "a doormat." On another level, an additional source of conflict was the possibility of autonomy, which aroused anxiety because of the threat of loss of still unresolved preoedipal object ties. Becoming successful meant giving up her fantasied hope of uniting with her mother in a regressive symbiotic relationship. Thus what might have been the most direct route toward autonomy—work—was itself blocked by the conceptual association of work with masculinity, as well as the fantasy of symbiosis.

Eventually this patient did progress toward autonomy using identification with her female psychiatrist in a variety of interesting ways. Once she described a dream in which the psychiatrist, in a therapy session, read to her report cards she (the psychiatrist) had received from patients. Many of the comments on the report cards were critical. The patient wondered how the psychiatrist could tolerate being criticized. In another dream, the psychiatrist spent the patient's entire therapy session on the telephone arranging for dates with various men, ignoring the patient. She wondered how a woman could work without being totally preoccupied with men.

Still later, in the course of psychotherapy, another dream illustrated how this patient was attempting to resolve her dilemma of independence and work equals masculinity. She had to present an oral report to her class (this had always, for her, been a source of tremendous anxiety). She went to the blackboard and drew a face in the lower-left corner and a map in the upper-right corner, connecting them with a line. This was accompanied by great relief and the realization that "this was all they wanted from me." At the time of the dream she was working on a portrait with a girl's face in one corner and a boy's face in the opposite corner; it reminded her of her and her brother and it was "like a comic strip where what the person is thinking is up in the corner." She thought that with the map, she could do what she needed to do to be successful, it would help her "find her way." The map did not have a gender; it was a neutral, conflict-free object in contrast to her brother, who was a reminder that to be successful one has to be male. This dream illustrated dramatically the mental shifts this patient was undergoing. Success in work, or even the ability to work at all, had been seen as an impossibility, as nothing in her experience had allowed her to believe that females could do this; it was something reserved for males only. With the realization that work could be a conflict-free function, there was a tremendous sense of mastery.

As pointed out by Anna Freud (1965), the completion of the developmental line from play to work requires control and modification of pregenital drive components, functioning according to the reality principle, and pleasure in ultimate results of activity. Erikson (1968) saw evolution of work goals and development of a work identity as ego-enhancing operations which further distanced the child from the confines of the preoedipal and oedipal conflicts. Although mastery of drives is essential in order to be able to work, work itself further aids in drive mastery.

I believe that for this patient the ability to work was crucial to the development of a stable sense of self and resolution of the separation-individuation process. Clearly a work identity was present in vestigial form at age sixteen, when she described her future goals in terms of a career. This notion of self as a successful college student and artist contrasted strikingly with the sense of failure and incompetence which permeated the rest of her personality. Experiencing success in work, although anxiety provoking, was initially less conflict laden than experiencing success in developing a social and sexual identity. Once a stable work identity was achieved, it facilitated her hatching from a symbiotic cocoon and provided a sharp boundary between herself and her mother.

As mentioned, psychoanalysts have emphasized the importance of intrapsychic conflict of masculine versus feminine trends, while sociologists point to conflict between social role expectations. Both schools agree about the existence of conflict but disagree about its origin, the sociologists seeing it as externally determined, the psychoanalysts, internally. Both imply an ideal of no conflict or resolution of conflict. It seems to me that this emphasis is, at best, unrealistic and, at worst, growth stunting for young women. The outcome can be premature closure, in which the adolescent feels that a firm commitment to one path or the other is the only solution. The feminist movement, in its emphasis on equal opportunities for women, often seemed to imply that it was possible for women to do everything and not experience conflict. Young women, finding they do experience conflict, may take this as a signal to abandon career goals. The cost of doing this may be considerable in the long run. Since in all likelihood today's young women will have to work to support themselves and/or their families for a portion of their lives, the failure to acquire necessary skills to compete in the job market will cost them financially. The cost in personal terms, while impossible to calculate mathematically, is equally important.

Recently, fears have been expressed that women's hard-won gains in employment opportunities will be lost, casualties of worsening economic conditions and social and psychological pressures. There is a danger that, as women perceive that they are being asked to become superwomen and are never told how, they will rebel against the unreality of it all. What is needed, along with support and encouragement for career goals, is the realistic awareness that conflict, while uncomfortable, is not best dealt with by avoidance. While it may not be possible to have it all, it should be possible to have some of each.

The emphasis on conflict as an undesirable, even pathological, state can obscure the positive aspects of duality of roles. The mother who works outside the home has, for all practical purposes in today's society, two careers. It is true that a woman who chooses career plus family may be pulled between demands of each; the need to invest energy toward the selfish goal of career advancement conflicts with the needs of others who depend on her. But she needs to know also that conflict between group needs and individual needs is part of all human existence; while the demands are great, there also is potential for a variety of satisfactions. As Erikson (1968) said, discussing Freud's dictum to love and to work, "When Freud said love he meant the generosity of intimacy as well as genital love; when he said work, he meant a general work productiveness which would not preoccupy the individual to the extent that he might lose his right or capacity to be a sexual and loving being."

Conclusions

There is still a danger that older female adolescents' anxiety related to work may be overlooked by therapists or considered to be of less significance than other issues. The importance of work as a means of gaining autonomy, a significant source of secondary narcissistic gains, and an expression of creativity is no less for adolescent females than for males. While the older male adolescent's parents usually express pride in his obtaining a job, the girl's parents often express concern that she is undertaking too much, endangering herself, or investing too much time in something not very important. Even worse, female adolescents may still be getting messages from their therapists that their career aspirations are simply "masculine strivings."

It is crucial for psychiatrists working with adolescent girls to be aware of these issues. Since there is a strong correlation between positive identification with the mother and self-satisfaction with one's own identity, adolescent girls presenting as patients are likely to have some difficulties in this area. The availability of alternative female models for identification becomes extremely important. The female therapist who can offer an example of the "good mother" along with a commitment to work is in a unique position to help the older female adolescent negotiate this difficult stage of the life cycle.

NOTE

1. Actually this is a myth. Current estimates suggest that the average American woman will spend a third of her adult years without a partner, although 95 percent of women marry at least once (Laws 1978).

REFERENCES

Almquist, E., and Angist, S. 1970. Career salience and atypicality of occupational choice among college women. *Journal of Marriage and the Family* 32:242–249.

Barrett, N. 1976. The economy ahead of us: will women have different roles? In J. Kreps, ed. *Women in the American Economy*. Englewood Cliffs, N.J.: Prentice-Hall.

Coleman, J. 1963. *The Adolescent Society*. New York: Free Press of Glencoe.

Deutsch, H. 1924. The psychology of woman in relation to the functions of reproduction. *International Journal of Psycho-Analysis* 6:405–419. In R. Fleiss, ed. *The Psychoanalytic Reader*. New York: International Universities Press, 1967.

Erikson, E. 1968. *Identity: Youth and Crisis*. New York: Norton.

Freud, A. 1965. *Normality and Pathology in Childhood: Assessments of Development*. New York: International Universities Press.

Harley, M. 1971. Some reflections on identity problems in prepuberty. In J. B. McDevitt and C. F. Settlage, eds. *Separation-Individuation: Essays in Honor of Margaret S. Mahler*. New York: International Universities Press.

Horner, M. 1970. Femininity and successful achievement: a basic inconsistency. In J. Bardwick, E. Douvan, M. Horner, and D. Gutman, eds. *Feminine Personality and Conflict*. Belmont, Calif.: Brooks-Cole.

Kreps, J., and Leaper, R. 1976. Home work, market work and the allocation of time. In J. Kreps, ed. *Women and the American Economy*. Englewood Cliffs, N.J.: Prentice-Hall.

Laws, J. 1978. *The Second X*. New York: Elsevier–North-Holland.

Matthews, F., and Tiedman, D. V. 1964. Attitudes toward career and marriage and the development of life style in young women. *Journal of Counseling Psychology* 11:375–384.

New York Times. 1980. Many young women now say they'd pick family over career (December 28).

Osterman, P. 1980. *Getting Started: The Youth Labor Market.* Cambridge, Mass.: MIT Press.

Pumpian-Mindlin, E. 1965. Omnipotentiality, youth and commitment. *Journal of the American Academy of Child Psychiatry* 4:1–18.

Rand, L., and Miller, A. 1972. A developmental cross-sectioning of women's careers and marriage attitudes and life-plans. *Journal of Vocational Behavior* 2:317–331.

Roper, B. S., and Labeff, E. 1977. Sex roles and feminism revisited: an intergenerational attitude comparison. *Journal of Marriage and the Family* 39:113–119.

Schrank, H., and Riley, J. 1976. Women in work organizations. In J. Kreps, ed. *Women in the American Economy.* Englewood Cliffs, N.J.: Prentice-Hall.

4 LEARNING TO HIDE: THE SOCIALIZATION OF THE GAY ADOLESCENT

A. DAMIEN MARTIN

Most literature on the gay adolescent deals with the causes and treatment of homosexuality. This chapter, however, will address itself to the process by which the gay person in general and the gay adolescent in particular are stigmatized within our society.

It is my contention that homosexuality is a normal variation in both sexual orientation and sexual behavior. Negative attitudes toward the homosexually oriented are primarily a result of homophobia, a prejudice similar in nature and dynamic to all other prejudices including anti-Semitism, racism, and sexism. Continued exposure to the prejudice results in a stigmatization of the homosexually oriented through which their social and personal identities are, to use Goffman's (1963) term, "spoiled." As a result, gay people become members of a minority group, a term defined by Allport (1958) as any segment of the population that suffers unjustified negative acts by the rest of society. These acts may range from mild discrimination to scapegoating. Gay people often demonstrate those traits that have been found in other minority groups, including obsessive concern with their stigma and state, denial of membership within the hated group, withdrawal, passivity, and aggression against their own group.

Most major differences between gay people and members of other minority groups occur because the gay person becomes a member of the group during adolescence rather than at birth. I am speaking here of the beginning of personal and social identity as a homosexually oriented person rather than of sexual orientation per se. Evidence indicates that the latter occurs much earlier than adolescence. As we shall see, the ensuing isolation creates unique problems for the gay individual.

Ideally, the gay adolescent should be able to reach what Troiden (1979) has called a "gay identity," the fusion of homosexual sexuality and emotionality into a meaningful whole. However, society's traditional view of homosexuality as a stigma prevents the easy attainment of such identity. Pain and suffering are inflicted on the very young, whom society is supposedly protecting, under the guise of preventing the spread of homosexuality or of treating the homosexual. For example, one author (Socarides 1978) stated, "Homosexual behavior through adolescence in the absence of anxiety, guilt or conflict together with perverted fantasies is an alarming sign. It is imperative to initiate therapy in order to create a conflict for the patient. . . ." In other words, conflict, guilt, and anxiety must be created where none existed. This is the essence of the stigmatization process.

Homophobia as a Prejudice

Allport (1958) defined prejudice as a negative attitude based on error and overgeneralization and described the acting out of prejudice in three interdependent stages: antilocution, discrimination, and violence. Antilocutions, verbal attacks against the group, can range from denigratory terms to elaborate pseudoscientific theories and research which serve as a foundation for discrimination and violence. Examples of pseudoscience as support for prejudice can be seen in the past use of physiognomy, phrenology, and anthropometry. In the nineteenth century, they provided "objective" evidence of the basic inferiority of Jews, blacks, women, and the homosexually oriented (Haller and Haller 1974; Mosse 1978). As part of this support, pseudoscience creates stereotypes. Thus, gay men are described as effeminate and lesbians as masculine, characteristics which make them unsuitable for the "hard" professions (Voth 1977), as "predatory" (Gilder 1979; Kardiner 1954), and as having overwhelming sexual appetites that interfere with the ability to have mature nonerotic relationships (Pattison and Pattison 1980). All of these charges, including the effeminacy of the male, were applied in the nineteenth century to groups considered to be racially inferior.

The most important antilocutionary themes are those that impute danger from the group. One of the more impressive indications of the intense antipathy toward gay people is the range of dangers attributed to them. As blacks and Jews were seen by racists to be dangerous to the purity of the race, criminals, or seducers, so too gay people are said to be a danger to the survival of the race (Socarides 1975), criminals, and seducers (Rupp 1980). They are accused of causing anorexia nervosa (Stearn 1962), crime in the streets (*Christian Anti-Communism Crusade* 1981), the Second World War (Podhoretz 1977), and the Holocaust (Jackman 1979) and are described as a danger to the family (Kardiner 1954; Socarides 1975), the state (Buchanan 1977), and even Western civilization.

These charges do not come solely from a lunatic fringe. Respected professionals often contribute to belief in the dangers of a hated group. Just as the pseudoscience of racism was an important part of the intellectual life of the nineteenth century (Mosse 1978), so too the underlying ideology supporting the stigmatization of the gay adolescent comes from all levels of society. One of the most destructive charges brought against the homosexually oriented is that they are somehow a danger to children. Voth (1977), a psychiatrist, states, "Homosexuality is as much a public health problem as any of the major diseases which have concerned public health officials and the medical profession. It is contrary to nature. . . . Little good can come to children from exposure to adults who are so disturbed as to become overtly homosexual."

Rupp (1980), in a text on forensic medicine and psychiatry, offered the following argument: "To be 35 in the 'gay world' is to be an 'old auntie' and many male homosexuals are always on the lookout for young proselytes. . . . When an inexperienced youth is wined and dined, flattered and fawned over, and finally seduced, the sex act itself may seem insignificant and the act repeated until it is finally learned and conditioned. Herein lies the pernicious and insidious evil of homosexuality."

The pernicious equation of homosexuality and danger to children does not emanate solely from the medical profession. Joseph Epstein (1970), a self-acknowledged liberal and an activist for civil rights, wrote the following introduction to an essay in which he detailed his fear and loathing for the gay person, especially the gay male.

In the beginning, I felt confusion, revulsion, and fear. I must have been ten years old when my father, who had read me stories out of a children's bible, out of Robin Hood, out of the Brothers Grimm, who carefully instructed me never to say the word "nigger," one night sat me down in our living room to explain that

54

there were "perverts" in the world. These were men with strange appetites, men whose minds were twisted, and I must be on the outlook for them—for myself, and even more for my little brother who was five years younger. There were not many such men in the world, but there were some and they might wish to "play" with my brother and me in ways which were unnatural. . . . I went to bed and dreamed about a tall thin man . . . who extended a bony index finger out to touch my little genitals. I awoke screaming.

He concluded his article with the expressed desire to see homosexuality wiped off the face of the earth.

When fears like this are legitimized and accepted without question, once stigma theory justifies it, discrimination against gay people is established. Qualified individuals are denied employment. Homosexually oriented teachers, clergymen, and physicians must hide their sexual identity. Aside from the effect on the professionals involved, this discrimination effectively denies suitable role models who can demonstrate to the gay adolescent by example, sharing, and teaching that the prejudices of society are false and that homosexuality does not automatically mean depravity, criminality, and degeneracy. Heterosexual adolescents have a multitude of role models for all possible social identities which may touch on their sexual orientation, but homosexual adolescents have no constructive models and indeed are led to believe that their sexual identity precludes other roles. This denial of role models is an essential part of the total stigmatization process. The young gay person is forbidden the opportunity to develop that personal identity which Erikson (1963) defined as "the sense of ego identity, then [which] is the accrued confidence that the inner sameness and continuity prepared in the past are matched by the sameness and continuity of one's meanings for others. . . ."

Social Identity

Each person is raised as a member of several in-groups. While difficult to define, the in-group has been described as one in which members use the term "we" with the same basic significance (Allport 1958). In-groups include the family, ethnic identification, religion, race, and so on. Each is a form of social identity and depends on categorization. While an efficient means of organizing and handling the overwhelming amount of information with which we are faced, categorization has within it the seeds of abuse and misuse.

Allport (1958) states: "Man . . . has a propensity to prejudice. This propensity lies in his normal and natural tendency to form generalizations, concepts, categories whose content represents an oversimplification of his world of experience. His rational categories keep close to first hand experience, but he is able to form irrational categories just as readily. In these, even a kernel of truth may be lacking, for they can be composed wholly of hearsay evidence, emotional projections and fantasy." The transformation from efficient information processing to dangerous oversimplification is an easy and all too frequent step. The moment we categorize people, we have lost important information about the individual while at the same time assigning much misinformation we believe we have about the group.

Goffman (1963) has called this assignment of character or characteristics "virtual social identity." It is based on expectations of behavior according to beliefs about the nature of the group rather than on actual behavior of the individual which Goffman calls "actual social identity." An individual can have a number of social identities, each defined by a single attribute and each carrying a separate virtual social identity. He may be at one and the same time a Roman Catholic, a male, a lawyer, a Nisei, and a husband. Each of these attributes has separate, distinct, and at times even contradictory expectations.

Sometimes an attribute by which an individual is assigned group membership is a stigma so discrediting that it in effect reduces or denies the individual's other social identities. Homosexuality is such a stigma in our society. It is so discrediting that the homosexually oriented person is denied social identities to which he is entitled. Some clerics say that one cannot be a Christian and homosexual. Even a category like one's identity as a full citizen is brought into question. For example, the homosexually oriented are regularly denied employment as "security risks." A U.S. Senate Committee (1950) recommended this action even though the committee was unable to cite a single case in which a homosexual American citizen had betrayed secrets because of blackmail. The denial of the right, some would even say the privilege, of serving in the armed forces is another example of denial of social identity as a citizen.

Sometimes the denial of the concomitance of a stigma attribute and another social identity is patently ludicrous. Howard Brown (1976), a physician and Public Health Administrator in New York who publicly announced his homosexuality, reported the following: "Shortly before I entered the army, in a moment of panic I took a train up to Cleveland to discuss my sexual dilemma with the aging chairman of the department of psychiatry at the medical school. He told me I couldn't possibly be a homosexual. I was going to become a doctor, wasn't I? Homosexuals didn't become doctors; they became hairdressers, interior decorators, that sort of thing. He explained away my urges as 'delayed adolescence.' "

The denial of other in-group memberships is more often tragic, especially when it involves the most basic societal in-group, the family. Discovery of an adolescent's homosexuality can cause guilt and fear in the parents, bring about the assignment or denial of blame, and result in a number of actions against the child ranging from enforced treatment to expulsion from the family unit. Many teenage prostitutes, male and female, are youngsters who have been disowned and evicted by their families because of homosexuality.

Every child learns not only what is expected of the various social identities he or she is being raised to but also what groups society abhors. In adolescence, young homosexually oriented persons are faced with the growing awareness that they may be among the most despised. They are forced to deal with the possibility that part of their actual social identity contradicts most of the other social identities to which they have believed they are entitled. As this realization becomes more pressing, they are faced with three possible choices: they can hide, they can attempt to change the stigma, or they can accept it.

Accepting homosexuality as normal would be optimal since it would make it possible for the adolescent to reach that fusion of sexuality and emotionality described as gay identity. However, acceptance, if it is ever attained, usually occurs only after much struggle and pain. For most, hiding and attempts to change are the strategies used to cope with their stigmatized status. Society does all in its power to reinforce these two strategies and thus prevents self-acceptance.

Hiding: The Discredited versus the Discreditable

The Greek word *stigma* originally referred to a visual sign of the negative status of the bearer. Generally imposed by the state, it often entailed branding or other ritual scarring. Stigma now can include attributes or signs that are not visible. When a stigma attribute is obvious, as in the case of the black, or even when made obvious by the forced wearing of the Star of David or the Pink Triangle in the concentration camps, the individuals can be considered as discredited. Those who can pass, however, and who choose to do so, become discreditable.

Actions against the discredited individual are usually obvious and direct. For the discreditable, however, the effects are less apparent, occurring within the individual and distorting the nature and depth of interpersonal relationships. The gay person can fall into either category.

A young male or female, seen respectively as too "effeminate" or too "masculine," or the young adolescent who has been caught indulging in homosexual behavior, is discredited with results that can include ostracism, violence, and forced attempts to change.

The presence of the "obvious" youngster can become a source of disruption for others as well. Within the family, the mother may emerge as protective and close binding, the father as distant and rejecting. Recently the Institute for the Protection of Lesbian and Gay Youth was called in by a settlement house in Brooklyn to help with the case of a fourteen-year-old black male publicly identified as homosexual because of effeminate mannerisms. Referred to the center as a consistent truant, he refused to attend school because of the verbal and physical abuse to which he had been continuously subjected. While at the settlement house the young man designed, directed, and executed a fashion show. What some saw as a real talent to be encouraged others saw as an example of effeminate behavior to be discouraged. Disagreement as to how to treat the young man caused much dissension among the staff and created further problems for the adolescent himself.

Isolation

Most adolescents are not that obvious and, as Goffman points out, the rewards for being normal are so great that those who can pass will. The gay adolescent who has opted for the "closet," a term derived from the "skeleton in the closet" metaphor, knows that in order to remain in certain settings and to maintain certain relationships, the fact of sexual orientation must be hidden. This strategy of deception distorts almost all relationships the adolescent may attempt to develop or maintain and creates an increasing sense of isolation. The adolescent realizes that his or her membership in the approved group, whether it be the team, the church, the classroom, or the family, is based on a lie.

This reinforces the belief that one is not truly a member of the group, even while membership within it is maintained.

Even in their homes youngsters are forced to act a role. Contrary to the current antilocution that argues that the homosexually oriented individual and homosexuality are a danger to the family, it is the fear and deception resulting from the need to dissemble that disrupt the family's integrity as a unit. Most adolescents, as their emphasis shifts from the home to peer socialization, feel a normal distancing between themselves and their parents. However, this distancing becomes abnormal for gay adolescents with the fear that their parents will discover their secret.

The socialization of the gay adolescent becomes a process of deception at all levels, with ability to play a role assuming primary significance. Techniques developed by the adolescent in this desperate attempt to hide are as varied as the individuals themselves. One young Roman Catholic male chose to date a young woman he knew was going to become a nun. With her, he could make an occasional obligatory sexual overture with the knowledge that she would say no. A young lesbian reported indulging in heavy petting as part of her hiding process, even though it frightened and disgusted her. She found it bearable only by fantasizing she was doing it with another girl.

A major aspect of the closet is the ever-present need to self-monitor. Unconscious and automatic behaviors, especially those relating to gender, are brought to the forefront of conscious attention. The way one walks, stands, talks, holds the wrist or hand become possible sources of disclosure. Clothing must be carefully considered, not just for style or group homogeneity but for the possibility that it may give something away. For years many gay men would not wear green and lesbians would not wear signet rings because each was considered to be a sign of homosexuality.

Possibilities for disclosure lie in the most prosaic situations. For example, many young males try to avoid gym class, not because of the sports involved but because they are afraid that they may get an erection in the showers. The heterosexual male adolescent can laugh off such an occurrence and can joke or even brag about it. The young gay male, however, must fear that it will reveal his stigma.

The process of deception may hinder the development of nonerotic friendships between members of the same sex. During this transition between childhood and adulthood, when it is difficult to separate feelings of friendship from erotic feelings, the young gay adolescent must be careful not to become too close for fear the closeness will be misunderstood on either side. This distancing from one's friends may be at the root of the belief that gay males are not able to have mature nonerotic relationships (Pattison and Pattison 1980), a belief that is contradicted by the data obtained in other studies (Bell and Weinberg 1978; Weinberg and Williams 1974). These data, however, deal with adult gay people and not adolescents. It is not that the gay adolescent cannot form friendships because of homosexuality, per se, but that stigmatization and the need to hide distort relationship formation.

The maintenance of a facade becomes all-pervasive. Each successive act of deception, each moment of monitoring what is unconscious and automatic for others, serves to reinforce the belief in one's difference and inferiority. Perry, Gawell, and Gibbon (1956) point out: "The awareness of inferiority means that one is unable to keep out of consciousness the formulation of some chronic feeling of the worst sort of insecurity, and this means that one suffers anxiety and perhaps even something worse . . . the fear that others can disrespect a person because of something he shows means that he is always insecure in his contact with other people; . . . now that represents an almost fatal deficiency of the self-system."

Like all stigmatized individuals, the gay adolescent needs a "sympathetic other." Centuries of discrimination preclude the presence of a gay adult role model to whom the adolescent can turn. Fears of ostracism, humiliation, and even violence deter the young person from seeking that other among peers. There are generally two sources open to gay adolescents troubled by fears, anxieties, pain, and especially isolation: they may turn to casual sexual contact with strangers, especially in the case of the young gay male, or they may ask for help from concerned professionals.

Casual sexual contact, at least for the young gay male, is common. For a few furtive moments he can achieve, not just a sexual release, but a lessening of the overpowering tensions of hiding. Forced by his fear of disclosure to have an obsessive concern with sexuality, the casual sexual contact becomes a means of compartmentalizing his life and separating sexual action from all aspects of his development. Rather than encouraging a fusion of sexuality and emotionality, the behavior further separates them. The setting, the danger, often the literal filth of the surroundings reinforce the belief that a homosexual orientation is sick, deviant, and despicable. The young person's sense of inferiority and worthlessness is intensified and, even worse, he grows to view his

60

partners in the same way, further lessening his chances of developing a network of sympathetic others that he can respect and rely on. Hatred for oneself and for one's group becomes a common unifying theme.

Public sexual activity by young males is well known. While condemned loudly and blamed on seductions by older men, as long as it remains hidden in restrooms, movie houses, parks, and beaches, little is done about it. Any attempt to provide the gay adolescent with an alternative is met with an immediate negative reaction. There are even vociferous attacks on sex education classes that present factual information about homosexuality and the homosexually oriented.

Roesler and Deisher (1972) have pointed out much of this behavior is age bound. They found that the earlier a young man "came out," that is, the earlier his first sexual experience, the more likely he was to have frequented parks, theaters, restrooms, and other known public meeting places. However, as the young men grew older and became legally able to go to gay bars, their involvement in such public encounters decreased. Since the gay bar is a primary social meeting place for young gay men, the male adolescent is unable to develop a social network of sympathetic others until he is about twenty-one years of age, and then only after he has been conditioned to respond to other gay males on a sexual level only. He often has not had the opportunity to develop courting behaviors other than direct sexual contact. Heterosexual adolescents learn to date and go through a series of societally ordained procedures with sexual contact as a possible end result. The young gay male often learns to start with the end result, sexual behavior, and then attempts to develop the relationship.

There are two possible outcomes to this depersonalization of sexual encounter. The gay adolescent who has learned to despise his sexual orientation may transfer his self-hatred to those who share his stigma. An alternative reaction may arise from the presence of concomitant emotions such as relief from the tension of hiding, pleasure at being able to "be oneself," the feeling that one is truly close to someone for the first time because one does not have to hide. These feelings may combine in a young adult who has not had the chance to socialize with other gay people to give an impression of intense closeness and involvement that is mistaken for love. This, too, is age related and may be a major factor in what appears to be the transitory nature of many homosexual affairs. Recent evidence indicates that there are many gay couples who develop deep and abiding relationships (Bell and Weinberg 1978). However, such attachments usually develop later for the

gay person because he or she learns at a later date those social interactions with peers that the heterosexual adolescent had the opportunity
to learn during the teenage years.

The young gay adolescent will often turn to a clergyman, physician,
or other professional for help. Too often these professionals share
society's stigma view of homosexuality and see the resolution of the
problem as the changing of sexual orientation. In so doing they exacer-
bate the sense of inferiority and increase the need and aptitude for
self-deception. This is especially true when it is believed that sexual
contact with the opposite sex, or even marriage, will be the answer to
the adolescent's problems. Such mistaken advice only intensifies what
Troiden (1979) has called the dissociation or signification stage of attaining a gay identity. In this stage, the presence of the homosexual
attribute is so ego dystonic for the individual that even overt homosexual behavior is interpreted as being something other than evidence of a
homosexual orientation. Typical examples are seen in the explanations
that the behavior was "something I would outgrow," "due to loneliness and lack of female companionship," or "sexual experimentation
and curiosity." Such dissociation is encouraged by people in the helping professions who believe that homosexuality is just a bad habit
(Kelly 1975) or a lack of "commitment to heterosexuality" (Pattison
and Pattison 1980).

This dissociation stage may last late into adulthood, in fact may
never be overcome, sometimes with tragic results. Humphreys's (1970)
finding that the majority of men who indulged in public sex in restrooms were married is probably best understood as a carryover of the
adolescent's inability to form a social network in which sexual partners
can be found. Recent reports concerning public officials who, though
caught in illicit homosexual behavior, denied their homosexuality and
cited their marriages as evidence of a heterosexual orientation are
further illustrative of this dissociation.

Gay Identity

Troiden (1979) has described a four-stage model for the attainment of
a gay identity. A consideration of this model may help us to understand
how we may help the young gay adolescent achieve the hoped-for
fusion of sexual identity and emotionality.

The first stage is sensitization, usually occurring before the age of
thirteen and between thirteen to seventeen. While Troiden sees this as

primarily the period in which one gains the experience that retrospectively is interpreted as homosexual, I propose that this is the
period in which the young person learns the virtual social identity of
the homosexual. The second stage, dissociation and signification,
arises from the need to reject the idea that the negative virtual social
identity assigned to the gay person applies to oneself. Stages 1 and 2
must be overcome before going on to stage 3, coming out, which is
divided into three parts: self-identification as homosexual; initial involvement in the homosexual subculture; and redefinition of homosexuality as a positive and viable life-style. Each part of stage 3 may be
reached separately and an individual may stop at any one. All three
parts are essential to achieve stage 4, the fusion of sexuality and emotionality.

Conclusions

Negative sensitization and the resulting dissociation can be changed
only if young people are exposed to alternatives to the present prejudicial attitudes toward the homosexually oriented.

The young person must have access to accurate information about
homosexuality and to the possibility of maintaining one's personal,
social, ethical, and professional integrity with the homosexual attribute. Greater attention should be paid in sex education curricula to
discussions of homosexuality as a normal variation of sexual orientation. In addition, suitable gay adult role models must be provided. To
achieve this important need, those who are homosexually oriented
must have the courage and strength to be open and public about their
sexual orientation. In addition, all professionals must work against
those discriminatory practices which make it necessary for the gay
adult to hide.

Equally important, there must be a concerted effort to provide gay
adolescents with the opportunity to have meaningful social environments in which they can develop their personal and social skills free
from fear of exposure and censure. These environments can range from
rap groups to ordinary social activities.

Gay adolescents themselves have identified their major problems as
arising from the need for secrecy and the disapproval of the straight
world (Roesler and Diesher 1972). The only way to eliminate the resulting pain and damage is to change the basis for the stigmatization
process, the prejudice of homophobia. Stigmatization of the gay ado-

lescent has evolved from centuries of misinformation and fear. Education through direct teaching and the example of role models will be the best way to attack discrimination at its root.

NOTE

I would like to acknowledge the help of Emery S. Hetrick and Harriet and Milton Klein for their suggestions and criticisms.

REFERENCES

Allport, G. 1958. *The Nature of Prejudice.* Garden City, N.Y.: Doubleday.

Bell, A. P., and Weinberg, M. S. 1978. *Homosexualities: A Study of Diversity among Men and Women.* New York: Simon & Schuster.

Brown, H. 1976. *Familiar Faces, Hidden Lives: The Story of Homosexual Men in America Today.* New York: Harcourt Brace Jovanovich.

Buchanan, P. 1977. Gay day: looking beyond the Miami Mauve Movement. *New York Daily News.* June 7.

Christian Anti-Communism Crusade. 1981. 21(1): 2–3.

Epstein, J. 1970. Homo/hetero: the struggle for sexual identity. *Harper's* 241:36–51.

Erikson, E. 1963. *Childhood and Society.* 2d ed. New York: Norton.

Gilder, G. 1979. Letters to the editor. *Commentary* 67(4): 8–9.

Goffman, E. 1963. *Stigma: Notes on the Management of Spoiled Identity.* Englewood Cliffs, N.J.: Prentice-Hall.

Haller, J., and Haller, R. 1974. *The Physician and Sexuality in Victorian America.* Urbana: University of Illinois Press.

Humphreys, L. 1970. *Tearoom Trade: Impersonal Sex in Public Places.* Chicago: Aldine.

Jackman, A. I. 1979. *The Paranoid Homosexual Basis of Antisemitism and Kindred Hatred.* New York: Vantage.

Kardiner, A. 1954. *Sex and Morality.* New York: Bobbs-Merrill.

Kelly, G. 1975. *The Political Struggle of Active Homosexuals to Gain Social Acceptance.* Chicago: Franciscan Herald Press.

Mosse, G. L. 1978. *Toward the Final Solution: A History of European Racism.* New York: Fertig.

Pattison, E. M., and Pattison, M. L. 1980. "Ex-Gays": religiously mediated change in homosexuals. *American Journal of Psychiatry* 137(12): 1553–1562.

Perry, H. S.; Gawell, M.; and Gibbon, M. 1956. *Clinical Studies in Psychiatry*. New York: Norton.

Podhoretz, N. 1977. The culture of appeasement. *Harper's* 255:25–32.

Roesler, T., and Deisher, R. 1972. Youthful male homosexuality. *Journal of the American Medical Association* 219(8): 1018–1023.

Rupp, J. C. 1980. Homosexually related deaths. In W. Curren, A. L. McGarry, and C. S. Petty, eds. *Modern Legal Medicine, Psychiatry and Forensic Science*. Philadelphia: Davis.

Socarides, C. 1975. *Beyond Sexual Freedom*. New York: Quadrangle.

Socarides, C. 1978. *Homosexuality*. New York: Aronson.

Stearn, J. 1962. *The Sixth Man*. New York: MacFadden.

Troiden, R. R. 1979. Becoming homosexual: a model of gay identity acquisition. *Psychiatry* 42:362–373.

U.S. Senate Committee. 1950. *Employment of homosexuals and other sex perverts in government*. Document no. 241. Washington, D.C.: Government Printing Office.

Voth, H. 1977. *The Castrated Family*. Kansas City, Mo.: Sheed, Andrews, & McMeel.

Weinberg, M., and Williams, C. 1974. *Male Homosexuals*. New York: Oxford University Press.

RUDOLPH G. RODEN AND MICHELLE M. RODEN

A minuscule percentage of European Jews survived the Holocaust of World War II by escaping, hiding, or facing the trauma of concentration camp. These survivors and their children, now scattered across the globe, share a number of characteristics and emotions which have permanently altered them. And although survivors of Nazi camps and their children may share similarities of traumatization with survivors of other catastrophes, certain aspects of their condition are unique.

The degree to which the survivor is traumatized depends to some extent on the nature of the life threat. Natural catastrophes such as floods, earthquakes, fire, explosions, hurricanes, and car accidents usually cause brief traumatization in which the victim may suffer fear, loss, and eventual feelings of abandonment. Prolonged traumatization usually develops from man-made catastrophes such as war; yet, in most cases, the victim still has some control over his environment or a stable role to cling to. The soldier is able to fight or defend himself, and even the prisoner of war has a special status. If he survives he can return to his home with honor and recognition. The liberated survivor has none of these.

As we are learning from Vietnam veterans, the survivor is particularly sensitive to social acceptance. The malevolent political oppression of the Nazi military regime and the unwillingness of the general population to accept anyone who seemed foreign or different either before or after incarceration were stresses for the Holocaust survivor that did not affect other types of survivors.

An ancient trend of anti-Jewish sentiment plagues the world to this day. For the French, the Slavs, and others, as well as for the Germans, Jews have always been the favorite minority for persecution. The re-

sultant Jewish paranoia, which has passed from generation to generation, traumatized the stereotypical Jew but also psychologically prepared him (Burnham 1980). Prisoners of concentration camps such as
those in the Communist bloc countries went through similar experiences, but since they were not as stereotyped as the Jews, the
traumatization took different forms (Borowitz 1979).

Because they could not return home after the war, the survivors'
only recourse was to emigrate to a new land and try to start a new life.
However, the effects of emigration—the uprooting, mourning for the
fatherland, inability to adapt, and feeling of rejection or persecution in
the new land—were also brutal. Families and family loyalties split, and
an unusually wide generation gap developed because the second generation is generally able to adapt more easily and assimilate to a new
environment.

Thus, feeling ostracized and isolated, the survivor is usually extra-
sensitive to and protective of his offspring, for they symbolize the
renewed meaning of life and the recreation of the new family or future
clan, and they represent all his hopes. These children, the survivors of
survivors—for it is difficult to live with a survivor—respond in various
ways.

There has been very little research on children of Nazi concentration
camp survivors, and what studies there are come to approximately the
same conclusions. The children are removed in place, time, and culture
from the parents' ordeal. Many are ignorant of the specifics of what
their parents went through, yet for them, just as for their parents, the
Holocaust is not a set of historical events safely locked in textbooks
and commemoration ceremonies. The tattoo on some survivors' arms
is very noticeable and shocking, and admiration for the parents is based
on the connotations of this tattoo. Many children are now making trips
to Israel and their parents' homeland in order to discover their true
identities as well as to know and understand the Holocaust.

Imagining situations that their parents describe, the children wonder
what they would have done in their places—whether they would have
had the luck and skill to survive. Some have dreams of running from
the Nazis or traveling in locked cattle cars. Many suffer from the
contrast between the comparative ease of their own lives and the suffering of their parents. "I haven't been tested enough," one woman
explained (Mostysser 1975).

A generation away, survivors of survivors share their parents' sense
of trauma. They possess as their own the emotions that grew out of

their parents' uprooting, persecution, and near extermination. Just as the survivors, members of the second generation feel an almost primordial pain and terror as well as a radical insecurity about their own worth and the sustaining power of their world. Moreover, irrational as it may seem, many feel guilty for not having suffered themselves and for not having prevented what happened. These emotions are carefully stored away from their daily comings and goings, but one can sense the feelings clearly enough as they speak of their parents' experiences in flat tones that could give way to chaotic emotions, even tears (Mostysser 1975).

For children of the Holocaust generation, raising a family has cosmic significance. In an attempt to remedy the damage of the Holocaust and assure that the deaths of the family predecessors and the rest of the six million victims were not in vain, they feel a sacred duty to have children. The children bear the names of deceased relatives, names that carry the responsibility for the lost life as well as their own.

The children of survivors often marry into families like their own. They continue to have recurrent fantasies, based more or less in reality, about different facets of concentration camps—shower heads, barbed wire, smokestacks, overcrowded trains, and so forth. They encounter major guilt that leaves them only two possible courses of action: either they must erase everything connected to their parents' history or they must live through it.

Beyond this anomalous identification, children of survivors are as varied in personalities, political views, and religious observance as the Jewish community as a whole. But out of their shared feelings arise pressures, conflicts, and ambivalence that make it possible to speak of them as a group.

A fair proportion of these children suffer some anomalies like hair pulling, nail biting, or thumb sucking. Their performance in school is generally above average. They are usually quite passive when confronted with open aggression. These children often show an unconscious denial of conflict with the immediate surrounding world. They seem to live out either the real experience some of their relatives underwent during the war or, more dramatically, the lives the relatives might have led had they been free.

In treating many children of refugees from Nazi camps, some Israeli psychiatrists (e.g., Davidson 1977) found that they often married hastily and focused all hope on their children. As parents, they proved overprotective but found it difficult to show love.

Upon visiting the United States, Davidson found that the problems here seemed worse than in Israel where there is nationwide support for refugees. He noted that in the United States the survivors were still aliens whose ordeal had never been recognized as part of a national experience.

The majority of the problems of the children of survivors occur at the same chronological age at which their parents were interned in the camps. This anniversary reaction occurs in 80 percent of the children of Holocaust survivors. The anniversary reaction, however, appears to be only one of a number of factors that set children of Holocaust survivors apart from others. Many present atypical diagnostic pictures, and a number have defied categorization. Many of those admitted to the hospitals, while seeming psychotic, were merely reenacting something in their parents' past. Such persons may present symptoms of paranoid schizophrenia: they are suspicious, distrustful, and delusional on occasion, but they do not respond to any of the drugs that usually affect the psychoses. Severe anxiety is also a common symptom. It may represent the fear of separation from parents. In the camps separation was usually final and meant death. Generally at this stage the children of survivors are pushed into the life position of overachievers.

Theories of Survivor Reaction

Numerous problems are encountered by the second generation and, consequently, an ample number of explanations for these problems have begun to take form. For example, the term "survivor syndrome" was first established by Niederland (1968), who realized that survivors share a common bond. However, survivor syndrome seems to be an extremely narrow and negative term. It does not take into account historical, cultural, and social considerations (Epstein 1979). Besides suffering trauma, concentration camp prisoners learned extraordinary survival skills, but the notion of survivor syndrome does not address itself to such beneficent effects. It seems to imply that only defective human mutants, intrinsically different from others in society, could result from the trauma.

Children of survivors know that they are far more complex. They are acutely aware that their parents are driven by an impetus toward life as well as death. In an attempt to justify their survival, the parents demand qualities of their children which are the accumulation of their expectations of all those who were murdered. The children, on the other hand, see their parents as sacred; they cannot express the aggression toward the parents that children usually express as they are growing up.

Sigal and Rakoff (1977) explained these differences chiefly as a result of parental preoccupation: survivors are an extremely preoccupied group, preoccupied with unending mourning of the loss of their siblings and with various psychological and physical illnesses that have beset them since the war. They regard their children's normal robust activities and need for control as an interference in their mourning process, as an extra burden imposed on their already taxed resources. As a result, survivors' children may become anxious and more disruptive. There are other reasons for the children's disruptive behavior. Survivor parents might unconsciously encourage aggressive behavior in their children, aggression they were never able to express toward their own dead families. Children of survivors tend to report greater feelings of alienation than children in a control group. Similarly, the survivors perceived their children to be disturbed more often than did the parents of the control group. Children of survivors appeared to be more dependent on their parents than the controls, which might be related to the children's fear of their own repressed aggression and of the outside world.

The difficulties become compounded in adolescence by the usual identity crises typical of that stage. Identifying with the parents would lead to loneliness, depression, and guilt for not living up to expectations that would have really awkward consequences (Epstein 1977).

Nearly all children of survivors have some problems, ranging from academic difficulties to stuttering, that differentiate them from the norm. Some of the children's problems seem to revolve around fantasies of what their parents did to survive as well as of their parents' persecutors. The degree to which family discussions of the Holocaust and their pre-Holocaust lives have been banned may contribute to the severity of the child's psychopathology by inhibiting the development of a secure identity.

The severity of their parents' wartime trauma and the size of the child's extended family appear to affect the child's predisposition to emotional problems (Epstein 1979). The child's conflict is intensified by overt comparisons made by the survivor: "I went through Auschwitz, and now you do this to me. How would you survive Auschwitz?" Yet the words are not really necessary. The empathy that children of survivors feel for their parents' suffering encourages them to be compliant and protective. They do not wish to cause their parents any more pain.

Like many of the survivors themselves, members of the second generation have a disparate image of themselves as Jews. The emotional component of this self-image involves pride and humiliation. They may feel vaguely ashamed of their parents' victimization and uncomfortable with their own relation to it. Their religious backgrounds are sparse and uncertain.

Survivors of survivors also inherit from their parents a fundamental insecurity about place. A number of individuals invoke the myth of the wandering Jew in order to describe their sense of uprootedness, yet the old and young are united in strategies of detachment (Schulweis 1979). Parents are excessively overprotective and constantly warn their children of impending danger, or they may use them as an audience in the relentless recounting of the terrifying memories. Many of the children have consequently become either moderately phobic or locked in combat with their parents as they try to throw off the smothering yoke. The parent may come to actively hate non-Jews, and the child rebels against this opinion by dating Gentiles or, even worse, Germans. Yet over all the emotional burdens the survivor places on his child weighs the spoken and unspoken communication that this child must provide meaning for the parent's empty life. The child is treated not as an individual but as a heavily invested symbol of the new world. High parental expectations are difficult for any college student, but the redemption of unhappy lives is well-nigh an impossibility; and so many students, even good ones, will give up in despair.

Conclusions

It is clear that the Holocaust experience is in many ways as difficult for members of the second generation to integrate into their lives as it is for those who actually suffered through it. Adjusting to the trauma of near genocide, even at secondhand, is nearly impossible. Those who have not lived through the experience of the Holocaust can never really understand, for those who have will never tell—not really, not completely. Between the memories of survivors and their portrayal in words, even their own, there exists an unbridgeable gulf. The past belongs to the dead and the survivors do not recognize themselves in the image and ideas which presumably depict them today (Wiesel 1976). They believe that only their survivors may come to know and understand the meaning of their lives. As Preston (1978) reflected about his adolescence,

71

To this day I feel my existence to be a miraculous thing, and I am often more serious about life than others. At the same time I tend to put things into [the] perspective of my parents' struggles, and find that today's problems are dwarfed by comparison. I wonder how many persons could make the kind of adjustment they made. While my parents could easily have been obsessed with death and possessed by hatred, I grew up in a home filled with life and love. My parents made close friends. They became the relatives we never knew. There was never a sense of loss in our family: only a sense of purpose.

NOTE

The research reported in this study was funded by a grant from the Harris and Eliza Kempner Fund.

REFERENCES

Borowitz, E. 1979. The changing forms of Jewish spirituality. *America* 140:346–349.

Burnham, H. 1980. The new wandering Jew. *Sh'ma: A Journal of Jewish Responsibility* 191:10–14.

Davidson, S. 1977. *Holocaust Children* 109:60–62.

Epstein, H. 1977. Holocaust. *New York Times Magazine* (June 19, 1977), pp. 14–19.

Epstein, H. 1979. *Children of the Holocaust*. New York: Putnam.

Mostysser, T. 1975. Growing up in America with a Holocaust heritage. *Jewish Student Press Service*.

Niederland, W. G. 1968. The psychiatric evaluation of emotional disorders in survivors of Nazi persecution. In H. Krystal, ed. *Massive Psychic Trauma*. New York: International Universities Press.

Preston, D. 1978. The Holocaust was about me. *Jewish Digest* (November), pp. 59–61.

Sigal, J. J., and Rakoff, V. 1977. Concentration camp survival. *Canadian Psychiatric Association* 16:393–397.

Schulweis, H. 1979. The prophet in a post-Holocaust age. *Jewish Digest* (September), pp. 3–7.

Wiesel, E. 1976. The ever mysterious Holocaust. *Jewish Digest* (April), pp. 37–39.

THE ADOLESCENT
IN LITERATURE

6   ASPECTS OF INTERNALIZATION AND INDIVIDUATION: JAMES JOYCE'S *PORTRAIT OF THE ARTIST AS A YOUNG MAN*

LEVON D. TASHJIAN

The question of identity remains a thorny problem of psychiatry. In part—but only in part—it has become debased and devalued as a term by an indiscriminate, ambiguous, inexact, and widespread usage by clinicians of all persuasions for all sorts of phenomena. It has passed into the vernacular to be used by adolescents of all ages to describe all sorts of minor and major ills, quandaries, and discontents. But even if we use more specific terminology—such as "separation-individuation process," "sense of self," the "self," "autonomy"—we are still left with the basic existential riddle of self-definition. By that I mean to describe that largely inner psychologic process wherein the individual—usually in his late teens or early twenties—coalesces his ontology, his unique and separate essence as a human being.

To be sure, there is a mass of solid and exciting work on the foundations of self-definition in children, especially Mahler's (1968) work on the separation-individuation process, which is indirectly applicable to our problem. There is also the work of Blos (1962) and Erikson (1959), among others, who look at theoretical problems of "identity formation" in adolescence. And, of course, there is the wealth of recent clinical work looking at that group of patients (borderline state) where there is the most critical failure at self-definition or individuation (especially Kernberg [1975] and Kohut [1977]). Therein, among other things, one sees an arrest in the borderline at that awkward, hyperconscious state of extreme vigilance and wariness and painful suffering that most adolescents pass through on the path to self-definition.

But we are still left with the problem of how one—with a reasonable constitution and a reasonable environment and a reasonable development—arrives at self-definition. What is the normative phenomenologic process whereby one takes one's baggage and garbage from the past and compresses it into a core that becomes the self? Is this an active or a passive process? Does one make it happen or does it just happen . . . or not happen? While James Joyce's *Portrait of the Artist as a Young Man* does not provide the answers, it does provide some clues to how one individual arrived at an extraordinary self-definition.

Joyce's *Portrait of the Artist as a Young Man* occupies an important position in twentieth-century literature. It is not only an exceptional novel in its own right, one that does stand on its own merits as a work of art, but it is a major link in the development of Joyce's unique and revolutionary vision that culminates in *Ulysses* and *Finnegans Wake.* Joyce moves away from naturalism—the "reality" of external life—to stream of consciousness—the private "reality of inner life." In *Portrait* we see this transition evolving, slowly transmuting. What seems objective is only apparent, and less important than how the perceiver subjectively perceives what is seemingly objective. This process is purified in *Ulysses,* that book which is the quintessence of our age's sensibility and, alas, is so rarefied in *Finnegans Wake* as to make it unreadable to all but a few.

Portrait also occupies an important place in psychoanalytic thought. Although Joyce derisively jeered any connection with or debt to Jung or Freud—"a certain Dr. Jung (the Swiss Tweedledum who is not to be confused with the Viennese Tweedledee, Dr. Freud)" (Ellman 1959)—he was working with the same material in artistic form that has been the proper concern of depth psychologists of our time. We acknowledge his feat of depicting primary process thinking. We are less aware of his tremendous contribution to unconscious thought patterns and to the way that the past lives, within the individual, within the present. Joyce said, "The past has no 'iron memorial aspect,' but implies 'a fluid succession of presents.' What we are to look for is not a fixed character, but an 'individuating rhythm' not 'an identificative paper but rather the curve of an emotion' " (Ellman 1959).

I choose in this chapter to focus our attention on one aspect of this work, that is, the development within an individual of his identity, of his personal consciousness, of his sense of self. This work is a frank and avowed autobiography which, "except for the incognito of its characters, . . . is based on a literal transcript of the first twenty years of Joyce's life. If anything, it is more candid than other autobiographies. It is distinguished from them by its emphasis on the emotional and intellectual adventures of its protagonist'' (Levin 1968). At the same time it is self-mocking and filled with ironic perceptions and conscious distortions and deflections. While Joyce's fictional account of his formative years jibes very closely with biographical studies (Ellman 1959) and commentaries by childhood contemporaries (Curran 1968), that is less important for our purposes than that it is a personal document of self-definition told not to record historical data about self, family, and others but to portray a true psychobiography about the emotional, intellectual, social, and artistic evolution of the self. And it is in this light that I will summarize the novel, knowingly leaving out much for the sake of developing my thesis.

The story begins in the nursery:

> Once upon a time and a very good time it was there was a moocow coming down along the road and this moocow that was coming down along the road met a nicens little boy named baby tuckoo. . . .
> His father told him that story: his father looked at him through a glass: he had a hairy face.

It quickly moves through infancy and early childhood to age seven where the protagonist, Stephen Dedalus, goes off to a private boarding school, Clongowes. At Clongowes, Stephen is young, frail, bewildered.

> He felt small and weak. When would he be like the fellows in poetry and rhetoric?

He experiences his first injustice when, having honestly broken his glasses and being unable to read, he is paddled by a strict Jesuit disciplinarian for presumably trying to put one over on him. His thoughts range from school to home and back to school. As befits a boy in the latency years, Stephen's thoughts have very little abstraction, are by and large concrete and limited in scope. Yet he hungers to learn.

> Words which he did not understand he said over and over to himself till he had learned them by heart: and through them he had

glimpses of the real world about him. The hour when he too would take part in the life of the world seemed drawing near and in secret he began to make ready for the great part which he felt awaited him the nature of which he only dimly apprehended.

He comes home, and does not return to Clongowes because of a sharp downturn in the family fortunes. His father, who started as an affluent businessman, stumbled and fell, dragging his family with him into not so genteel poverty. He drank and became a blowhard. And Stephen reacted by shutting him out.

The question of honour here raised was, like all such questions, trivial to him. While his mind had been pursuing its intangible phantoms and turning in irresolution from such pursuit he had heard about him the constant voices of his father and of his masters, urging him to be a gentleman above all things and urging him to be a good catholic above all things. These voices had now come to be hollowsounding in his ears. When the gymnasium had been opened he had heard another voice urging him to be strong and manly and healthy and when the movement towards national revival had begun to be felt in the college yet another voice had bidden him be true to his country and help to raise up her fallen language and tradition. In the profane world, as he foresaw, a worldly voice would bid him raise up his father's fallen state by his labours and, meanwhile, the voice of his school comrades urged him to be a decent fellow, to shield others from blame or to beg them off and to do his best to get free days for the school. And it was the din of all these hollowsounding voices that made him halt irresolutely in the pursuit of phantoms. He gave them ear only for a time but he was happy only when he was far from them, beyond their call, alone or in the company of phantasmal comrades.

His awakening is quickened by his father's downfall. At the age of fifteen he wins a school prize and attempts to use the money to help the family. But it quickly passes. And, in the awakening, he turns to his sexual and carnal desires.

He burned to appease the fierce longings of his heart before which everything else was idle and alien. He cared little that he was in mortal sin, that his life had grown to be a tissue of subterfuge and falsehood. Beside the savage desire within him to realise the enormities which he brooded on nothing was sacred. He bore cynically with the shameful details of his secret riots in which he exulted to defile with patience whatever image had attracted his eyes. By day and by night he moved among distorted images of the outer world. A figure that had seemed to him by day demure and innocent came towards him by night through the winding darkness of sleep, her face transfigured by a lecherous cunning, her eyes bright with brutish joy. Only the morning pained him with its dim memory of dark orgiastic riot, its keen and humiliating sense of transgression.

And he has his first sex with a prostitute.

Looking at these data with Mahler's (1968) schema (as metaphoric paradigm) in mind, it is clear that Stephen enters the first subphase of his adolescent separation-individuation process—that of differentiation—in part because of his disillusionment toward his father and the dissolution of the family fortune, in part because of the awakening of his sexual desires. With his first sexual experience, he moves quickly into the second subphase—practicing—and experiences an exhilarating freedom.

> From the evil seed of lust all the other deadly sins had sprung forth: pride in himself and contempt of others, covetousness in using money for the purchase of unlawful pleasure, envy of those whose vices he could not reach to and calumnious murmurings against the pious, gluttonous enjoyment of food, the dull glowering anger amid which he brooded upon his longing, the swamp of spiritual and bodily sloth in which his whole being had sunk.

This freedom, alas, is short-lived. At a religious retreat he hears a Jesuit priest describe, in most exquisite and painful detail, the physical and spiritual pains of hell, eternal damnation. Of these the greatest pains are spiritual, namely, the pain of loss and separation and the pain of conscience, guilt.

Stephen, physically and spiritually shaken by this picture of his damnation, has a change of heart. In his repentance he makes a partial rapprochement with his mother and with not his real father but God the Father: "It was better never to have sinned, to have remained always a child, for God loved little children and suffered them to come to him." He becomes scrupulous, ascetic, and compulsively pious, so much so that he receives a calling from his priest-teacher who tells him, "No angel . . . has the power of a priest of God." He entertains and almost accepts a role that will give him order, status, power, and influence but will rob him of the possession of his own self: "The wisdom of the priest's appeal did not touch him to the quick. He was destined to learn his own wisdom apart from others or to learn the wisdom of others himself wandering among the snares of the world."

Soon afterward he enters the university and strongly flouts his mother's wishes that he enter the church. He has a vision, while with his school chums at the beach, of himself as an artificer, a creator. He begins to delineate his own destiny and to get a strong, unswerving sense of the course in life he must and will chart. But when he returns home he is struck by the barren, dreary reality of existence and how he is bound there.

Thus he continues his course toward individuation, torn by his inspirations and his ties to home. Each one of his separations, up to now, has left him progressively more isolated. Though the loneliness pains him, he pushes on. His ultimate challenge, the last hurdle, is his mother. He refuses to take Easter communion for her, partly because of his superstitions about a religion he no longer believes in, partly because it would be an act of bad faith. In dialogue, with his friend Cranley, he says:

> You have asked me what I would do and what I would not do. I will tell you what I will do and what I will not do. I will not serve that in which I no longer believe. Whether it call itself my home, my fatherland or my church: and I will try to express myself in some work of life or art as freely as I can and as wholly as I can, using for my defense the only arms I allow myself to use—silence, exile, and cunning.

Suddenly and quietly, without warning, the style changes. From a measured, reasoned, full, and round language it becomes staccato, fragmented, episodic. In the form of diary notes, Joyce has taken us completely out of the naturalistic order and plunged us into Stephen's interior monologue. He has individuated. These last few pages bristle with an excitement, an impatience to get on with learning and beginning. They culminate in the last two notes:

> 26 April: Mother is putting my new secondhand clothes in order. She prays now, she says, that I may learn in my own life and away from home and friends what the heart is and what it feels. Amen. So

be it. Welcome, O life! I go to encounter for the millionth time the reality of experience and to forge in the smithy of my soul the uncreated conscience of my race.

27 April: Old father, old artificer, stand me now and ever in good stead.

Discussion

Thus we see, in sketchy summary, the broad picture of Stephen's surge toward individuation, an individuation marked by a hypertrophied need for separateness. Certainly it is more separateness than most of us attain, but perhaps not more than many of us would wish for. With the separateness came loneliness and pain, but also power and strength. Young Joyce bewildered the Irish literary set, then in full renaissance. Tall, thin, handsome, and striking in his bizarre and studiedly disheveled dress, his arrogance offended while, at the same time, his genius, as yet largely untapped, attracted. Yeats wondered why he spent time with this "wild genius" who, instead of repaying his kindness with deference, was critical, challenging, and acted as if he were the equal of his master (Ellman 1959).

In this surge toward individuation we can clearly see the four sub-phases of the separation-individuation process: *differentiation* clearly brought on by a disillusionment with his father and by the kindling of his own sexual desires; *practicing* sexually, arrogantly in defiance of all authority, experiencing "an intoxicating sense of triumph over his past and . . . addicted to this state of apparent liberation" (Blos 1962); *rapprochement* brought about by fear of damnation (eternal separation and guilt) with a return to the home and the church; and, finally, a slow, steady *consolidation of individuality*, gradually teasing, dissecting away the infantile symbiotic bonds. We see his ego at work, always at work even when he is passive. And it is this active, relentless, searching strength and courage that lead him to have a greater belief in himself and sense of his destiny.

He meets Erikson's (1959) criteria for having a shaped and full "ego identity": he certainly has a "conscious sense of individual identity." He shows "an unconscious striving for a continuity of personal character." There is much evidence of "the silent doings of ego synthesis." We must, however, stretch a point to say that he maintained "an inner solidarity with a group's ideals and identity." For, while he rejected his family, friends, and, indeed, all Irish society to move into a voluntary lifelong exile on the Continent, he wrote only about Dublin, about himself, family, and friends. Yet he maintained inner solidarity with a larger, more universal group—the group of creators, artists, artificers, makers. His nom de plume—Dedalus (Stephen *Hero* in an earlier version)—is deliberate, symbolic. Daedalus, the architect, inventer, artist, built a labyrinth on Crete for Minos, was imprisoned in that labyrinth, and escaped from that labyrinth on wings. Dedalus-Joyce, the writer, constructs labyrinths of his past as he struggles to escape from them. Thus we see a reworking in his life and writings of his struggles for separation and longing for reunion. He rejects his past as he retains it. And in retaining his past he rejects it.

But there is something missing. While we can see the landmarks of Stephen's process of self-definition, and the end result, we still have not explained how he was able to stalk his way through the labyrinth of his own adolescence and survive. Why did he not get lost? Why did he not give up and return home? Why did he not realize that his adolescent fantasy was grandiose, bordering on being delusional? We have a sense of his constitutional givens—his need to master, to forever churn and be active, his searching mind. We know, as much as we know about most people, of his early life and development and his infantile object ties. Yet we still must accept on faith his passage through adolescence but have difficulty in delineating the phenomenology of this passage.

Here Joyce can help us, not only understand his own passage, but perhaps gain some clues to conceptualize those critical nodal points which, day in and day out, are so necessary for any adolescent in ordering and integrating his disparate and diverse experiences into an inner psychic vision, an entity. And that lies in his concept of epiphany, which is a galvanizing force that illumines and enlightens. Internally, an epiphany is a "manifestation or appearance of some divine or superhuman being," a very religious term, associated with the coming of Christ. Like many a well-schooled Jesuit turned apostate, he gives up the faith but maintains the thought. To quote Ellmann (1959) further:

> The epiphany did not mean for Joyce the manifestation of the Godhead, the showing forth of Christ to the Magi, although that is a useful metaphor for what he had in mind. The epiphany was the sudden "revelation of the whatness of a thing; the moment in which the 'soul of the commonest object . . . seems to us radiant.' "

An epiphany is a special kind of insight that has a private symbolism not necessarily understandable to the world at large. It is Proust's madeleine triggering a flood of associations and reminiscences. It may be clarifying, but just as often it is ambiguous or untranslatable into logical (secondary process) thought. Epiphanies are associational, ordering, combining, and recombining to the inner mind. They are the nuances, the noting of seemingly irrelevant and trivial details, oblique and ironic insights that seem utterly without meaning.

We are familiar with the epiphanies when they are out of control, as in our psychotic patients. Sometimes we are startled by them, sometimes we seek to understand them and thus communicate with their maker. But we are not so used to thinking of them as normative shaping devices when they are in control and work in the service of the ego. As such they are the mortar which helps to seal the building blocks of experience. They differentiate, separate figure from ground, and serve to integrate as they separate.

Portrait of the Artist as a Young Man is filled with such epiphanies, many of which pass unnoticed by the casual reader. The climaxes of each episode, save for the final leaving, are muffled rather than dramatic. Some are passionless, others filled with passion. Some convey the flavor of ecstatic experience, but all serve, for Stephen, a personal and very private synthesizing function which assimilates and orders the external world within the self, thus strengthening and ennobling the self, building toward separateness and individuation.

Conclusions

As a psychobiographical document, *Portrait* illustrates in a frank and complete way the complexities of the separation-individuation process and the evolutionary development of a unique identity. The work is an excellent case study to complement the theories of Mahler, Blos, and Erikson, among others, being concerned with the private emotional and intellectual strivings of the protagonist, rather than with a depiction of some kind of historical reality. As such the reader is with the protagonist at each step of the shaping of his "self" and can experience, at the same time being able to analyze that experience, the formation of his unique identity. Further, Joyce's concept of epiphany—a religious term he uses to describe the artistic process—can be very helpful in understanding the psychological process of assimilation of identifications and external realities, of internalization and reworking of these data to the end of defining one's own self.

REFERENCES

Blos, P. 1972. *On Adolescence*. New York: Free Press.
Curran, C. P. 1968. *James Joyce Remembered*. New York: Oxford University Press.
Ellman, R. 1959. *James Joyce*. New York: Oxford University Press.
Erikson, E. 1959. *Identity and the Life Cycle*. New York: International Universities Press.
Joyce, J. 1916. *Portrait of the Artist as a Young Man*. New York: Viking, 1964.
Kernberg, O. 1975. *Borderline Conditions and Pathological Narcissism*. New York: Aronson.
Kohut, H. 1977. *The Restoration of the Self*. New York: International Universities Press.
Levin, H. 1968. *James Joyce: A Critical Introduction*. Norfolk, Conn.: New Directions.
Mahler, M. 1968. *Human Symbiosis and the Vicissitudes of Individuation*. New York: International Universities Press.

7 THE POSTADOLESCENT CRISIS OF JOHN STUART MILL

JON A. SHAW

John Stuart Mill was one of the great English philosophers of the nineteenth century. As a young man of twenty, he experienced a profound postadolescent crisis which he was later to describe in his autobiography. The pre-Freudian account of this episode resulted, I believe, in an unusually candid and graphic portrayal of this experience. This chapter will attempt to explore this crisis within the context of our present understanding of this phase of development. Particular attention will be given to those facets of his life which represent not only the intrinsic conflicts of this phase of development but also those particular tasks whose resolution is required for the consolidation of mature character formation. Specifically, this refers to his struggles to loosen his infantile ties, to consolidate a sexual identity, to establish an enduring sense of identity, and to master an infantile trauma.

Mill (1806–1873) was a child prodigy and the son of James Mill, a philosopher and disciple of Jeremy Bentham. He experienced one of the most intense and relentless educations ever perpetrated on a son by a father. His *Autobiography* (1887) is most notable in its delineation of this early educational experience. He received instruction in Greek when he was three. By the time he was eight, he had read the first six dialogues of Plato, the whole of Herodotus, and had undertaken the study of Latin. He writes, "My father in all his teaching, demanded of me, not only the utmost that I could do, but much that I could by no possibility have done." The boy studied and prepared all his lessons at the same table as his father. "I was forced to have recourse to him for the meaning of every word which I did not know" (p. 6).

One of the son's childhood memories is of early morning walks with his father. This earliest recollection of green fields and wild flowers is mingled with the recollection of the account he gave daily to his father of what he had read the previous day. Father would offer him ideas and explanations regarding civilization, government, morality, and mental cultivation, which he then required his son to restate to him in his own words. He was not allowed to read children's books, have playthings, or associate with other boys. His father was bent on his escaping the corrupting influence which boys exercise over boys, particularly their vulgar modes of thought and feeling.

When John was twelve years of age, he wrote a history of the Roman government and first displayed his lifelong interest in revolution and his concern for the emancipation of the individual from tyrannical government. Mill noted that the ". . . struggles between the patricians and the plebians . . . engrossed all the interest in my mind" (p. 13).

Lest he forget, his father would tell him that whatever he knew more than others could not be ascribed to any merit in him, but to the unusual advantage which was his in having a father who was able to teach and so willingly to give the necessary trouble and time to him. The son's dependency on his father is reflected in his comment: "I thought for myself almost from the first and occasionally thought differently from him, though for a long time only on minor points and making his opinion the ultimate standard" (p. 29).

The autobiography of John Stuart Mill is unique in that not once among all the pages of his writing is there a reference or thought given to his mother. One is left with the impression of a child without a mother. The only hint that there might be a mother is a reference to eight younger siblings. Yet the influence of this unknown woman, cruelly scorned by his father and no less scorned by her son, had, I believe, a profound impact on his choice of a woman and his devotion to the cause of women in general. In an early draft of his autobiography, he had indicted his mother for not being warmhearted. However, on closer scrutiny, it becomes evident that he indicts her particularly for her passivity and unassertiveness in demanding respect and obedience—a fault not possessed by his father. His mother was in his mind not "man enough." He had little sensitivity to his mother's plight in providing for nine children in an impoverished family where she was devalued by the father as a stupid housemaid.

While J. S. Mill ignored his relationship with his mother, he recounted in detail the unfolding of his relationship with his father, though not fully realizing the full extent to which this relationship determined so much of his later life. Mill writes of his father, "I was always too much in awe of him to be otherwise than extremely subdued and quiet in his presence" (p. 34).

The father reportedly had little belief in pleasure and dismissed feelings as irrelevant. He displayed little tenderness toward his children. His son writes that his father "resembled most Englishmen in being ashamed of the signs of feeling and by the absence of demonstration, starving the feelings themselves" (p. 52). The father's behavior toward his son was determined by his belief in the tabula rasa and by the doctrine of association. Since experience determines all, the object of praise and blame should be the encouragement of right conduct and the discouragement of wrong conduct.

From the time Mill was fifteen he had defined his object in life as being a reformer of the world. His conception of happiness was identified with this goal. His internal adolescent struggles and conflicts were externalized in social reforms which served both as an extension of his father's beliefs and values and as a not-too-subtle disavowal of recognized authority. All this continued until his twentieth year when he underwent a profound mental crisis. Years later, Mill wrote a poignant account of this postadolescent experience which served as a turning point in his psychic life.

It was the autumn of 1826. I was in a dull state of nerves, such as everybody is occasionally liable to; unsusceptible to enjoyment or pleasurable excitement; one of those moods when what is pleasurable at other times, becomes insipid or indifferent. . . . In this frame of mind it occurred to me to put the question directly to myself: "Suppose that all your objects in life were realized; that all the changes in institutions and opinions which you are looking forward to, could be completely effected at this very instant; would this be a great joy and happiness to you?" And an irrepressible self-consciousness distinctly answered, "No." At this my heart sank within me; the whole foundation on which my life was constructed fell down. All my happiness was to have been found in the continual pursuit of this end. The end had ceased to charm, and how could there ever again be any interest in the means? I seemed to have nothing to live for. [P. 133]

In vain he sought relief from his favorite books, but he now read them without feeling. He felt unable to confide his grief to anyone. He did not love anyone sufficiently to make confiding his grief a necessity. He felt his distress was neither interesting nor respectable.

> My father to whom it would have been natural for me to have recourse in any practical difficulties was the last person to whom, in such a case as this, I looked for help. Everything convinced me that he had no knowledge of any such mental states as I was suffering from and that even if he could be made to understand it he was not the physician who could heal it. . . . My education which was wholly his work had been conducted without any regard to the possibility of its ending in this result; and I saw no use in giving him the pain of thinking that his plan had failed when the failure was probably irremediable and at all events beyond the power of his remedies. [P. 135]

How desperately the son had to struggle against the wish to tell his father that he, the father, had failed him. The inability to discuss his distress with his father reveals how deeply he felt betrayed by him. He writes, "I was left stranded at the commencement of my voyage, with a well-equipped ship and a rudder, but no sail; without any real desire for the ends which I had been so carefully fitted out to work for. . . . There seems no power in nature sufficient to begin the formulation of my character anew. . ." (p. 139). Two lines from Coleridge read at a later date he thought best described his mental state at that time: "Work without hope draws nectar in a sieve, and hope without an object cannot live" (p. 140).

It is clear that a boy's idealized love and admiration for his father had been sorely challenged. His father's teachings as a way of life had been seriously questioned. It was the father as the love object of his life who had been lost. He had sought to emulate and please his father and had, alas, discovered that this did not bring happiness. He sank into a heavy melancholy and performed his duties mechanically and by mere force of habit.

Mill's profound depression, lethargy, and paralysis of will were the result of a profound guilt and a profound loss. Levi (1945) has suggested that his mental crisis was brought on primarily by the repression of his hatred and death wishes against his father. In his mind he had committed parricide. A *parricide* is "a person who murders either or both of his parents or someone else who stands to him in a somewhat similar relationship" (*Webster's* 1980). It was parental authority that had been

murdered. The bond between child and parent had been violated. He felt
he could no longer rely on his father as the omnipotent and omniscient
guide in his life. By evolving his own autonomy, he had, indeed, psy-
chically killed his father. He had usurped his father's responsibility and
competence in directing his life. Loewald (1979) writes, "Insofar as
humans strive for emancipation and individuation, as well as for object
love, parricide on the plane of psychic action is a developmental necessity." The unconscious murdering of one's father leaves one guilty and
calls for atonement.

After six months, a fortuitous event brought "a small ray of light in
upon the gloom"—an event puzzling in its curative effect, yet so clearly
confirming that the thought he had in his mind (unconscious murder of
his father) subsequently altered his mental state. He notes, "I was
reading accidentally, 'Marmontel's Memoires' and came to the passage
which relates his father's death, the distressed position of the family,
and the sudden inspiration by which he, Marmontel, then a mere boy,
felt and made them feel that he would be everything to them . . . that he
would supply the place of all that they had lost." At that moment, Mill
noted that "a vivid conception of the scene and its feelings came over me
and I was moved to tears. . . . From this moment my burden grew lighter.
The oppression of the thought that all feeling was dead within me was
gone. I was no longer hopeless; I was not a stick or stone. I had still it
seemed some of the material out of which all worth of character and all
happiness are made. . . . Thus the cloud gradually drew off and I again
enjoyed life. . . . I never again was as miserable as I had been" (p. 141).

The reading of the history of another man who had survived the death
of his father and yet had resolved to continue seemed to have galvanized
him to live his own life. Like the other boy, perhaps, he could supply the
place of all that had been lost. It was not just the mitigation of guilt that
comes with the shared experience of an unconscious parricide that
enabled him to suddenly appropriate his own desires and impulses, to
orchestrate his own life, but it was also the shared experience of having
mourned a lost and once excessively loved object. This brings into focus
the comment by Blos (1979) that "the resolution of the negative Oedipus
complex is the task of adolescence." The coming to terms with the
homosexual component of pubertal sexuality represents one of the
determinants of the postadolescence crisis. Sexual identity is predicated
on the completion of this process.

Blos (1968) has observed that the adolescent process comes to an end
and character formation is consolidated when four developmental challenges have been encountered, integrated, and synthesized. First is the

second individuation process or the loosening of the infantile object ties, that is, the disengagement of libidinal and aggressive cathexis from the internalized infantile objects; second, the establishment of a sexual identity which is predicated on the resolution of the positive and negative oedipal components and the capacity to enter into a nonincestual relationship characterized by some degree of novelty; third, the establishment of a sense of ego continuity in which one experiences the self in terms of one's values, perceptions, and essence as having continuity and sameness in time, confirmed by the self and others; and fourth, one that is frequently ignored and very paramount in the life of John Stuart Mill, is the process of working through and resolving the infantile trauma. It is apparent that these four challenges intrinsic to the postadolescent crisis are interwoven into the oedipal tapestry, and their particular resolutions provide the stamp of character.

The recapitulation theory of adolescence has recently been modified (Blos 1979). According to this earlier view, the regressive reexperiencing of early infantile sexuality is initiated by the biological event of puberty. Yet, there is increasing clinical evidence that there is no definitive resolution of the Oedipus complex at the end of the phallic phase but, rather, a suspension of a conflictual constellation. Adolescence represents the continuation of the childhood struggle with the Oedipus complex. Nevertheless, oedipal issues reemerge at adolescence with regularity and a new level of intensity. Their resolution and transformation represent one, if not the essential, aspect of adolescence. This is monitored by an ego which has greatly expanded in its synthetic, integrative, defensive, and adaptive capacities and which necessarily alters the adolescent's experiencing of his oedipal conflicts.

The Oedipus complex refers to both the positive and negative components. The positive oedipal dimension refers to the love relationship with the parent of the opposite sex. The negative oedipal component refers to the child's love relationship with the parent of the same sex. It is the positive oedipal component that falls under repression or finds its partial resolution through identification and the regulatory influences of the superego at the termination of the phallic phase. The negative oedipal component continues throughout childhood. Blos (1968) notes that the state of bisexuality is tolerated in the prelatency child without the catastrophic disharmony that is experienced at puberty.

At puberty the inappropriate nature of the infantile negative oedipal strivings reaches an impasse. The sexual tie to the parent of the same sex has to be severed.

As long as Mill idealized his father and the father represented what he wished to be, his attachment was a narcissistic tie in which Mill assumed the role of a passive extension of his father. His attachment, therefore, was a negative oedipal attachment in which he renounced his own ambitions and strivings for autonomy. The renunciation of his autonomy represented a passive submission to father. His mental crisis represented the symbolic struggle to attain autonomy and independence from his father. As we will see, he was partially successful in this endeavor.

His second individuation process was clearly initiated with the loosening of the infantile ties. The libido invested in the father becomes desexualized with subsequent elaboration of the narcissistic structure of the adult ego ideal. The ego ideal as the heir of the negative oedipal complex represents the internalization of the idealized aspects of the father. As we shall see, Mill's ego ideal is later externalized onto Harriet Taylor as a love object representing predominantly a narcissistic object choice.

Character has its origin in conflict. Character formation aims at the resolution of conflict through the integration and synthetic functions of the ego. Blos (1968) notes, "The high noon of this integrative achievement lies in the terminal period of adolescence when the enormous instability of psychic and somatic function gradually gives way to an organized and integrated mode of operation."

The working through of the mourning process associated with the loss of the idealized father results in an increasing capacity for self-determination, a more realistic self-appraisal with greater acceptance of the limitations of the self and others.

Mill noted that as a consequence of his mental crisis he experienced "two very marked effects on his opinions and character." First, he never wavered in his conviction that happiness is the test of all rules, conduct, and the end of life. He recognized that only those are happy who have their minds fixed on some other objects than their own happiness. Second, he stated,

I for the first time gave its proper place, among the prime necessities of human well-being, to the internal culture of the individual . . . the cultivation of the feelings became one of the cardinal points in my ethical and philosophical creed. . . . I began to find meaning in the things which I had read or heard about the importance of poetry and art as instruments of human culture. [P. 143]

He felt bitterly ashamed about an earlier essay in which, like an extension of his father, he had cynically attacked all sentiment and emotion. He discovered the poetry of Wordsworth. He drank deep from its sentiments and experienced new feelings; he became a lover of nature and a collector of botanical specimens. One might wonder if this exultant love of Wordsworth, whose poetry resonates with a mystical love of nature in which is embodied the poet's love of his mother lost in death, was not, in part, the resurrection of Mill's early love for a once kind, bountiful, and now forgotten mother. As Packe (1954) observed in his biography, "Time and again from this time forward he dragged reason along behind his sympathies; time and again he acted extravagantly from his passions and found a flawless chain of reasoning to justify it afterwards."

Soon afterward he would be able to realize "that there was really something fundamentally erroneous in my father's conception of philosophical method." He writes,

> My father's tone of thought and feeling, I now felt myself at a great distance from; greater indeed than a full and calm explanation and reconsideration on both sides might have shown to exist in reality. But my father was not one with whom calm and full explanations on fundamental points of doctrine could be expected, at least with one whom he might consider as . . . a deserter from his standard . . . I did not always tell him how different. I expected no good, but only pain to both of us from discussing our differences. [P. 179]

Throughout his life, Mill's philosophy would be concerned with the individual's relationship to authority. He would be called the Saint of Liberalism, the greatest nineteenth-century symbol of spiritual liberality and intellectual reasonableness. Aiken (1957) states, "Mill's passionate and complex defense of liberty is perhaps the most powerful and imaginative defense that has ever been made of the open society and the ideal of self-development."

From the time he was twelve he had slowly evolved a passionate interest in revolution—first, it had been the struggle between the plebians and the patricians; then, as an adolescent, it had been the voracious reading of every book he could find on the French Revolution. Now, as a young man, he clearly separated himself from his father's dislike of violence. In a long letter in October 1881, he expressed his views in favor of revolution: "I should not care though a revolution were to exterminate every person in Great Britain and Ireland who has 500 pounds a year. Many very amiable persons would perish, but what is the world the better for such amiable persons" (Packe 1954). Mill's espousal of humanism and individualism became ever more apparent. With the death of James Mill it even became more predominant. "So long as James Mill lived, the heretical humanism so offensive to the stricter Benthamites had been held in check. Now that he was gone, all that was changed" (Packe 1954). The resolution of an infantile conflict and the mastering of a childhood trauma would become ego-syntonic and become a life's task woven into the fabric of his character structure.

Greenacre (1967) defines the childhood traumatic situation as "any condition which seems definitely unfavorable, noxious or drastically injurious to the development of the young individual." As Freud (1906) observed, "The etiology of the neuroses comprises everything which can act in a detrimental manner upon the processes serving the sexual function." Blos (1968) maintained that "trauma is a universal human condition during infancy and early childhood, leaving even under the most favorable circumstances a residue." It seems to me that the summation of the patterning of Mill's experience with an intrusive, omnipresent, demanding, and controlling father and a mother with "frozen sensibilities" represented an early trauma. As Mill wrote, "I grew up in the absence of love and in the presence of fear" (Packe 1954).

It is apparent that adolescence, even with its second chance at resolving infantile conflicts through a regressive process, now monitored by an intact ego with its synthetic and integrative capacities, fails to eliminate all the residues of the pathogenic developmental experience. The adolescent, unable to master the early trauma, assimilates it into his character structure, making it ego-syntonic, and renders it into a life task.

Freud (1939) distinguished between the negative and positive effect of trauma. The negative reactions have the aim that "nothing of the forgotten trauma shall be remembered and nothing repeated." These reactions lead to character formation characterized by avoidance, phobias, compulsions, and inhibitions. The positive reactions to trauma are characterized by "attempts to bring the trauma into operation once again—that is, to remember the forgotten experience . . . to make it real, to experience a repetition of it . . . to revive it in an analogous relationship with someone else. . . . These efforts . . . may be taken up into what passes as a normal ego and as permanent trends in it, may lend it unalterable character traits" (Freud 1939). We will see the consequence of Mill's attempt to resolve his trauma in his choice of a woman as a life's companion and in the tapestry of his philosophy.

John Stuart Mill's philosophical concerns represented a continuous working through of his relationship with his father. In an article (Mill 1831) called "Spirit of the Age," Mill pointed out the anomalies and evils characteristic of the transition from a system of opinions which had worn out, to another only in process of being formed. Is this an ongoing externalization of his own adolescent crisis? In a moment of insight, he noted, "The destiny of mankind in general was ever in my thoughts, could not be separated from my own. I felt that the flaw in my life must be a flaw in life itself" (Mill 1887). He would constantly vacillate between the doctrine of philosophical necessity in which "I was scientifically proved to be the helpless slave of antecedent circumstances; as if my character and that of all others had been formed for us by agencies beyond our control and was wholly out of our own power" and his wish to believe that "although our character is formed by circumstances, our own desires can do much to shape those circumstances; and that what is really inspiriting and enobling in the doctrine of free will is the conviction that we have real power over the formation of our own character; that our will by influencing some of our circumstances can modify our future habits."

Aiken (1957) wrote that Mill believed that the "primary social factor in modern life which blocks the way of individual and collective well-being is the widespread interference of institutions, formal and informal, with individual self-government." This seems to represent an externalization of his own lifelong struggle for self-development and emancipation from his internalized father. His concern with the powerful influences of antecedent experiences on individual self-development is still evident in his essay "Nature," published posthumously. Mill noted that "whatever man does to improve his condition is . . . a thwarting of the spontaneous order of nature, and caused new and unprecedented attempts at improvement to be generally thought of as uncomplimentary . . . and very probably offensive to the powerful beings." Here, again, we see the little boy concerned that he might be a deserter from his father's standards, afraid to make his differences of opinion known to him. In the same essay, he goes on to state, "there still exists a vague notion [that] we should be guided by nature's own ways; that they are God's work, and as such perfect; that man cannot rival their unapproachable excellence, and can best show his skill and piety by attempting in however an imperfect way, to reproduce their likeness." Those who contradict nature's scheme "are afraid of incurring the charge of impiety by saying anything which might be held to disparage the works of the creator's power," just as he had been afraid of the charge of impiety by saying anything which might be held to disparage his father's work.

In his autobiography, Mill would still refer to his father's history of India with a sense of awe, "Though I perceive deficiencies in it now as compared with a perfect standard, I still think of it as, if not the most, one of the most instructive histories ever written." This by a man who had read all the classical historians. Like his father, Mill would live out his life as a bureaucrat working in the same office as his father, initially as his subordinate, and at the age of fifty, assuming the position held so long by his father, the Examiner of India Correspondence. He remained his father's son. At the time of his father's death he would note, "He left as my knowledge extends, no equal among men and but one among women." This made reference to the woman he later married, with whom, in many ways, he would re-create the early relationship with his father.

Adolescence often precipitates the crystallization of those conflicts which become the tasks of adulthood. Certainly Mill's subsequent choice of a love object resonated with his ongoing struggle to resolve the oedipal conflict, particularly the resolution of the negative oedipal conflict. Encompassed in this struggle is his lifelong conflict between his wish to submit passively to authority and his wish to emancipate himself from it. In his choice of a wife, he would relive the experience with his father. Without the threat of homosexuality, he would be able to passively submit to a woman.

It is clear that whatever Mill felt for his mother, in his conscious awareness these feelings were tinged with scorn and contempt. Packe (1954) noted in his biography that "his love for his mother, mangled in their chilly home, became an incoherent pity so intense that all feeling being unbearable he had no feeling left for her at all." He later notes that in her last days, "having been scorned for thirty years by an icy and ungenerous husband, she now found herself despised by her equally icy eldest son."

Mill's scorn and devaluation of his mother reflected the father's values. He was never to make an independent judgment in this regard. His model for the ideal beloved would be predicated on the early idealized and valued image of the incisive and omniscient father. Freud, in his intuitive genius, observed as much on his reading of Mill's autobiography. His comment is worth quoting: "Mill's autobiography is so prudish or so ethereal that one could never gather from it that human beings consist of men and women and that this distinction is the most significant one that exists. In his whole presentation it never emerges that women are different beings . . . '' (Jones 1953).

It is evident that Mill's ideal-beloved had to have elements of bisexuality. He writes, ''But the women, of all I have known, who possessed the highest measure of what are considered feminine qualities, have combined with them more of the highest masculine qualities than I have ever seen in but one or two men, and those one or two men were also in many respects almost women'' (Packe 1954).

Yet, the influence of his mother lingered underneath the surface. His first love, Harriet Baring, who did not return his affections, and his chosen wife to be, Harriet Taylor, would both bear the first name of his mother, Harriet Burrow.

The oedipal character of his love for Harriet Taylor was evident in that she clearly belonged to another and would remain another man's wife for twenty years. She was described as vivacious; capable of consuming violence either of love or of indignation; and possessing majestic pride, grace, beauty, and large dark eyes with a look of quiet command in them (Packe 1954). She and Mill would continue a platonic liaison known and tolerated by her husband, stimulating scandalous ridicule which would result in loss of friends. Even after their marriage their sexual relationship would remain true to their platonic ideal.

Packe (1954) writes, ''All revolved around Harriet and Harriet was very spoilt. Two men were devoted to her; both were distinguished, and one was rich. She managed the household of one and the philosophy of the other.'' Mill's own qualities of overtolerance, passivity, and his readiness to overvalue others' capacities resulted in submission to her ideas and the force of her personality. ''When Harriet required him to deny his main political belief, he meekly answered: 'This is probably the only progress we have always been making, by thinking sufficiently I shall probably come to think the same—as is always the case, I believe always when we think long enough''' (Packe 1954).

In little things as well as great he followed where she led. He did not hesitate to change his views. He became opposed to the secret ballot and a supporter of capital punishment. Every major work subsequent to their marriage bore her imprint. Although she did not write them she suggested, approved, and dictated parts of them verbatim. He felt his capacity exhausted compared with the obvious genius of Harriet. In a letter to Harriet he wrote, ''I am fit to be one wheel in an engine, not to be the self moving engine itself, a real majestic intellect, not to say moral nature, like yours, I can only look up to and admire'' (Packe 1954).

Conclusions

John Stuart Mill negotiated his postadolescent crisis and achieved partial resolution of his conflicts. He acquired an increasing stabilization of his ego functions and interests as well as an extension of his conflict-free sphere of the ego. There was a partial consolidation of his sexual position, a clearer defined sense of self, and a greater sense of autonomy and self-direction. Yet, no infantile conflict is ever completely resolved and, like the tide, it always has to be reckoned with one more time. His philosophy and his life would be a continuation and a disavowal of his father's life and philosophy. Like the primal horde that rose up and slew the father and then, unable to bear his absence, re-created him in the form of the Totem, so John Stuart Mill found and re-created the special relationship he once shared with his father in the personage of Harriet. He remained his father's son. His whole philosophy and the pattern of his life would be an ongoing struggle between the individual struggling for self-development and autonomy and the passive wish to be the powerful extension of another.

Aiken, H. 1957. *The Age of Idealogy*. New York: Braziller.

Blos, P. 1968. Character formation in adolescence. *Psychoanalytic Study of the Child* 23:245–263.

Blos, P. 1979. Modifications in the classical psychoanalytic model of adolescence. In *The Adolescent Passage*. New York: International Universities Press.

Freud, S. 1906. My views on the part played by sexuality in the etiology of the neuroses. *Standard Edition* 7:279. London: Hogarth, 1964.

Freud, S. 1939. Moses and monotheism. *Standard Edition* 23:75–76. London: Hogarth, 1964.

Greenacre, P. 1967. The influence of infantile trauma on genetic patterns. In *Emotional Growth*. New York: International Universities Press.

Jones, E. 1953. *The Life and Work of Sigmund Freud*. Vol. 1. New York: Basic.

Levi, A. W. 1945. The mental crisis of John Stuart Mill. *Psychoanalytic Review* 32:86–101.

Loewald, H. 1979. The waning of the Oedipus complex. *Journal of the American Psychoanalytic Association* 27(4): 751–755.

Mill, J. S. 1831. Spirit of the age. In G. Himmelfarb, ed. *Essays on Politics and Culture*. Garden City, N.Y.: Doubleday, 1962.

Mill, J. S. 1887. *Autobiography*. New York: Henry Holt.

Packe, M. 1954. *The Life of John Stuart Mill*. New York: Macmillan.

Webster's New Twentieth Century Dictionary Unabridged. 1980.

8 THE STUDY OF LIVES: DISCUSSION OF TASHJIAN AND SHAW

AARON H. ESMAN

I am pleased to have been given the opportunity to discuss these two exceptionally interesting papers. They are of particular value in demonstrating the reciprocal contributions of psychoanalytic developmental theory and the study of lives. Psychoanalytic developmental theory provides us with a framework for the examination and understanding of the autobiographic reflections of such outstanding contributors to our cultural heritage as John Stuart Mill and James Joyce; on the other hand, their self-revelations represent a useful body of data through which our developmental theories can be refined and sharpened by application that avoids the perils of reductionism and "wild analysis."

Dr. Shaw's discussion of the postadolescent crisis of John Stuart Mill is a sensitive and illuminating study of an extraordinary father-son relationship and its developmental vicissitudes. It would appear that Dr. Shaw was unaware of a previous exploration of Mill's developmental crisis by Anthony (1970) in which attention was directed primarily to the depressive symptomatology manifested by Mill at the time of his breakdown. Like Dr. Shaw, Anthony was particularly struck by the absence of reference to the mother in Mill's autobiography; it represents a glaring gap in the data necessary for a full understanding of Mill's psychological development.

Nonetheless, it is clear that James Mill was the major figure in his son's intellectual development and provided him with an object for ambivalent identification, which may, in my view, have constituted a major factor in the genesis of his creativity. What came to be of critical importance in Mill's affective life was his experience of disillusionment in his idealized father in late adolescence and his struggle to come to terms with this disillusionment and its consequent disruption of his ego ideal and the structure of his internal object relations. As Dr. Shaw points out, Blos (1974) has described this process of disillusionment as a major feature of normal mid- to late-adolescent development in Western culture. It plays a central role in the taming of unrealistic omnipotence strivings and in the genesis of realistic self-esteem. The preservation of idealized representations of an omnipotent parent figure can seriously stifle autonomous development and contribute to lifelong feelings of inadequacy, born of the effort to achieve unattainable goals. It is one of the perils inherent in being the child of the rich and powerful.

In Mill's case the abrupt destruction of the idealized, internalized father image was, as Dr. Shaw shows, fraught with feelings of patricidal guilt and a profound sense of loss. His mourning process, facilitated by his "chance" encounter with the memoirs of Marmontel, permitted Mill to restructure not only his ideals but the cognitive system that had been organized around them through the massive incorporation of his father's thought. It was as though Mill went through rapidly, belatedly, and pathologically what many intelligent and reflective adolescents experience gradually and over an extended period of time—that is, the reassessment of internalized values and the reconstitution of an autonomous value system that accompanies the gradual process of object removal characteristic of adolescents. In his reworking of the traumatic experience of the loss of the introjected representation of his idealized father, Mill achieved not merely a repetition but ultimately a mastery of what had initially appeared as a passively experienced psychic catastrophe.

As a result Mill became, as Dr. Shaw points out, the apostle of liberty, the living expression of man's struggles against irrational patriarchal authority. It is good to be reminded of his contribution to the ideal of liberty that forms the base, not only of our political system, but also of psychoanalysis itself. Freud was profoundly interested in the work of John Stuart Mill and, indeed, translated Mill's writings into German during his medical student years. It is fascinating to reflect, as Anthony does, on the contrast between Mill's and Freud's responses to the influence of their fathers in their lives. To quote Anthony:

> With Mill, he fell ill when he became aware that the realization of his father's aims in life would not satisfy him, and he regained his

AARON H. ESMAN

mental health . . . when he understood that the death of the father brought with it the growth of identity, autonomy and responsibility for the son. In contrast, Freud's own self-analysis of his father's influence on his life led to the formulation of the Oedipus complex but brought no depressive breakdown in its track.

Dr. Shaw succeeds brilliantly in doing what Mill conspicuously failed to do—that is, in bringing Mill's mother to life. One can add little to his ingenious reconstruction of the manifestly oedipal character of Mill's relationship to the various Harriets in his life, except to suggest that his subservient self-castrative posture with his wife may have represented, not only a reenactment of his early passive submissiveness toward his father, but a self-punitive masochism imposed on himself for having achieved the ultimate oedipal victory—not only to have killed his father, but to have married his mother. No wonder that, as Dr. Shaw points out, he came in the end to believe in capital punishment.

Dr. Tashjian's paper was of particular interest to me because, coincidentally, I have recently had occasion to reread *A Portrait of the Artist as a Young Man* in connection with my own teaching activities. Joyce's (1916) book is one of those cultural monuments which, like youth itself in George Bernard Shaw's epigram, is wasted on the young. To reread it in one's maturity is to be overwhelmed by the power of its imagery, the magic of its language, and the miraculous evocativeness of its recreation of adolescent experience.

Dr. Tashjian has focused in his essay on the late-adolescent segment of Joyce's barely fictionalized autobiography—on, that is, the consolidation of his sense of self, his identity, and his character. Joyce himself put it as cogently as anyone could possibly do in his oft-quoted statement of his determination "to encounter for the millionth time the reality of experience and to forge in the smithy of my soul the uncreated conscience of my race." In this he gives expression not only to the consolidation of his self-organization but also the recognition of the continuity of his experience with that of the culture from which he sprang. He exemplifies here, then, Erikson's concept of identity as a Janus-faced structure, looking inward at intrapsychic organization and outward at psychosocial integration.

I was interested in Dr. Tashjian's proposed parallels between the subphases of adolescence and those of the separation-individuation process as described by Mahler. I too have suggested such analogies (Esman 1980), and I agree that they are useful so long as we remember that they are analogies rather than identities. The adolescent is not really recapitulating separation-individuation any more than he is really recapitulating the oedipal configuration. He is a different organism, with a far more complex psychic organization, and we risk over-simplification if we apply the Mahlerian model of the toddler's development too literally to the adolescent process.

In the *Portrait*, Joyce describes with agonizing sensitivity the struggles of a mid-adolescent coming to terms with his sexual awakening and the anguish generated by its conflict with his religious upbringing. As though in direct illustration of Anna Freud's (1958) description of adolescent turmoil, Joyce's alter ego, Stephen Dedalus, oscillates between abandoned sensual indulgence in masturbation and intercourse with prostitutes and self-tormenting asceticism, self-abnegation, reinforcement of his religious vows, and self-punitive confessions. I know of no more poignant description of this struggle in a sensitive adolescent wrestling with the reorganization of his superego than that offered by Joyce.

Dr. Tashjian emphasizes the role of what Joyce referred to as "epiphanies" in the ultimate consolidation of the self-organization. Such experiences, which are in some ways equivalent to religious experiences of revelation, have been frequently described by those who enjoy both literary talent and a particular kind of psychic organization characterized by a certain fluidity of boundaries and an exceptional openness to and tolerance of primary process phenomena. There are a number of cognate psychological phenomena that relate to these epiphanies. These would include the so-called aha-erlebnis, or flash of awareness that follows the lifting of a repression in analysis; or the sudden creative insight exemplified by Kekule's famous dream of the benzene ring; or, in a more ominous vein, the crystallization of a paranoid delusional system which brings a kind of order to a preexisting psychic chaos. It is fair to say that such experiences are not open to most, and that it is the unusual adolescent who is favored with such moments of revelation. When they do occur, as with Joyce, William James, the Buddha, and a host of lesser artists and mystics, they are of crucial organizing significance, but the rest of us seem to struggle along in a more pedestrian way with a gradual reshaping of ego ideal, reorganization of identification systems, and adaptation of early superego rigidities to the demands of life in the real world that ultimately lead to the formation of the adult character of the nongenius.

Both chapters discussed here deal with a situation in which I have had a recent interest. Joyce and Mill were both uncommonly creative and productive individuals. In both cases their characters were decisively shaped by a relationship with a father who played a prominent role in their intellectual development. With Mill, of course, we know the story. In Joyce's case the situation was somewhat more subtle, but Joyce's father was clearly a man of considerable intellect who strongly encouraged his pursuit of classical education, who was an active Irish patriot and a pronounced religious skeptic. Although Joyce's relationship with his father was ambivalent, he clearly modeled himself on him in a number of areas, including his dandyism and his manifest interest in the rich communicative power of the English language.

In a recent study of those rare individuals who have achieved significant creative work during their adolescent years, I have found a uniform pattern of such an intense formative relationship with a father who has served as the primary educator and shaper of the potential genius's early development. Mozart, Schubert, Raphael, and Picasso all exemplify this pattern. I do not suggest that this is a necessary condition for the development of creative potential. I have indicated explicitly in other places (Esman 1979) the wide diversity of developmental pathways to creativity. Still, it is worth some additional study to determine the extent to which this particular pattern of identification with a powerful, supportive paternal figure constitutes one of the more favorable routes to its early flowering. Certainly for Joyce this pattern was a recurring theme in his work, not only in the *Portrait* but in *Ulysses* (1922), where precisely such a relationship is established between young Stephen and Leopold Bloom, respectively the Telemachus and Odysseus of Joyce's recreation of the Homeric classic. And it was, I suspect, this link that enabled Joyce to wander through what Dr. Tashjian aptly calls "the labyrinth of his adolescence" without losing his way. His adolescent fantasy was, after all, not so grandiose or delusional. He did, in his own way, through the magic of language, remake the world—or, at least, the way in which we experience it.

As Dr. Tashjian points out, Joyce would have been explicit in his repudiation of any connection between his self-explorations and those deriving from psychoanalysis, whether of the Freudian or Jungian sort. It is of interest to note, however, that one of Joyce's close friends during the years in Trieste when he was struggling with the *Portrait of the Artist* was a man named Ettore Schmitz, who became famous in later years as the author of the first psychoanalytic novel, *Confessions of Zeno,* under the pseudonym "Italo Svevo" (1923). Svevo was related by marriage to the late Edoardo Weiss, who later immigrated to Chicago and became an important figure in American psychoanalytic life. Joyce must certainly have been aware of Svevo's interest in psychoanalysis and of his (fruitless) efforts at self-analysis (Weiss, personal communication, 1981), nor could he have been totally oblivious to the excitement about psychoanalytic thought that was prevalent in intellectual circles in Trieste (which was, after all, at that time a part of the Austro-Hungarian Empire and therefore in constant communication with Vienna) and later in Zurich, where much of *Ulysses* was written.

Svevo confirms, however, Joyce's assertions that he was not significantly influenced by psychoanalysis in his development of the stream of consciousness technique in his fiction. To quote Svevo (1927), "Joyce's works, therefore, cannot be considered a triumph of psychoanalysis, but I am convinced that they can be the subject of its study. They are nothing but a piece of life of great importance just because it has been brought to light, not deformed by any pedantic science, but vigorously hewn with quickening inspiration. And it is my hope that some thoroughly competent psychoanalyst may arise to give us a study of his books, which are life itself, a life rich and heartfelt and recorded with a naturalness of one who has lived and suffered what he writes. They are as worthy of study, but with a difference, as that poor *Gradiva* of Jensen's, which Freud himself honored with his celebrated comments."

Dr. Tashjian has, I think, begun to undertake the work Svevo anticipated in these remarks. It must be apparent that Dr. Tashjian's chapter has opened the door to endless reflections on the subject of Joyce's inexhaustible masterpiece. I thank him for giving me the opportunity to indulge in such ruminations, and encourage all of you to enjoy for yourselves the incomparable experience of rereading this unparalleled example of what the Germans call a *Bildungsroman*. To Dr. Shaw and to Dr. Tashjian I express my appreciation for the stimulus their chapters have given me. It has been a pleasure to think and write about their work.

REFERENCES

Anthony, E. J. 1970. Two contrasting types of adolescent depression. *Journal of the American Psychoanalytic Association* 18:841–859.
Blos, P. 1974. The genealogy of the ego ideal. *Psychoanalytic Study of the Child* 29:43–88!

Esman, A. H. 1979. The nature of the artistic gift. *American Imago* 36: 305–312.

Esman, A. H. 1980. Adolescent psychopathology and the rapprochement phenomenon. *Adolescent Psychiatry* 8:320–331.

Freud, A. 1958. Adolescence. *Psychoanalytic Study of the Child* 13:255–278.

Joyce, J. 1916. *A Portrait of the Artist as a Young Man*. New York: Viking, 1964.

Joyce, J. 1922. *Ulysses*. New York: Vintage, 1961.

Svevo, I. 1923. *Confessions of Zeno*. New York: Vintage, 1958.

Svevo, I. 1927. *James Joyce*. New York: New Directions, 1950.

9 ROMEO AND JULIET: THE TRAGIC SELF IN ADOLESCENCE

HYMAN L. MUSLIN

Where does the tragedy lie in the lives of Romeo and Juliet? The legend of Romeo and Juliet is a presentation, in Shakespeare's version, as well as earlier versions, of a tale of two adolescents in love reacting to the unempathic self-absorption of their elders, and ultimately their own, by giving up their lives. While it is clear that the psychological meanings within the play can be understood from a variety of psychoanalytic vantage points, the attempt in this chapter is to evolve a psychoanalytic critique based on the views of self psychology.

The Romeo and Juliet legend of lovers whose love leads to separation and destruction has a long history. Perhaps its origins can be traced indirectly to a story of Pyramus and Thisbe of Ovid and the second century A.D. story of Xenophon of Ephesus. The basis on which Shakespeare built his play is the Arthur Brooke poem, "Romeus and Juliet," an adaptation from Boisteau and first published in 1562 (Dowden 1930). Shakespeare in his version of the tragedy departed from Brooke in several particulars; the time of the play is reduced from five months to five days, Juliet is fourteen not sixteen. However, Shakespeare's most significant contribution to the Romeo and Juliet legend was in transforming the story—as he had so often done in the past—from a simple tale of two lovers in tragic circumstances to a complex psychological drama.

Shakespeare's Romeo and Juliet

Our introduction to the tragedy is in the overview given by the chorus that the play is concerned with the ill-destined lovers whose death finally ends the civil strife between two feuding families. The implication is that these two young people were unfortunate in finding each other since their love sealed their destiny. We are first introduced to Romeo in a state of despair reacting to the rejection by the chaste Rosaline who, it turns out, is a member of the Capulet family. Romeo's parents, Lord and Lady Montague, are concerned about Romeo's "black and portentous" mood but, significantly, have not been able to persuade their son to reveal the cause of his sorrows. Thus, they encourage Benvolio to engage Romeo in conversation so as to obtain a "true shrift" (true confession):

> BENVOLIO: Alas that Love, so gentle in his view, should
> be so tyrannous and rough in proof!
> ROMEO: Alas that love, whose view is muffled still,
> Should without eyes see pathways to his will!
>
> [act 1, sc. 1]

Romeo is urged to join his comrades at a festival at the house of the enemy, the Capulet mansion, where he will meet Juliet for the first time. We have been informed, just prior to this scene, that Juliet is being thought of and prepared for a potential marriage with Count Paris.

Our first introduction to Juliet reveals her being urged by her mother to consider the prospect of marriage. Her father has already spoken to Paris and cautioned him to approach her gently. At this stage in the play, Lord Capulet relates that his consent will be limited by her own wishes:

> But woo her, gentle Paris, get her heart;
> My will to her consent is but a part.
> And she agreed, within her scope of choice
> Lies my consent and fair according voice.
>
> [act 1, sc. 2]

Her mother, on the other hand, speaks directly to Juliet of marriage and Paris:

> WIFE: Marry, that "marry" is the very theme
> I came to talk of. Tell me, daughter Juliet
> How stands your disposition to be married?
> JULIET: It is an honor that I dream not of.
>
> [act 1, sc. 3]

Unswayed by her daughter's remarks, Lady Capulet persists in her wishes to have Juliet consider the suit of Paris and encourages her to examine his many virtues. Juliet replies:

> I'll look to like, if looking liking move;
> But no more deep will I endart mine eye
> Than your consent gives strength to make it fly.
>
> [act 1, sc. 3]

These lines reveal Shakespeare's characterization of Lady Capulet as a singleminded mother, insensitive to her daughter's self-development. Her father, although reluctant at first to discuss marriage, gives Paris permission to pursue his suit without attempting to ascertain Juliet's interests. Our initial introduction to Juliet thus portrays her in an environment marked by unempathic elders, seemingly (even though sympathetically, as in the case of her father) unresponsive to her lack of interest in the issues of marriage and separation from the family. Thus the scene is prepared for the next movement in the play—the instant engagement of Romeo and Juliet. The two lovers are in a state of self-vulnerability, each reacting to adolescent events that have interfered with their emotional equilibrium.

The initial contact takes place in a manner characteristic of a merging process. Romeo, vulnerable as he is since his defeat with Rosaline, on seeing Juliet at the Capulets' feast, immediately reveals that she is regarded by him as being the essence of perfection:

> Did my heart love till now? Forswear it, sight!
> For I ne'er saw true beauty till this night.
>
> [act 1, sc. 5]

At the Capulet family ball, after engaging in some defensive repartee, Juliet allows Romeo to kiss her and soon after reveals that she too has become consumed with the notion that Romeo is indispensable for her survival:

> My only love, sprung from my only hate!
> Too early seen unknown, and known too late!
> Prodigious birth to love it is to me
> That I must love a loathed enemy.
>
> [act 1, sc. 5]

The famous balcony scene now ensues with the two thunderstruck lovers. To Romeo, Juliet is the sun, a saint, an angel. He wishes to be the glove on her hand that he might touch her cheek; he stands immediately ready to give up his offensive name since he could not endure a rejection from her eyes. Nothing and no one can cause him to be deflected from his love of her, as he says:

> I am no pilot, yet, wert thou as far
> As that vast washed with the farthest sea,
> I would adventure for such merchandise.
>
> [act 2, sc. 2]

On Juliet's part, she too has become immersed in the merger, urging him to give up his offending name:

> And for that name, which is no part of thee
> Take all myself.
>
> [act 2, sc. 2]

Juliet now declares that, on her part, she would relinquish her family ties for Romeo. To her, Romeo is perfection, the "god of my idolatry." Juliet's self is so filled with the tension of the merger and perhaps the ultimate consequences of her love—separation from her family—that she complains that it is like lightning and may disappear, that it is "too rash, too unadvise, too sudden." Together they express the wish to be each other's "prisoner-bird" so as not to have any distance between each other. This instant union can perhaps best be described as a self/selfobject twinship merger in which one needs the other to feel intact. The other is experienced as Kohut (1977) described, "the carrier of the infantile greatness and exhibitionism."

Juliet and Romeo now make plans for their marriage in a manner befitting their membership in families opposed to one another. While it seems reasonable that the two must pursue their love affair in secret, we are led to suspect that a more definitive reason for secrecy lies in the age-old conviction that their families would not support their strivings for autonomy. An arranged marriage, as was being pursued by Lord and Lady Capulet with Paris, provides a measure of continuing control over the parties involved and maintains the illusion that a genuine separation is not to take place.

Shakespeare gives evidence in several instances that the family feud was waning. Benvolio's attempt at conciliation between the two warring families at the beginning of the play is one of several indications that the family feud is dying. Rosaline, the first love of Romeo, is the niece of Capulet, a fact which did not seem to deter Romeo. In urging Romeo to go to the Capulets' feast, both Mercutio and Benvolio were unconcerned over going to the enemy's lair; later, when Romeo pursues Juliet, they were not concerned in leaving Romeo in the Capulets' compound. Lord Capulet's comments add further evidence that the feud was resolving:

> But Montague is bound as well as I,
> In penalty alike; and 'tis not hard, I think,
> For men so old as we to keep the peace.

To which Paris agrees and says:

> Of honorable reckoning are you both
> And pity 'tis you lived at odds so long.
>
> [act 1, sc. 2]

Save for the presence of Tybalt, the archvillain of the piece, perhaps negotiation would have been permitted between all concerned parties if the two lovers had entreated their respective families to consider their petition for marriage and felt safe in this petitioning. However, empathy—in their view—was missing from the side of their elders.

One can view the material to this point as a matter of adolescents in rebellion against the mores of their elders. The fact of their being from enemy camps would serve to intensify their romantic strivings and would serve as well as an act of defiance against established patterns of behavior. From another point of view, the protagonist, Romeo, is caught up in a play in which he cannot control his strivings to seek out and capture a woman in a forbidden house—an oedipal drama.

A corollary of this point of view would conceive of the master of the opposing camp to Romeo, Lord Capulet, as the displaced father figure from his own father, Lord Montague. Romeo's and Juliet's passion for each other could be conceived as yet further displacement reactions, this time from their original oedipal objects. Although these views are compelling, the material to this point can perhaps be most fruitfully viewed as instances of a self/selfobject unit in formation between Romeo and Juliet and taking place in an environment that is not responsive to their needs.

110

HYMAN L. MUSLIN

Pursuing the line of the play, directly after the secret marriage in Friar Laurence's cell, the tragic killing of Mercutio by Tybalt occurs, followed by Romeo—resuming his Montague identity—killing the villain Tybalt and immediately being banished from Verona by the prince. The good friar arranges for the newlyweds to spend one night together before Romeo has to leave for his place of exile. Directly after the love tryst with Romeo, Juliet is informed that her father has laid plans for marriage with Paris. She begs her mother for delay, without informing her of her marriage, now consummated, with Romeo.

Her mother rejects her entreaties and instead tells her father of Juliet's resistance to marriage. Lord Capulet storms at her defiance:

> Hang thee, young baggage! disobedient wretch!
> I tell thee what—get thee to church a Thursday
> Or never after look me in the face.
>
> [act 3, sc. 5]

A raging Lord Capulet is yet another invention of Shakespeare. His rage at Juliet is clearly overdetermined, in part derived from his reaction to her impending separation as a bride-to-be. Capulet's discomfiture and explosion—so intense that his wife and all others at the scene are taken aback—can be readily understood as the ubiquitous response of the father about to relinquish ownership of one of his prized females. Juliet's resistance to his commands then serves to ignite his rage at the victor, Paris, now displaced onto Juliet who becomes the disloyal wretch whom he curses without restraint. From another point of view, we are witnessing Capulet's narcissistic rage at the imminent threat to a self/selfobject dyad he has struggled to maintain. When Capulet first attempts to fend off Paris's wishes to marry Juliet, he pleads her immaturity but also alludes to his feeling for her as "the hopeful lady of my earth." Thus, when Capulet protests that he is enraged, since Juliet is thwarting his long-term plan for her marriage, we know that this is not the case. Capulet had actually made a "desperate tender" (a rash offer) to Paris, an impulsive act representing an attempt to overcome his resistance to separation by a flight into action.

Juliet's despair intensifies as she seeks comfort from her trusted nurse who also disappoints her:

> Faith, here it is.
> Romeo is banisht; and all the world to nothing
> That he dares ne'er come back to challenge you;

111

Or if he do, it needs must be by stealth.
Then, since the case so stands as now it doth,
I think it best you married with the County.
O, he's a lovely gentleman!

[act 3, sc. 5]

And so Juliet takes herself to the benevolent friar and unfolds her
bitterness at her destiny. The friar's advice is to take a potion that will
allow her to feign death for forty-two hours. He will manage to inform
Romeo of the scheme, and when she awakens she and Romeo will flee
to Mantua. Seemingly, the friar has joined forces with the lovers from
the beginning of their relationship, but always on the side of their
maintaining secrecy, that is, viewing their mission as requiring stealth
but never viewing the marriage as an act to be supported. Thus he does
not encourage them to discuss their plans with their elders—indeed, he
supports their conviction that their actions are to be maintained in
secrecy.

Romeo's interactions with his elders, the Montagues, are not reported. However, Romeo's confidante after the tragedy of the slaying
of Tybalt is also the trusted friar. There is no turning to his parents in
an attempt to get support. Further, he never informs his parents of his
love for a member of the enemy camp.

The drama quickly unfolds into mass tragedy directly after the secret
marriage takes place. At the end four people are dead, the families are
in mourning, and the friar is exposed for his share in the tragedy. The
secret merger between the two lovers has revealed itself to be a vol-
cano of destructiveness. The Montagues and Capulets are not aware
and have never been apprised of the liaison between Romeo and Juliet.
Romeo, who has now killed Tybalt and Paris, takes his life to be followed by his Juliet. The lovers and their parents have never had to
confront the psychological separation from each other.

Adolescent Love

Romeo and Juliet in Shakespeare's drama display a paradigmatic
form of love in adolescents in an early love encounter. It has in the
main the characteristics of what Kohut (1977) has called a self/self-
object twinship merger; each one of the dyad is experienced as necessary for the other's self-integrity. They each stand ready to relinquish
past ties and renounce distance between each other.

Perhaps another ubiquitous aspect of adolescent love that is high-lighted in the tragedy is conflict over autonomy. The young lovers while pursuing their wishes for autonomy in one way—they plan marriage—in another reveal their fear of autonomy by maintaining their liaison in secrecy. From the viewpoint of the self, what is at stake here is the dissolution of the self/selfobject ties of childhood with one's parents, and thus a relationship is entered into with reluctance and trepidation. In modern times, a variant of the Romeo-Juliet secret liaison continues in the living-together arrangements of adolescents and young adults on college campuses and throughout our society. These arrangements are commonly kept secret from the respective families, but not from peers, even though they may continue for long periods of time. From this perspective, the need for secrecy is due to the fear of confronting the self/selfobject ties between the adolescent or young adult and their families. Still another modern commonplace variant of the Romeo-Juliet secret liaison is the reluctance of some couples to marry, with an anxiety outbreak when marriage is finally agreed to even though the relationship is of several years' duration.

As alluded to earlier, tragedies such as this one have been described in the literature through the centuries, although various elements of the plot have been different. The common elements have been the tale of two lovers whose relationship cannot be maintained for a variety of reasons. However, the central obstacle, in my view, is a reflection in each of these romantic tragedies of the ubiquitous conflict in adolescents of their quest for and a fear of greater selfhood. Thus the two features of adolescent love highlighted in Shakespeare's tragedy—from the viewpoint of self psychology—may be considered as ubiquitous features of adolescent development. Symbolically, Romeo and Juliet can be considered as adolescents self-reacting to a flawed selfobject milieu, the fused Montagues and Capulets.

The psychological milieu in which Romeo and Juliet's love unfolded was one in which neither of the sets of parents could recognize and respond to their children's messages. Perhaps to emphasize this parent-adolescent gap, Shakespeare has a frustrated Lord Montague at the outset of the play entreat Benvolio to ferret out and ameliorate his son's distress. Further, on several occasions, the Capulets cannot appreciate Juliet's manifest distress. Thus Shakespeare's *Romeo and Juliet* highlights a familiar occurrence in the lives of adolescents and their elders—the phenomenon of self-absorbed parents unable to respond to their children's strivings for greater selfhood.

Lady Capulet is cast as the unempathic mother, interested solely in procuring a distinguished person as a son-in-law. To Juliet's dismay, to Juliet's pleas, she does not respond except with contempt. Her lack of empathy with her only daughter is perhaps most clearly revealed when she has to turn to Nurse to find out Juliet's age. Lady Capulet's interactions with Juliet can be understood as evidence of her wish to be rid of a rival for the affections of Lord Capulet. However, the central element in her responses to her daughter is the manifest absence of concern for the fourteen-year-old's anguish.

> JULIET: Is there no pity sitting in the clouds
> That sees into the bottom of my grief?
> O sweet my mother, cast me not away!
> Delay this marriage for a month, a week;
> Or if you do not, make the bridal bed
> In that dim monument where Tybalt lies.
> LADY: Talk not to me, for I'll not speak a word.
> Do as thou wilt, for I have done with thee.
>
> [act 3, sc. 5]

Lord Capulet, from the outset of the tragedy, demonstrated an intense bond with Juliet. When Capulet does initiate the marriage plans it is clearly an impulsive act, born of conflict. For the moment, his flight into action serves to disavow his needs to maintain his ties with Juliet. Shortly thereafter, when Juliet rejects her father's plans for her, Capulet's facade of joy is dismantled and his underlying rage at his rejecting daughter is revealed. This rage evoked by the impending dissolution of his bond to her represents a narcissistic rage reaction in response to the break-up of a self/selfobject bond. Juliet has apparently been experienced by Capulet as a source of nurturance, a selfobject, important or necessary for his cohesiveness. He has, after all, referred to her as "the hopeful lady of my earth." Thus, in relation to the impending marriage, Juliet by accepting Paris will no longer be his—the ultimate rejection. Indeed, when Juliet seemingly accedes to his wishes and asks for forgiveness his equilibrium is restored. Once again she and he are bound together, there is no more rejection in the surround, and the old self/selfobject ties are restored.

Capulet's reactions to Juliet—the reluctance to consider separation and later the rage at the imminent separation—point to a phenomenon familiar to students of the family, the parent who has invested a child with the qualities of a selfobject nurturer. These self/selfobject ties between parent and child ordinarily occur when the spouses cannot function effectively in their relatedness and turn to one of their children for support. When the child or adolescent, in harmony with its own developmental needs, resists the parental appeal and goes its own way (academic pursuits, marriage), it may be experienced by the parent as a narcissistic wound with ensuing rage at the rejecting child. Thus, when Capulet tells Paris to wait for two more years for Juliet's hand and Paris in rebuttal says that women younger than she are made happy mothers, Capulet says, ''And too soon marred are those so early made.''

These lines seem to refer to Capulet's wife who was a mother at fourteen and, therefore, in Capulet's eyes "marred," that is, a marred mate and the reason why his relationship with Juliet needs to be maintained without interruption by a marriage. Shakespeare has portrayed in his drama a crucial period of emotional development in the lives of adolescents and their parents. The Montagues and Capulets can be understood as parents who cannot rise to the true parental attitude: to serve as selfobjects for the child during the period of their adolescence when their selves are undergoing transformation toward greater autonomy. In fact, the parents' need from their children is to hold back the passage of time since their children serve as sources of support to them.

While most literary critics have described the imperfections in the play in terms of the poet's youthful intemperances, they also have been appreciative of Shakespeare's success in forming the characters of Romeo and Juliet (Brown 1949; Bullough 1957; Harris 1909). Thus Granville-Barker (1946) admired Shakespeare's ability to evolve the character of Romeo. ''This Romeo, when he had achieved him, must have stood to Shakespeare as an assurance that he could now mold a tragic figure strong enough to carry a whole play wherever he might want to.'' A whole host of critics, while calling attention to the flaws in the play centering around Shakespeare's excesses of language and inadequate realization of some of the characters (for example, Lord Capulet), were nonetheless taken with the beauty of the language and genuine quality of the tragedy. Coleridge (1957) was impressed with Shakespeare's empathic awareness of the process of love starting with ''that sense of imperfection, that yearning to combine itself with something lovely.''

Conclusions

Psychoanalytic critics have commented only rarely on this play of Shakespeare's. While Menninger (1938) described the impulsiveness of the self-destructive aspects of the tragedy, Reik (1944) noted the theme of romantic love and the wish to seek and find one's ideal of oneself. Holland (1963) described the unconscious mechanism of reversal in the famous emperor dream in act 5 which transposes subsequent events; thus instead of Romeo's death, shortly to be dramatized, Romeo will be found by his lady, revived by kisses, and be transformed to an emperor. Cox (1976) and Faber (1972) have contributed papers on the miscarried adolescent process revealed in the play and the attempt to form relationships with nonincestuous objects which, when frustrated, resulted in suicide. Most recently, Kernberg (1980) commented on the nature of adolescent sexuality and the complex mechanisms (disavowal, projection) necessary to maintain the love bonds against the eruption of aggression.

Perhaps the nature of this work—two tragic adolescents alienated from parents with a mutuality of empathic failure—has inhibited both literary and psychoanalytic critics from pursuing a more systematic study of *Romeo and Juliet*. Indeed, in the seventeenth century, two versions were played, one with a happy ending, one with the original ending (Dowden 1930). Shakespeare's capacity to involve the audience in this and other tragic tales evokes the wish to offer new solutions to adolescents and their caretakers.

REFERENCES

Brown, I. 1949. *Shakespeare*. Garden City, N.Y.: Doubleday.
Bullough, G. 1957. *Narrative and Dramatic Sources of Shakespeare*. London: Routledge & Kegan Paul.
Chambers, E. K. 1930. *William Shakespeare: A Study of Fact and Problems*. Oxford: Clarendon.
Cox, M. 1976. Adolescent process in *Romeo and Juliet*. *Psychoanalytic Review* 63:379–389.
Dowden, E. 1930. *The Works of Shakespeare*. Indianapolis: Bobbs-Merrill.
Faber, M. D. 1972. The adolescent suicides of Romeo and Juliet. *Psychoanalytic Review* 59:169–181.

Fliess, R. 1957. *Erogenicity and Libido*. New York: International Universities Press.

Granville-Barker, H. 1946. *Prefaces to Shakespeare*. Princeton, N.J.: Princeton University Press.

Harris, F. 1909. *The Man Shakespeare and His Tragic Life-Story*. London: Boni.

Hawkes, T. 1959. *Coleridge's Writings on Shakespeare*. New York: Capricorn.

Holland, N. N. 1963. Romeo's dream and the paradox of literary realism. In M. D. Faber, ed. *The Design Within*. New York: Science House, 1970.

Holland, N. N. 1966. *Psychoanalysis and Shakespeare*. New York: McGraw-Hill.

Jonas, M. 1921. *Romeo and Juliet*. London: Davis & Oioli.

Kernberg, O. F. 1980. Adolescent sexuality in the light of group processes. *Psychoanalytic Quarterly* 49:27–47.

Kittridge, G. L. 1940, *The Tragedy of Romeo and Juliet by William Shakespeare*. Boston: Ginn.

Kohut, H. 1977. *The Restoration of the Self*. New York: International Universities Press.

Menninger, K. 1938. *Man against Himself*. New York: Harcourt Brace.

Pace-Sanfelice, G. 1869. *The Original Story of Romeo and Juliet by Luigi da Porto*. Cambridge, Mass: n.p.

Reik, T. 1944. *A Psychologist Looks at Love*. New York: Farrer & Rinehart.

Vredenburgh, J. L. 1957. The character of the incest object. *American Imago* 14:45–52.

Waters, W. G. 1895. *The Novellino of Masuccio*. London: n.p.

Wright, L. B. 1959. *The Tragedy of Romeo and Juliet by William Shakespeare*. Folger Library ed. New York: Pocket.

PART II

DEVELOPMENTAL ISSUES AND ADOLESCENT PROCESS

EDITORS' INTRODUCTION

Increasingly, adolescent character formation is being acknowledged as a resultant of complex psychodynamic, social, and biological factors. The capacity for symbolic logic and increased cognitive skills aid in the deidealization of parents in the development of a cohesive sense of self. The chapters in this part not only focus on the normal adolescent task of self-transformation and achievement of sexual identity but also describe developmental arrest resulting in adolescent violence and despair, triggered by a felt sense of meaninglessness in the adolescent's existence.

Melvin Lewis, in developing a model of a biopsychosocial matrix, reexamines the concept of character in adolescents and the kinds of societal factors that might influence the adolescent's psychic structure, and discusses violence and depression in adolescents. He sees character as including a biological component, a developmental level, and a social context resulting in personality formation. Lewis concludes that there is no simple link between societal factors and the psychic structure of an adolescent, but believes psychodynamic, social, and biological factors all affect psychic structure in complex, interactive ways.

Sol Nichtern examines the sociocultural and psychodynamic aspects of aggression and violence in adolescents. He notes a large increase in the death rate of adolescents and discusses some of the factors contributing to these developments: early exposure to violence and changes within the family structure resulting in a growing social instability. Personality fragmentation during adolescence may evoke a generalized excitatory state that makes aggression a naturally occurring phenomenon. The intensity and degree of regression determine the nature and severity of the violence. Types of violent adolescents discussed include those reflecting an early loss of object relatedness and manifesting elements of depersonalization and dehumanization, those engaged in the pursuit of object constancy with anxiety stemming from the possible loss of object relatedness, those characterized by behavior reflecting the preservation of the self by compulsive preoccupation with ideological activity, and those manifesting occasional violence with the sudden appearance of immature patterns. Nichtern calls for stability and order in ourselves, our families, and the institutions of our society.

Richard C. Marohn, Ellen Locke, Ronald Rosenthal, and Glenn Curtiss study violent death in juvenile delinquents and consider the relationships among suicide, homicide, and accidental death. In those adolescents who suffered violent deaths they found sexual abuse, early father loss, severe parental discord, parental rejection, sexual difficulties, disturbed peer relationships, chronic truancy, and a history of suicide attempts. The authors conclude that behaviorally disordered adolescents should be evaluated for self-destructive tendencies in order to understand the extent to which they are at risk of violent death.

Ernest S. Wolf explores the need of adolescents for selfobjects, a psychological function performed by an object for the self and its development. The maintenance of the self's cohesion and self-expression rather than sexuality is seen as the main motivator of psychological development. Wolf believes that new insights into the surrounding world and its associated selfobject milieu, made possible by the leap in cognitive capacity, force the self into a restructuring during adolescence. He discusses such adolescent tasks as transformation of the self, deidealization of parental selfobjects, achievement of cohesiveness, and construction of symbolic selfobjects. Wolf concludes that it is not the intensity of the physiological upheaval leading to puberty that is the adolescent's main conflict but, rather, the quality of empathic responsiveness and understanding that the youngster receives from a self-supporting selfobject ambience.

Joseph D. Lichtenberg examines developmental continuities and transformations that exist between infancy and adolescence. He discusses eating, sleeping, and eliminating; socializing, play, and work; sexuality; and thrills and risks as examples of biophysiological regulation, social and sensual experiences, interactive behavior, perceptual-cognitive developments, regulation of bodily sensation, and affectively charged behavioral patterns. Lichtenberg observes that, when an adolescent resolves a disturbance that has persisted from an earlier period, he does so under entirely different circumstances and with fully formed body schemata, controls, and defense mechanisms. When an adolescent works to achieve goals and values, he builds on those internalized from childhood but is equipped with the capacity for symbolic logic, one of the major transformations from infancy, and a cohesive sense of self that must be expanded in its range and skills.

Mary C. Lamia studies the revision and relationship between the adolescent's self- and object representations and their manifestations in conscious and unconscious attitudes toward the opposite sex. She found that the attempt by the adolescent male to cope with his own anxiety about sexuality leads to distorted notions about female sexuality and interferes with his understanding of the female psyche. Lamia believes that sexism is not merely a product of culture but has its roots in the unconscious foundations of beliefs upon which the male's development is based.

Adrian Sondheimer explores the sexual concerns of mid adolescents and the use of the mental health professional as a sexual educator in the schools. The value of the psychiatrist himself teaching sexual education is discussed and illustrated as a facet of mental health consultation. Sondheimer describes the content of the sessions with students, their questions, and the general basis for his responses.

Helene Cooper Jackson explores aspects of moral and adolescent development that relate to understanding the Vietnam veteran's experience of combat stress and postcombat adjustment. These veterans present a severity of disorganization in their internal and external lives that is inconsistent with their relatively benign, premorbid personalities, and they reflect a nihilistic philosophy, a mood of despair over the emptiness or triviality of human existence. Jackson states that her study revealed evidence of developmental arrest caused by the residual stress of combat trauma. She describes a group treatment approach designed to reestablish developmental growth.

10 ADOLESCENT PSYCHIC STRUCTURE AND SOCIETAL INFLUENCES: A BIOPSYCHOSOCIAL MODEL

MELVIN LEWIS

The recent emphasis on a comprehensive biopsychosocial viewpoint of behavior suggests that we should reexamine the concept of character in childhood and adolescence in this light. I shall therefore discuss, first, some thoughts on character in general in adolescents as a reflection or, so to speak, precipitate of the adolescent's psychic structure; second, the kinds of powerful societal factors that might influence the balance of the adolescent's dynamic psychic structure; and, third, I shall use violence in adolescents and adolescent depression as paradigms for a model of the biopsychosocial matrix within which the brain, the mind, and society interact.

Character in Adolescence

Character generally refers to a relatively stable individual pattern of ego functions, often manifested in response to stress. In the past a distinction has been made between character and symptom neurosis. The symptom neuroses were said to be the result of specific conflicts and the specific defenses mobilized to deal with those conflicts.

Character as a concept has strong roots in psychoanalysis. Yet surprisingly, Freud wrote little about character; in fact his most important statements can be easily summarized. They include the following ideas: First, the "formula for the way in which character in its final shape is formed out of the constituent instincts [was simply that] the permanent character traits are either unchanged prolongations of the

125

original instincts, or sublimations of those instincts, or reaction-formations against them" (Freud 1908, p. 175). What Freud described as a person's character was built up to a considerable extent "from the material of sexual excitations and is composed of instincts that have been fixed since childhood, of constructions achieved by means of sublimation, and of other constructions, employed for effectively holding in check perverse impulses which have been recognized as being unutilizable" (Freud 1905, pp. 238–239). In the case of some character traits, he thought he could trace a connection with particular erotogenic components. Thus, obstinacy, thrift, and orderliness arose from an "exploitation of anal eroticism," while ambition was determined by a "strong urethralerotic disposition" (Freud 1905, p. 239).[1] Freud drew a sharp distinction between character and neurosis, stating flatly that "the failure of repression and the return of the repressed—which are peculiar to the mechanism of neurosis—are absent in the formation of character. In the latter, repression either does not come into action or smoothly achieves its aim of replacing the repressed by reaction-formations and sublimations . . ." (Freud 1913, p. 323). What created character was "first and foremost . . . the incorporation of the former parental agency as a superego, which is no doubt its most important and decisive portion, and, further, identifications with the two parents of the later period and with other influential figures, and similar identifications formed as precipitates of abandoned object-relations. . . . [Other] contributions to the construction of character . . . [include] the reaction-formations which the ego acquires" (Freud 1933, p. 91). In essence, Freud summed up his views by saying that "the character of the ego is a precipitant of abandoned object-cathexes and that it contains the history of those object-choices" (Freud 1923, p. 29).

Nowadays we would have to say that this psychoanalytic concept of fixed derivatives from defenses against early drives is no longer sufficient to account for character. Nor is Reich's (1933) later description of "character armor" sufficient. (Interestingly, Reich himself still thought that "the continuing actual conflicts between instinct and outer world give it [the character armor] its strength and continued reason for existence" [p. 146], meaning essentially that it still continued to have the exclusively defensive function from which he thought it derived.)

Even the more recent ideas on the so-called narcissistic character do not do justice to what we are talking about today.

In one view (Kohut 1971, 1980), the patient has a disorder of his or her sense of self, arising during the separation-individuation phase (especially the so-called rapprochement phase) of development when their parents responded to them inadequately. The disordered sense of self may be perpetuated either as a draining and persistent regressive need to seek a kind of accepting, affirming mirror of the child's sense of omnipotence or grandiosity or as a tendency to overidealize another person and merge with that person. Such persons have little tolerance either for the less than ideal nature of others or for their own defects. They require perfection in others. They are easily overwhelmed and are often chronically enraged—a rage that may be projected in the course of a projective identification. They may turn to drugs or other kinds of self-stimulating activities. Recurrent bouts of depression, low self-esteem, and preoccupation with bodily functions are common. Separations are difficult.

In another view (Kernberg 1975), the patient has a grandiose self, again arising during the separation-individuation phase but as a defense against early splitting of rage and envy directed toward internalized object representations. This may persist as a constant tendency toward splitting, seen often as rapid shifts between overidealization and devaluation of the object.

Neither view has been reliably documented or validated, and in neither view, it should be noted, is there sufficient attention paid to biological and social factors. We now know that many factors other than ego defenses contribute to character, including biological and social factors. For example, biological factors start with the genetic programming for survival available to the neonate, the intactness of the central nervous system, the infant's individual level of activity, his or her intelligence, the biological guarantee of the semiotic function, and the "goodness of fit" (Chess 1980) between the child's temperament and the environment. One other biological concept that is particularly important is the notion of discontinuity, suggesting that entirely new stages emerge as a consequence of maturation. Nor does the biology of character development stop there. Myelenation and hormonal changes continue during adolescence, again only to be influenced in turn by psychosocial factors.

One can also take a cognitive-developmental view of character, especially of certain character traits, such as honesty and moral thinking. For example, Piaget (1932), and later Kohlberg (1964) and others, have viewed moral development in the context of the major stages of cognitive development. Piaget essentially conceptualized a progressive decentering in moral thinking as the child advances through pre-operational, concrete operational, and formal operations. At the pre-operational stage, the child's morality is that of constraints—rules of behavior are viewed as natural laws handed on to the child by his or her parents. Violation brings retribution or unquestioned punishment, and no account is taken of motives. At the concrete operational stage, rules of behavior become a matter of mutual acceptance, with complete equality of treatment, but no account is taken of special circumstances. At the stage of formal operations, the morality is that of cooperation, and rules can be constructed as required by the heads of the group, so long as they can be agreed upon. Motives are now taken into account, and circumstances may temper the administration of justice.

Kohlberg essentially elaborated on Piaget's ideas, and again suggested a developmental interpretation of children's moral responses at different ages. That is, the stages of moral thinking in the child might represent the child's effort to make sense out of his or her experience in a complex social world, each stage arising sequentially from its predecessors. In this way the stages of moral thinking represent an invariant developmental sequence, each stage of moral thought depending upon earlier attainment of each preceding stage and each involving a restructuring and displacement of previous stages of thought. While the content of moral thought might well be influenced by the mores of the historical moment, as we saw in the 1960s, and perhaps are seeing now in the 1980s, the form seems to be biologically guaranteed.

In the light of these new biological and cognitive perspectives, should we drop the term "character"? Interestingly, the word "character" does not occur anywhere in DSM III; instead, the term "personality" is used, as either a personality trait or a personality disorder. However, in truth, a personality trait in DSM III amounts to a character trait, since it is defined as an enduring pattern of perceiving, relating to, and thinking about the environment and oneself, and it becomes a personality disorder when the trait becomes inflexible and maladaptive and causes either subjective distress or impairment in social or occupational functioning.

Any redefinition must now more fully take into account the biological component, the developmental level of the individual whose style we are describing, and the social context and influence. If we do redefine character, or personality, in a biopsychosocial way, some interesting questions arise. For example, is there a continuity, or can one have a discontinuity in a characteristic style of behavior in relation to different developmental phases and different societal conditions? Clinically we sometimes see amazing changes of character, often at mid-life.

Many people have noticed the frequent associations between certain personality traits and certain symptoms, for example, the academic scholar who develops an obsessive disorder, or the rigidly obsessional person who develops paranoid delusions. We might, therefore, think of symptoms and personality as temporal and spatial expressions (that is, varying with time and place, as well as being focal and generalized respectively) of a personal style of functioning. The particular style, we presume, is formed as a result of biopsychosocial factors during development and pervades perception, attention, cognition, feelings, and so on in specific ways and in a specific context. If this is so, we should be able to describe specific behavior (personality) items, note how they cluster, define the conditions under which they occur, search for their antecedents, and follow their course over time.

Achenbach (1980), for example, recently cluster analyzed children's overall profile patterns obtained from large samples of disturbed children and used this as a basis for categorization.

However, while theoretically we should be able to devise a typology of character, I suspect there will be almost as many types as there are people—for example, impulse-ridden character, obsessive-compulsive character, phobic character, hysterical character, depressive character, passive-aggressive character, borderline character, schizoid character, narcissistic character, sadomasochistic character, antisocial character, as-if character, and paranoid character (Meissner 1980).

How should we classify the child or adolescent with a noncharacter—that is, the adolescent we used to label as having a borderline personality? In this disorder the adolescent's behavior is characterized by unpredictability and marked fluctuations. Such an adolescent has immature and poor social relationships. He or she may have severe temper tantrums during which he or she is out of contact with reality and acts as if he or she were warding off an attacker—that is, the child or adolescent becomes quite paranoid and regressed. The behavior is like that of a younger child; when the adolescent feels unloved he or she will either withdraw or become hostile and aggressive. Such an adolescent has a small reality span. He tries to control the person he is struggling to stay attached to, in part to maintain his hold on reality. He is often obsessional and has difficulty in thinking abstractly. In fact, the presence of a thought disorder, however fluctuating, may be central. Often there is an associated disorder of mood (especially depression), of behavior (which may be disorganized, aggressive, withdrawn, or bizarre), or perception (delusions, hallucinations). Interestingly, one often finds signs of organicity in these adolescents, and in some cases there may be a genetic factor.

From the point of view of standard psychoanalytic theory, there is an instability of inner representation in the borderline child or adolescent, and as a result the inner world appears to invade, color, and even at times obliterate a true perception of the external world as far as the child or adolescent is concerned; reality testing is lost at these times. Unstable primitive defenses (such as projection and identification) and impaired reality testing prevail. Primary process is all too evident. The borderline child or adolescent also manages to make the therapist feel a regressive pull toward a similar chaotic and archaic level of functioning.

This clinical picture, however, is not fixed. Much depends on the age of the child or adolescent and the degree of structure in the adolescent's environment. Thus, it is perhaps more accurate to view such an adolescent as suffering from a pervasive developmental disorder, with biological, psychological, and social influences, rather than as a fixed "borderline personality."

Genetic influences, neurotransmitter regulatory disturbances, environmental conditions, and developmental phase affect multiple functions of the individual—including his or her perceptual, cognitive, attentional, and emotional behavior, as well as his or her motivations— resulting in a behavior characteristic for that individual. Thus, even if the term "personality" is now preferred, it should be qualified by an account of the impact of each of these factors, in much the same way that we no longer talk of maternal deprivation as a simple, one-to-one phenomenon but are aware now of the many variables that affect the outcome of different kinds and degrees of deprivations at different times.

Societal Factors

We can, I think, identify a number of important societal factors that our clinical experience leads us to believe have a major influence on the balance of psychic structure. As a clinician I am struck by the force of certain societal stresses, either in their direct effect upon character development, symptom formation, and the emergence of psychiatric disorder or in their indirect effect through the lowering of thresholds or the heightening of adult (parent)–adolescent distrust and conflict.

The list of social stresses includes: unemployment and poverty, which affect the self-esteem and physical health of the adolescent; social policy, mediated through legislation and court decisions, affecting such matters as abortion, adoption, child placement, and custody with all their serious consequences; racial discrimination, notably in education and in the disposition of the violent adolescent, with sometimes disastrous results; inadequate medical care, from poor antenatal care to inadequate treatment of disease, including venereal disease, leading to impoverished bodies and minds; changing family structure, notably as a result of divorce which may increase the adolescent's sensitivity to separation anxiety and heighten his or her reluctance to the kind of commitment required in a marriage; historical events and contexts, such as the upheaval of the 1960s that was accompanied by uprisings on campuses across the country; and population shifts in our cities and the impact of instant communication.

Whatever the number of factors, it is important to note that these factors seldom stand alone; more often they coexist in some degree. In fact, their very multiplicity creates compounding and confounding variables. As a result, many of these factors give rise to multiple determined disorders, beginning with the genetic inheritance and the ill effects of malnutrition and trauma on brain development itself.

In order to look at some of these relationships (that is, the relationships between some of these multiple antecedent factors and certain clinical disorders in adolescents), I must first attempt to define the word "antecedent," since it is not as unambiguous as one might think. An antecedent is simply a preceding event. It does not have to be invariably present, nor must it be uniquely present. In saying that, I mean to emphasize that if I refer here to a prior event during the childhood of a disturbed adolescent, that is not to be immediately equated with the etiology of that adolescent's condition (the error of *post hoc ergo propter hoc*). Before an antecedent can be regarded as part of the etiology of a condition, there must be a valid demonstration of a relationship between prior and subsequent events.

As we look at antecedents, including social factors, sometimes found in association with certain kinds of adolescent psychic structures and disorders, I hope to draw some tentative conclusions about the likelihood that some of these antecedents may be truly part of the etiology of these conditions.

This brings me to several other conventional assumptions implied in this general notion of childhood antecedents, including societal factors, to adolescent disorders: first, that psychopathology is always formed in early childhood; second, that a kind of crystallization occurs in the elementary school years; third, that without treatment these warpings will manifest themselves later as the symptomatology found with certain psychiatric disorders of adulthood; and fourth, that the earlier the treatment the better the prognosis.

The fact is, in my opinion, that probably none of these assumptions is universally true. The ultimate assumption, of course, is that we should be able to predict outcome. Interestingly, Freud (1920) thought that prediction is impossible; the best we can do, he thought, was to reconstruct in retrospect. Which view is correct?

As usual, the answer is both, depending on the circumstances. Let me digress for a moment to address the question of how well we can predict. If we look at some of the work on early prediction, particularly that on normal cognitive functioning and emotional development, some interesting observations can be made.

Looking first at cognitive functioning, Anderson, Harris, Werner, and Gallistel (1959) found that the best and most consistent predictor among early childhood (age two to five years) measures of normal young adult (age thirty) adjustment was IQ. Second to IQ as a predictor, and almost as good, was the socioeconomic status and cultural richness of the parental home. Both predictors, that is, IQ and socioeconomic status/cultural richness, were better than some thirty-eight measures investigated. Here at once, then, a societal factor appears to be at work. However, it is also possible that all of these investigations may be saying nothing more than that we do not have as good tests for personality as we do for IQ and socioeconomic and educational status.

More recently, Kagan made the startling statement that there is little support for the view that the behavior of the one- or two-year-old provides a clear picture of the adult behavioral profile and that differences among infants in activity, irritability, and affectivity do not predict profiles during later childhood, and, more specifically, social class may be a more important determinant in the long run than individual mothering patterns, at least as far as intellectual functioning is concerned (Kagan 1978; Kagan, Kearsley, and Zelazo 1978).

But is this always true? Let us turn for a moment to emotional development. A number of studies, of which the Robbins (1966) study is an outstanding representative, suggest that: (*a*) children who are referred to child guidance clinics for emotional problems, but who do not have cognitive or antisocial behavior problems, are almost as likely to become well adults as a random sample of the population; (*b*) the gross childhood behavior of normal adults and neurotic adults is indistinguishable; and (*c*) children with cognitive defects and antisocial behavior who later become psychotic may or may not have emotional symptoms as children. That is, the presence of emotional symptoms adds little to the predictive power of early antisocial behavior or cognitive defects.

It begins to appear, then, that few antecedents, including societal factors, during childhood are either specific for, or predictive of, later development during adolescence. Yet we know that there are genetic factors, prenatal and perinatal factors, and later traumatic, psychological, and social factors that seem to be present in conditions, beginning with the almost unimaginable hazard of not being conceived at all.

There is, for example, evidence for genetic factors in schizophrenia, manic-depressive illness, and some forms of attention deficit disorders (ADD) and mental retardation (MR). The effects of malnutrition, drug or radiation toxicity, and illness, during the prenatal period as well as later, are increasingly being reported in such conditions as attention deficit disorders, mental retardation, and certain forms of learning disorders. Loss, separation, and deprivation have been noted repeatedly in the early history of children who have affectionless character disorders and borderline personalities and who later may become violent juvenile delinquents, as well as in children who become depressed.

What, then, makes the difference? Let us now look at two specific disorders: first, serious delinquency in adolescents and, second, depression in adolescents.

DELINQUENCY AND VIOLENCE AS PARADIGMS

Robbins (1966), as mentioned, compared 524 children seen in a child guidance clinic with 100 matched normal children in a local school. Her study found that children referred to the clinic for such complaints as temper tantrums, learning problems, sleep and eating problems, and speech problems did not differ much from the control group when seen as adults thirty years later. That is, shyness, seclusiveness, nervousness, tantrums, insomnia, fears, tics, and speech problems, for example, were not related to later psychiatric disorder.

However, children referred to the clinic for antisocial behavior did

133

differ from the control group thirty years later, and the more severe the early antisocial behavior was during childhood, the more disturbed was the later adult adjustment. Among the children referred to the clinic for antisocial behavior, most of them had been held back in first grade; their problems became obvious by the age of seven years; and the most common referral symptoms were theft, incorrigible behavior, truancy, runaway, bad friends, school discipline problems, and sexual activity including promiscuity. (Truancy and poor school performance were almost universally present in presociopathic children.)

Interestingly, in many of the families of children referred for anti-social behavior, the father was sociopathic or alcoholic and the homes were impoverished or broken. In short, the best single predictor of adult sociopathy was the degree of childhood antisocial behavior, es-pecially in six- to eleven-year-olds. Robbins stated that serious anti-social behavior was "a particularly ominous childhood pattern," but factors such as poverty, slums, maternal deprivation, foster home or orphanage placement, or even a sociopathic mother did not predict adult sociopathy. However, if a child had a sociopathic or alcoholic father and was also sent to a correctional institution, the prognosis for the child was poor.

Robbins was essentially taking issue with the so-called culture of poverty hypothesis for sociopathy. She believed it was the other way around: that is, children with antisocial behavior and sociopathic fathers simply fail to rise socioeconomically. Robbins concluded that antisocial behavior predicts class status more than class status predicts antisocial behavior. This is an important conclusion, because it warns us against the too facile incrimination of social factors as a determinant of adolescent disorder.

More recently, Lewis, Shanok, and Balla (1979) found that a sample of nonincarcerated delinquent children had more serious medical his-tories than a matched group of their nondelinquent peers. The de-linquent group reported more hospital visits, accidents, and illnesses and were more likely to have sustained head injury and abuse than the nondelinquent group. More recently still, in a controlled study of eighty-four incarcerated juvenile delinquents, Lewis (1981) found "an especially high prevalence of perinatal difficulties, head and face trauma, and child abuse in the medical histories of seriously de-linquent, incarcerated children."

Lewis concluded that there seemed to be identifiable biopsychoso-cial factors that contribute to violent delinquency. The combination of trauma to the central nervous system; parental psychopathology, often expressed through incredible physical and psychological abuse; and social deprivation, particularly as manifested by failure to recognize and treat psychiatric illness and/or central nervous system dysfunction in lower socioeconomic children, creates the kind of serious, often violent, delinquent acts so prevalent in our society today.

This suggests that a single factor—for example, brain damage, social deprivation, or vulnerability to psychosis—is insufficient to engender violent delinquency. Unfortunately, often the combination of familial vulnerability, trauma to the central nervous system, physical and psychological abuse from a parent, and social deprivation is sufficient to create the violent young offender, and this combination of factors occurs frequently. Here, then, is a sophisticated concept of societal factors acting in combination as a part of a complex etiological system.

DEPRESSION

Loss and deprivation have long been held to be important antecedents to depression. Jacobson, Fasman, and DiMascio (1975) studied 461 depressed women (347 inpatients and 114 outpatients) aged eighteen to sixty years, and compared them with a control group of 198 normal women. Surprisingly, their findings "revealed no association of adult depression with overt childhood loss events, but did provide evidence to support an association of depriving childrearing processes with adult depression. The findings also suggested that a relationship existed between the degree of depriving childrearing experience with the severity of the adult illness as measured by hospital status." What was particularly noteworthy was the greater incidence of "separation of parents, more frequent psychiatric illness of parents, and a more deprived childrearing milieu," deprivation being defined as "the lack, loss, or absence of an emotionally sustaining relationship prior to adolescence."

Deprivation can occur in at least four major ways (Langmeir and Matejeck 1975): Stimulus deprivation, in which there is a lack of sensory and motor stimulation, particularly at the earliest stages of life; cognitive deprivation, in which the environment fails to provide sufficient structure, organization, and reasonable predictability of events, making it difficult for the child to make sense out of his or her experience, particularly in terms of his or her behavior and the responses from the environment; attachment deprivation, in which there

135

is a failure of the reliable presence and responsiveness of a person to whom the child can focus his perceptual, cognitive, and affective activities, this failure leading to a failure to become attached; and social deprivation, in which the absence of adequate socialization experiences gives rise to a series of impairments, including learning difficulties, a deformed value system, and impaired facility for the performance of social functions and roles.

All of these social or environmental forms of deprivation may affect the outcome of personality development in the adolescent. Thus it would seem that many childhood and adolescent depressions are associated with the antecedent of apparent insufficient human contact induced by a variety of societal and family conditions.

If the effects of insufficient positive human interaction were exclusively psychological, one might expect depressions to yield to replacement therapy in the form of an ongoing psychotherapeutic relationship. Indeed, many depressions do resolve with psychotherapy alone. These depressions we retrospectively tend to call "reactive" depressions and find an immediate psychological precursor to which to attribute the disorder.

Unfortunately, many depressions continue even after the psychodynamic issues of loss, anger, and low self-esteem have been well analyzed and understood or the social conditions rectified. Such ongoing intense depressive states often yield quite dramatically to antidepressant medication when psychotherapeutic intervention alone has been ineffective. In cases where there is no family history of depression to suggest a genetic predisposition, the question arises whether certain kinds of antecedent cognitive, emotional, or sensory deprivation at particular times of development, or antecedent but ongoing deprivation of a particular quality or intensity, may permanently alter the biochemical functions of the human organism and result in a chronic or recurrent dysphoric state recalcitrant to psychotherapy alone and resistant also to environmental change.

Mandell (1976) hypothesized a psychologically induced altered biochemical state to account for this persistent condition. He suggested that this could conceivably arise because the developing nervous system of the young infant is particularly vulnerable to impingement on its biochemical balance. Thus, if a depletion of monoamine transmitters occurs in response, say, to an early and persistent psychological loss, aggravated perhaps by such societal influences as isolation and deprivation, that altered biochemical state may then become the so-called normal, permanent biochemical state for that individual throughout his or her life. Any subsequent return to a more gratifying or stimulating social environment would then be perceived as though that were the deviant and temporary state of mind, in the sense that the prevailing tendency of the biochemical response would remain in the direction of returning to the previously acquired and permanent depressive baseline state.

Here perhaps we can see the beginnings of a connection among genetic vulnerability, societal influences, psychodynamic forces, and biological mechanisms resulting in this case in an alteration of mood. This is an especially promising and exciting direction for future research, particularly in depressive illness in children and adolescents; it also represents a biopsychosocial paradigm within a developmental frame of reference that may apply to other disorders that presently defy our understanding.

Conclusions

The examples described illustrate the importance of taking this complex viewpoint of the causes of behavior and make the point that there is no simple link between societal factors and the psychic structure of an adolescent. Psychodynamic factors, social factors, and biological factors do affect psychic structure and behavior, but only in complex, interactive ways. This is an important direction for future research. We have moved beyond the single theory model and must now embrace a complex biopsychosocial model until someone in the tradition of Darwin, Freud, or Watson and Crick has the genius to conceive of a superordinate general theory of human behavior.

NOTE

1. Footnote added 1920.

REFERENCES

Achenbach, T. M. 1980. DSM-III in light of empirical research on the classification of child psychopathology. *Journal of the American Academy of Child Psychiatry* 19:395–412.

Anderson, J. E.; Harris, D. R.; Werner, E.; and Gallistel, E. 1959. *A*

Study of Children's Adjustment over Time. Minneapolis: Institute of Child Development and Welfare.

Chess, S. 1980. Temperament and character development in childhood. Paper read at Fifth Annual Child Psychiatry Symposium, Character in Childhood, Tufts University School of Medicine, Boston, November 7, 1980.

Freud, S. 1905. Three essays on the theory of sexuality. *Standard Edition* 7:123–343. London: Hogarth, 1953.

Freud, S. 1908. Character and anal eroticism. *Standard Edition* 9:167–175. London: Hogarth, 1957.

Freud, S. 1913. The disposition to obsessional neurosis. *Standard Edition* 12:313–326. London: Hogarth, 1958.

Freud, S. 1920. The psychogenesis of a case of homosexuality in a woman. *Standard Edition* 18:167–169. London: Hogarth, 1955.

Freud, S. 1923. The ego and the id. *Standard Edition* 19:3–68. London: Hogarth, 1961.

Freud, S. 1933. New introductory lectures on psycho-analysis. *Standard Edition* 22:3–184. London: Hogarth, 1964.

Jacobson, S.; Fasman, J.; and DiMascio, A. 1975. Deprivation in the childhood of depressed women. *Journal of Nervous and Mental Diseases* 160:5–14.

Kagan, J. 1978. *The Growth of the Child: Reflections on Human Development*. New York: Norton.

Kagan, J.; Kearsley, R. B.; and Zelazo, P. R. 1978. *Infancy: Its Place in Human Development*. Cambridge, Mass.: Harvard University Press.

Kernberg, O. 1975. *Borderline Conditions and Pathological Narcissism*. New York: Aronson.

Kohlberg, L. 1964. Development of moral character and moral ideology. In M. L. Hoffman and L. W. Hoffman, eds. *Review of Child Development Research*. Vol. 1. New York: Russell Sage.

Kohut, H. 1971. *The Analysis of the Self*. New York: International Universities Press.

Kohut, H. 1980. Self psychology: reflections on the present and future. Paper read at Boston Psychoanalytic Association Symposium on Reflections on Self Psychology, Boston, November 2, 1980.

Langmeir, J., and Matejeck, Z. 1975. *Psychological Deprivation in Childhood*. New York: Halsted.

Lewis, D. O. 1981. *Vulnerabilities to Delinquency*. New York: Spectrum.

Lewis, D. O.; Shanok, S.; and Balla, D. 1979. Perinatal difficulties, head and face trauma, and child abuse in the medical histories of serious youthful offenders. *American Journal of Psychiatry* 136:419–423.

Mandell, A. J. 1976. Neurobiological mechanism of adaptation in relation to models of psychobiological development. In E. Schopler and R. J. Reichler, eds. *Psychopathology and Child Development*. New York: Plenum.

Meissner, W. W. 1980. Theories of personality and psychopathology: classical psychoanalysis. In H. Kaplan, A. Freedman, and B. Sadock, eds. *Comprehensive Textbook of Psychiatry III*. Baltimore: Williams & Wilkins.

Piaget, J. 1932. The moral judgment of the child. In H. E. Gruber and J. J. Vonecke, eds. *The Essential Piaget*. New York: Basic, 1977.

Reich, W. 1933. *Character Analysis*. New York: Orgone Institute Press, 1949.

Robbins, W. N. 1966. *Deviant Children Grown Up*. Baltimore: Williams & Wilkins.

11 THE SOCIOCULTURAL AND PSYCHODYNAMIC ASPECTS OF THE ACTING-OUT AND VIOLENT ADOLESCENT

SOL NICHTERN

Aggression and violence are portrayed vividly within adolescent behavior because of the special characteristics of adolescence. Adolescence, a developmental stage between childhood and maturity, is accompanied by a predictable fragmentation of personality stemming from the necessary psychic reorganization. This fragmentation introduces a temporary loss of the psychological self and activates regressive behavior as an adaptive maneuver directed at preserving or reconstituting the self. Regression may result in loss of impulse control, confusion of thoughts, breakdown in values, distortion of feelings, and, when combined with some of the sociocultural determinants affecting adolescence, in different forms of acting out and violence. These may extend from irrational psychotic acts to seemingly purposeful incidents of murder and suicide; to acts of violence whose outcome may be determined by happenstance; and to more prevalent acts of delinquency, drug usage, sexual promiscuity, fire setting, physical assaults, and truancy.

Sociocultural Aspects

Since the ultimate result of violence to human beings is death, an examination of death statistics among the young should illuminate some of the characteristics of their violence. Studying the death rates in the United States (Hollinger 1978, 1979; Stevens 1981), we find that from 1960 to 1978 the overall death rate had been reduced by 20 percent. However, during the same period the death rate among adolescents (fifteen to twenty-four years of age) increased by 11 percent, largely as a result of automobile accidents, murder, and suicide. In 1980 the major causes of death among our young were the motor vehicle, with a death rate among white youths of forty-two per 100,000 and nonwhite youths of twenty-six per 100,000; homicide, with a death rate among white youths of seven per 100,000 and nonwhite youths of forty-two per 100,000; accidents (other than motor vehicles), with a death rate among white and nonwhite of twenty per 100,000; suicide, with a death rate of twelve per 100,000 for white youths and ten per 100,000 for nonwhite youths; and cancer and heart disease, with death rates among both white and nonwhite groups of five per 100,000.

The decrease in the overall national death rate, accompanied by the increase in the death rate among youths, suggests the existence of significant sociocultural determinants within their acts of violence. Further light is shed on the nature of this violence by examining the differences within their death rates. The suicide rate for whites and nonwhites approaches parity and is two times as great as the death rate from natural causes. The death rate from accidents is four times as great as the death rate from natural causes. Then a significant difference appears between white and nonwhite youths. The death rate among nonwhite youths for homicide jumps to eight times the death rate from natural causes—the same as the death rate among white youths from motor vehicle accidents.

These differences suggest some of the features of aggression and violence among adolescents. They give recognition to the motor vehicle as an instrument of violence and suggest that its greater availability to the better financially positioned white youths may make it their instrument of homicidal violence. Accounting for the difference in homicide and motor vehicle death rates between whites and nonwhites introduces the possibility that there may be no real difference between white and nonwhite adolescents in terms of aggressive drives and highlights adolescents in general and their special problems with control of impulse.

If homicide is viewed as violent behavior stemming from aggression directed outward and suicide as violent behavior directed inward, their higher incidence among adolescents supports the proposition that aggression is an important part of the adolescent stage of development. However, it should be noted that suicide and homicide rates doubled during the period 1961–1975 while there was little change in the death rate due to accidents. This special kind of rapid escalation suggests sociocultural factors rather than those developmentally determined. This period did coincide with the Vietnam War which stands out as a confused, unpopular, and ill-defined conflict imposed upon our young. Aggression became a way of life for an entire generation. It was the first major war that was fought within our homes as a television war. It was brought into the very growth experience of children who remembered the daily body count and the constant visual imagery of violence. Such exposure to violence on a repeated daily basis during the early stages of development cannot be dismissed as an innocent process but may have served as a preconditioning system to a developmental stage characterized by its own aggression.

During this same period, other major social changes occurred within the family introducing new conditions for child rearing and child development. The construct of family had been altered by increased mobility leading to the dislocation of ties needed for communication of clearly defined values. The inclusion of the female of childbearing age into the work force resulted in many more children being reared by multiple surrogate parents, adding further confusion and subtle distortions to relationships and feelings. The breakdown of the family unit became an established phenomenon. The exploding divorce rate resulted in one out of two children being reared within family units containing only one or no biological parent and a dramatic increase in the number of single-parent families. The number of children born out of wedlock to adolescent females increased dramatically. All of these have contributed to the growing social instability of the family that consequently has major effects on stages of life having their own developmental instability—childhood and adolescence.

Psychodynamic Aspects

Disturbances of adolescence reflect arrests or regressions of maturationally produced sequences of thoughts, feelings, behaviors, and conflicts generated by the developmental progression toward maturity. The conflictual state of adolescent behavior is simultaneously undifferentiated and differentiating, organismic and selectively responsive, dominated by intellectualism and determined by sexual drive, reflexive in nature with the need to gratify impulse, hyperreactive to environmental stimuli, mixing fantasy and reality, dominated by a shifting perception serving to disrupt basic object constancy, possessed by an uncertain identity, influenced by an affective response system of a recurrent depressive and aggressive attitude related to object loss, vacillating between introjective and projective thinking, and having a capacity for regression that makes the adolescent vulnerable to stress and unpredictable in response.

Much of the behavior of adolescence is related to expected personality fragmentation and its accompanying regression. The extent of the regression correlates with the achieved level of personality development, that is, ego organization. However, regression always brings back early determined functions such as object relatedness and object constancy. Sensorimotor organization serves to organize impulse so that we can perceive and respond to ourselves and our environment. Our early interactions reinforce this perception and response system so that a constancy is introduced permitting us to experience the same set of circumstances in the same manner. Thus, object relatedness and object constancy are established early as the base for perceptions and responses. The primary object of this system is the self. The personality fragmentation of adolescence introduces loss of the self as a significant object. This loss stimulates further regression while evoking a generalized inhibitory state designed to arrest further fragmentation as an adaptive maneuver directed at preserving or reconstituting the self. This inhibitory process makes depression a characteristic of adolescence and should be recognized as a naturally occurring phenomenon (the depressive stance of adolescence). Just as often, the loss of self may evoke a generalized excitatory state designed to preserve or reconstitute the self. This excitatory process makes aggression another characteristic of adolescence and should also be recognized as a naturally occurring phenomenon (the aggressive stance of adolescence). The intensity and degree of regression determine the nature and severity of the depression or aggression. Thus, depression and aggression are present universally within adolescence. The severe forms leading to overt violence can be identified and grouped.

Types of Violent Adolescents

The most severe forms of violence seen in adolescents reflect an early loss of object relatedness. These aggressive, violent acts appear to be irrational and have elements of depersonalization and dehumanization along with complete loss of control over impulse. Often the thought processes are unrelated to the acts of aggression. The

143

magical omnipotence of archaic thinking is evident. The violence is accompanied by a high risk of destruction to life as a result of the accompanying nonfeeling and depersonalized state. Suicidal or homicidal behavior is deliberate, purposeful, and too often successful under these circumstances (for example, immolation).

Another type of adolescent violence is characterized by aggressive behavior reflecting the pursuit of object constancy with anxiety stemming from the possible loss of object relatedness. There are fluctuations of mood, withdrawal, and immobilizing anxiety. These are accompanied by a gross sense of inadequacy with only minimal depersonalization. The anxiety may be internalized or externalized. Homicide, suicide, self-destructive behavior, or somaticization (anorexia, accident proneness, or self-mutilation) may occur. Behavior appears to be directed at reestablishing object constancy through self-stimulation or recruiting symbiotic attachments. The self-stimulating behavior is visible but frequently its significance is unrecognized. It is often mutilating or life threatening, and recurrent and more destructive when ignored. Much aggressive behavior appears to be directed toward achieving some degree of object constancy through fixation of impulse onto the self or some substitute object. Thus, paranoid or delusional systems are common. The pattern of the appearance of aggressive behavior is gradual and accompanied by all sorts of rationalizations. On closer examination, a well-entrenched symbiotic relationship and a preexisting pattern of separation anxiety in childhood can be identified. The demand for maturity within the adolescent period becomes a severe stress to the well-established and entrenched symbiotic system and activates the aggressive state toward others (homicide) or toward the self (suicide or self-destructive behavior).

Another type of aggressive violence within adolescence is characterized by behavior reflecting the preservation of the constancy of the self by purposeful activity. Object relatedness and object constancy are well established. Impulse is channeled into the recruitment of activities designed to reinforce the existence of the self and to relieve anxiety engendered by any threat to its existence. There is an aggressive over-investment in all of the behavioral components of adolescence to the point of violence. Contemporary group interests and activities (fashions, culturally determined social and political interests, drug usage, sexual behavior) are recruited and exaggerated for the reinforcement of the self whose existence is threatened within the developmental process by personality fragmentation occurring during adolescence. There is little attempt to control impulse, and the need for instant gratification is evident in the search for sensations and self-stimulation. Affective responses appear to be inhibited or suppressed. Thought processes are sometimes distorted, diminished, or overflowing with content. The magical omnipotence of archaic thinking is represented by compulsive preoccupation with ideology (religious beliefs, conception, causes, revolution, war, death). There is the danger of self-destruction through martyrdom. There is excessive physical activity and aggressive behavior designed to achieve visibility and recognition of the self. The accompanying lack of controls sometimes assumes the proportions of contagion to others. Destructive behavior is recruited for the cause and purpose of making the self significant. Interventions are difficult because the aggression is ego-syntonic and designed to reinforce the self. Social and group processes are the interventions of choice.

A final type of adolescent aggression resulting in occasional violence can be identified as reactive and is characterized by the integrity of the self. Behavior correlates to affect and is in response to identifiable circumstances. This type represents a continuous adaptation to the changes taking place within adolescent development. There are fluctuating levels of activities and mood. There is a more direct relationship between cause and effect within the aggressive behavior. There is the sudden appearance of immature patterns and then rapid reconstitution. Serious regression occurs rarely. Violence is accompanied by poor judgment, transient problems with coping, withdrawal, and mood swings. Insights leading to constructive changes of life-style and better coping mechanisms are frequently helpful.

Conclusions

The nature and severity of the violence of adolescents are determined by the place, the time, and the circumstances as much as the internal forces at work. Unless this is understood, there is a tendency to consider violence a special characteristic of adolescent aggression when it should be recognized more appropriately as the result of the blending of sociocultural forces with the essence of adolescence—the variable, changing, unpredictable nature of a human being in transition.

If we are to look at adolescents' behavior as the focal point of violence, we do them and ourselves an injustice. For they are us. They are our prototype. They mirror all that we are and all that we created in our society and culture. If we recognize adolescents as violent, we must recognize ourselves as violent. If we call adolescents promiscuous, we must recognize ourselves as promiscuous. If we call adolescents acting out, we must see our own forms of acting out. And if we see adolescents as self-destructive, we must see our own self-destructiveness and begin to give our young the opportunity to escape the acting-out violence of our society. We must control our impulses by bringing order and stability to ourselves, our families, and the institutions of our society. We must offer our young the opportunity to grow and mature by permitting and encouraging them to separate and to achieve their own identity without intensifying their conflicts with our own.

REFERENCES

Hollinger, P. 1978. Adolescent suicide: an epidemiological study of recent trends. *American Journal of Psychiatry* 135(6): 754–756.

Hollinger, P. 1979. Violent deaths among the young: recent trends in suicide, homicide, and accidents. *American Journal of Psychiatry* 136(9): 1144–1147.

Stevens, W. K. 1981. Youth and violence: a look at four lost lives. *New York Times* (January 25).

12 JUVENILE DELINQUENTS AND VIOLENT DEATH

RICHARD C. MAROHN, ELLEN M. LOCKE, RONALD ROSENTHAL,
AND GLENN CURTISS

Suicide, homicide, and accidental death are not unrelated. They have been conceptualized and studied in the aggregate as violent death. In a recent series of epidemiological studies, Hollinger (1977, 1978, 1979, 1980) has cited violent deaths among the young as worthy of special attention. While the mortality rates for violent death among all age groups combined have tended to decrease, they have increased regularly among the younger age group. In 1975, the rate of violent death among fifteen- to twenty-four-year-olds was higher than ever previously recorded, claiming eight times as many lives as the next two leading causes of death—malignant neoplasms and major cardiovascular disease—combined.

Consistently, mortality rates for accidents are higher than those for homicide and mortality rates for homicide are higher than those for suicide. While the rates for accidents and homicides have tended to remain fairly stable, those for suicide among youths have risen steadily, increasing 131 percent during the years 1961–1975. Accidents and homicide claim more black, and suicide more white, victims. All three causes of death affect males more than females, but females do outnumber males in the frequency of attempted rather than completed suicides.

Various relationships between suicide and homicide have been described in the literature. For example, it has been noted that individuals often express both suicidal and homicidal impulses and that homicide followed by suicide is not uncommon (Finch and Poznanski 1971). Perpetrators of successful and attempted presidential assassinations

147

have frequently been found to reveal strong suicidal intent (Weinstein and Lyerly 1969). MacDonald (1967) reported that individuals admitted to a psychiatric hospital on the basis of expressed homicidal intent were found on follow-up to have a high suicide rate. Wolfgang (1959), investigating 588 consecutive criminal homicides in Philadelphia, found that 26 percent had been victim precipitated and represented suicides. Wolfgang's data suggest a victim profile of a black male who has a previous arrest record, often for assaults against persons. This supports the notion that aggressive criminal offenders are at increased risk for suicide.

Several empirical investigators of accidental deaths have led to the conclusion that accident proneness and risk taking may reflect depression and/or rage, and that they afford a means of acting out self-destructive tendencies (Litman, Curphey, Schneidman, Farberow, and Tabachnick 1963; Porterfield 1960; Schrut 1964; Tabachnick, Litman, Osman, Jones, Cohn, Kaspar, and Moffat 1966). Car accidents have received particular attention. Selzer and Payne (1962) reported that suicide and car accidents were correlated to the extent that adults with serious suicidal tendencies were twice as likely to have car accidents as adults without them. MacDonald (1964) stressed that wrecking a car at high speeds allows violent discharge of great anger and noted that 25 percent of his inpatient sample had driven their cars into other vehicles. Shaffer et al. (1977) have also commented on the personality characteristics of high-risk drivers, which they labeled "socially obstreperous." Conger, Gaskill, Glad, Hassel, Rainey, Sawrey, and Turrell (1959) stressed the poor control of hostility, low tolerance for tension, dependency, egocentricity, and unreflectiveness among males involved in fatal crashes. Tillman and Hobbs (1949) found that high-risk drivers were often those who could not tolerate and were in chronic revolt against authority. They were further characterized by antisocial attitudes, impulsivity, distractibility, and relational and fiscal irresponsibility.

Collectively, these reports link impulsive and antisocial personality patterns with accident proneness and victim-precipitated homicide. To the extent that dynamic processes underlie both the general behavioral patterns as well as the specific risk-taking behaviors of these individuals, some authors (for example, Tabachnick 1975) have suggested that violent deaths may result from "subintentioned," self-destructive, or suicidal impulses.

Freud (1920), Menninger (1938), and others of the early psychoanalytic community had drawn theoretical links among the

148

phenomena of suicide, homicide, and fatal accidents long before there were any broadly based epidemiological data to support their theories. Freud proposed that suicide begins with a death wish toward a hated or lost object, for which one feels guilty and which is then directed back at the self. Menninger stated that suicide is "a death in which are combined in one person the murderer and the murdered." He also described the complexity of self-destructive impulses, which may comprise a wish to kill undesirable features of identifications within the self, a wish to be killed, a masochistic desire to atone, and/or a wish to die to obtain reunion with a loved one. Thus, suicide may be a form of murder, or murder a form of suicide, when the victim represents the murderer in the latter's unconscious. Freud (1901) and Menninger (1935) also speculated that many serious or fatal accidents were atypical forms of suicide.

More recent data suggest that the theorized relationship between suicide and aggression requires modification if it is to be of predictive value, particularly where adolescent suicide is concerned (Eisenthal 1967). A number of reports have presented evidence which challenges the hypothesis that inhibition of aggression is a distinctive and characteristic response of suicidal individuals (Lester 1967; Lewis, Shanok, Balla, and Bard 1980; Litman et al. 1963; McCandless 1968; Schrut 1964). To the extent that psychoanalytic theory may have fostered the impression that suicide and homicide were almost mutually exclusive phenomena (so that aggression is discharged either against the self or against others), it is not consistent with much of the recent literature describing deaths among adolescents. Litman (1967) has argued that aggression and guilt have been overemphasized as components of suicide and that the helpless, dependent, and libidinal elements have been underemphasized. Several authors (Margolin and Teicher 1968; Schneer, Kay, and Brozovsky 1961; Schrut 1968) have linked adolescent suicidal behavior to disturbances in the oedipal development and the resulting deficits in sexual identity and superego formation. Schneer et al. (1961) have reported their conclusion that virtually all adolescent suicidal behavior, regardless of the conscious ideation or precipitating event, derives from an overwhelming crisis in sexual development and at the service of controlling aggressive urges. For some of these youths—that significant minority whose mothers were depressed during the child's infancy and/or whose fathers were not present during the initial oedipal phase—the recapitulation of the oedipal crisis during adolescence may revive unbearable memories of old frustrations and further tax the already vulnerable ego's ability to hold in

149

check the "brittle alliance between aggression and libido" (Eisen 1976) which they acquired during early childhood.

It may be readily seen that disturbances in aggressive and libidinal development arise in the context of disturbed family relationships. As Litman (1967) has pointed out, for many adolescents "the suicidal drama produces not so much guilt for the unconscious wish of the child to murder the parent, but rather a reaction of abandonment on the part of the child to the parents' unconscious wish for the child's death." A growing body of reports indicates that the role of hostility toward the child on the part of significant others may be as important in adolescent suicide as the role of the adolescent's hostility turned inward (Eisen 1976; Glaser 1965; Margolin and Teicher 1968; Rosenbaum and Richman 1970; Sabbath 1969; Schrut 1968). Parents are often found to have an intense ambivalence toward these children and to regard them as "expendable" (Sabbath 1969). A notable incidence of physical (Lewis, Shanok, Pincus, and Glaser 1979) or sexual abuse, including incest (Bigras, Gauthier, Bouchard, and Tasse 1966; Kaufman, Peck, and Tagiuri 1954), has also been found in the early histories of violent and self-destructive adolescents.

The contribution to suicidal vulnerability of having experienced abuse is multiple and complex. First, physical abuse may cause central nervous system damage and thus contribute to impulsivity, attention disorders, and learning disabilities, all of which have been significantly correlated with overt violent behavior (Lewis et al. 1979, 1980; Spellacy 1977). Second, abuse produces rage against the abusing parent and may lead to identification with the aggressor, to displacement in homicidal rage toward others, or to retroflexed aggression against the self. Finally, it provides a model to follow. Evidence thus far tends to show that the aggressive, hostile, and delinquent or violently acting-out adolescent is at no less risk for intentioned, and is possibly at greater risk for subintentioned suicide than more clinically depressed youth (Otto 1964; Schrut 1968, 1974; Shaffer 1974). Therefore, Rosenbaum and Richman (1970) have advised that, when assessing any destructive or self-destructive behavior, it is important to consider not only "whom did the patient really want to kill, or wish to have dead, or to suffer?" but also "who wished the patient to die, disappear, or go away?"

Among all adolescents, overt intentionality or a clear "wish to die" is probably less frequent than among adults (Kovacs and Beck 1977; Otto 1964). The adolescent's concern with power and powerlessness, his reluctance to admit limitations, his impulsivity, lack of judgment, proclivity toward recklessness, and the exacerbation of these qualities through abuse of drugs (Jalali, Jalali, Crocetti, and Turner 1981) or alcohol (Caine 1978) no doubt play a part in a certain number of violent deaths resulting among youths with no clearly observable wish to die. However, Teicher and Jacobs (1966, 1977) have stressed that, while the act of taking one's life may be impulsive, the decision to do so, particularly among adolescents, often is not. Of their sample of twenty adolescent suicide attempters, the large majority were found to have no previous history of "irrational acts" and had been viewed by parents, siblings, peers, and teachers as functioning in a "rational manner." They had been subject to a long series of problems formed through escalating situational stress, and these factors had combined to bring about a progressive social isolation which in turn became "the problem" and inhibited the adolescent's access to helping services and relationships. They concluded that a significant majority of their adolescent sample had considered the suicide attempt in advance, and from the perspective of the youth, had weighed it rationally and selected it after more "conventional" problem-solving techniques—such as rebelling, withdrawing, running away from home, physical violence, or psychosomatic symptoms—had failed.

Considering the complexity of factors which influence adolescent suicide, how can we begin to predict suicide potential? Certainly the clinician should carefully assess the nature of aggressive and libidinal issues. In addition, a number of situational variables have been shown to relate to the likelihood of attempting suicide. When compared to those of normal adolescents, the histories of presuicidal adolescents have shown a higher incidence of child abuse, parent loss, parental discord, broken homes, one-parent families, social dislocation resulting in frequent changes of residence and of school, absence from school for other than academic reasons, disturbed peer relations, and history of suicide or suicide attempt on the part of a parent or significant other. However, when compared with other emotionally disturbed adolescents, the distinguishing and predictive characteristics of suicidal youths are fewer than might be expected. Only two variables—loss of a parent before age twelve and parental discord specifically concerning divorce—have been found to differentiate the groups significantly (Stanley and Barter 1970). Since current situational factors may also contribute to suicide potential, it may well be that we are not yet equipped to predict which of these may represent suicide-triggering events (Beck, Resnick, and Lettieri 1974; Rosen 1954). Given the further possibility of subintentioned suicide as a factor in violent death, we may do well to heed Neuringer's (1975) advice that every emotionally disturbed adolescent be seen to be at risk of violent death.

Since 1969, the Adolescent Program of the Illinois State Psychiatric Institute has attempted to study, understand, and treat adolescents with behavior disorders, many of whom could be referred to as "juvenile delinquents," whether known as such to the authorities or undetected.[1] This work has resulted in a number of research studies and treatment recommendations in numerous publications and presentations (Marohn 1974, 1977, 1980; Marohn, Dalle-Molle, McCarter, and Linn 1980; Marohn, Dalle-Molle, Offer, and Ostrov 1973; Marohn, Offer, and Ostrov 1971; Marohn, Offer, Ostrov, and Trujillo 1979; Offer, Marohn, and Ostrov 1975, 1979; Ostrov, Offer, and Marohn 1976).[2]

Of the initial fifty-six subjects reported on by Offer et al. (1979) interviewed about a year and a half after discharge from the hospital, forty-three (75 percent) reported doing quite well. A ten-year follow-up study is now in progress and by replicating instruments used at the time of admission is attempting to determine something about the natural history of the behaviorally disordered adolescent: Does borderline pathology persist as borderline pathology? Do aspects of the treatment approach, such as helping young people develop a capacity to introspect, persist into later adolescent and adult life? Do these adolescent delinquents turn into adult criminals? Do they become emotionally disturbed or unhappy adults without necessarily presenting a criminal history? The ten-year follow-up study is now in its beginning stages and will be reported on more extensively later. What is striking, however, is that although not all of the fifty-six subjects have been located, at least five of them have died violent deaths since their discharge from the program. Two met death through murder, one died through a suicide, and one was killed in an automobile accident. The fifth appears to have been an accidental homicide. One subject died very shortly after discharge from the program and the other four in recent years.

Five Instances of Violent Death

CASE EXAMPLE 1

Fran, a fourteen-year-old white girl, was admitted to the program after being referred by her private psychiatrist. She was referred because, since age thirteen, she had been running away from home, with steadily increasing frequency and periods of time. She had been deemed an "incorrigible" runaway by the court, which had placed her in the detention home immediately prior to her hospitalization. Although white, Fran would invariably head for black ghetto areas of the city and seemed to have developed a strong identification with that culture. She had adopted a black dialect, for which she was sometimes ridiculed by black patients on the unit. She was a gifted and prolific writer, yet all of her work—short stories, songs, poems, and novels—displayed themes of depression and featured characters who were black, Mexican, or Puerto Rican. Her idealization of these cultural groups was horrifying to her upper-middle-class parents, as was her sexual activity, which they reported to have begun when Fran was in the seventh grade. Just prior to admission, she was known to have been dating a twenty-nine-year-old divorced black male, with whom she stayed while on runaway and from whom she contracted gonorrhea.

Fran's early developmental history was not adequately obtained because her parents refused to cooperate with both treatment and research procedures, despite their initial agreement to do so. However, material from the juvenile court indicated that her milestones were within normal limits and that there was no significant medical history. Her parents reported that she had a "good disposition" as a child—that is, she was outgoing, cooperative, and very bright. Despite her behavioral problems, she always did well academically, having been an excellent student through the sixth grade. Fran confirmed that she was a "do-gooder for thirteen years," and although she eventually strove to reject that image of herself, she continued to be regarded as a highly intelligent and talented girl of great promise.

There was evidence that both parents had deep and chronic psychological disturbances. Mother, an erratic and emotionally cold woman, had a severe problem with alcohol and often would be incoherent. In addition, she was paranoid and assaultive, with an impulsive and violent temper. Father was viewed as having a rigidly defended, obsessive compulsive personality, which rendered him extremely cold and withdrawn. Both parents were highly ambivalent toward their daughter, while mother was often openly rejecting. Fran represented, to others as well as to herself,

that her runaway behavior was closely connected to these problems at home; that is, she felt that the problem for focus should be
not her own behavior, but that of her parents.

At the hospital, Fran presented as tough, hardened, and unafraid; she was depressed and pessimistic but also defiant and
evasive. Her parents would not visit the unit, although a foster
parent did spend a considerable amount of time with her. As it
became apparent that her parents' refusal to cooperate was solidly
entrenched, we determined that there was little potential for Fran
to benefit from the Adolescent Program. We believed it would be
more important for her to continue in treatment with her trainee-
therapist, who was moving to another unit and arranged for Fran
to transfer at the same time. However, before this plan could be
implemented, she ran away from the hospital. She called the unit
on one occasion but refused to return, and exactly one month after
having run away, she was murdered by her boyfriend. The murder
was described in considerable detail in the local newspapers: as
she knelt before her lover, pleading for her life, she was shot
twice. Her boyfriend was arrested, convicted, and sentenced.

Fran's elopement from the hospital may well have represented a
suicidal equivalent—an acting out of the despair and rage she felt toward her parents, whose refusal to participate in our program represented their final rejection of their daughter. Faced with this abandonment, Fran may consciously or unconsciously have determined to separate from her parents in a most negativistic way; rejecting in her turn
the milieu of her upper-middle-class family, fleeing to the lower-class
ghetto, seeking and cementing a relationship with an older man. We
also must consider that she may have experienced abandonment by,
and rage against, the Adolescent Program when forced to choose between continuing in the program or continuing with her therapist.

CASE EXAMPLE 2

Nick, a thirteen-year-old white boy, was referred to the program
by his private psychiatrist, who had been treating him because of
repeated episodes of delinquency: running away, vandalism,
breaking and entering, and window peeping. These symptoms represented only the latest incidents in a long-standing history of
problem behavior—Nick's mother reported that he had always

been depressed, very difficult to discipline, and hyperactive at home. Although the hyperactivity quieted somewhat following the prescription of amphetamines, he continued to be restless, inattentive, and uncooperative at school. As a young child, he vandalized the neighborhood, set fires, and stole from friends and relatives.

Nick had been sexually abused as an infant by his natural father, the revelation of whose sexually perverse behavior with other neighborhood children occasioned the parents' divorce when Nick was two. This aspect of his early history seemed to have significant impact on his later development, both intrapsychically and interpersonally. His mother reported that she became extremely anxious and unavailable to her children for three years following the divorce. She turned to Nick to meet her emotional needs and developed inappropriate and impossible expectations of performance from him. At the same time, she conveyed to him the likelihood that he was irreparably damaged, both organically and in his personality development. She shared with him the fact that he had been sexually abused and would often state to him her opinion that this made him fundamentally different from other children. Her expectation was that he would "probably turn out just like his father." Mother remarried when Nick was six, and although his stepfather tried desperately to establish a relationship with him, he was unable to do so. As a result, Nick came to identify himself with his sexually abusive father. He felt that he was incapable of establishing any kind of meaningful or mature heterosexual relationship and believed himself tainted and damaged, much as his mother would frequently describe him to be. He was seldom able to form supportive peer relationships, perceiving that others "could not stand me," and so resorted to presenting himself as a clown in order to engage with peers and to mask the lurid aggressive fantasies with which he was often obsessed.

Nick was hospitalized for about a year, and although he was extremely hyperactive and impulsive, he did make some gains during the course of his stay. It was clearly demonstrated through a double blind study that he profited from the prescription of stimulants. His prognosis at discharge was deemed good, based on his improved ability to relate to others, to present himself in a more appealing and positive fashion, and to maintain islands of ego strength.

During a follow-up interview about sixteen months after discharge, Nick seemed to be less anxious and more mature, no longer presenting himself as a clown. At the time of the interview, he was involved in another treatment program, where he had been hospitalized for approximately one year. He reported that he was benefiting from the program, although he had run away twice during that time. His delinquent behavior had considerably diminished, although he had been arrested for burglary, jaywalking, and hitchhiking while on runaway. Though he felt that interpersonal relationships still posed great difficulty for him, he had maintained some positive self-regard, offering as evidence the facts that he understood himself better, had stopped swearing, and took better care of his personal hygiene. Family therapy sessions had also helped him to feel closer to his mother and stepfather and had improved their communication. Nick stated that there were some staff members at ISPI to whom he continued to feel particularly close, but he also expressed some negative feelings about the treatment program; for example, he wished it had allowed more freedom of movement. He predicted that ten years from the time of the interview, he would be living happily and well in society, would have a wife, and would be employed as a carpenter like his stepfather.

Between the time of his discharge and his death some nine years later, Nick had continued to require treatment. He had been in halfway houses, had become psychotic, paranoid, and severely suicidal on a number of occasions, slashing himself and requiring emergency treatment. He was involved for a long time in a daycare program for chronic psychotic patients but continued to have a difficult adjustment. He finally burglarized a store, stole some food, and was sentenced to two years in the state correctional system, his pleas of defense on the basis of mental illness having been set aside by the court. Once in the correctional system, however, he was referred to a specialized program for the criminally insane because he was judged to be "paranoid and psychotic." He was housed on an intensive care unit, which received new inmates and provided the suicidal precautions which Nick gave evidence of needing. On one occasion, he had tied a string around his neck and attached the other end to a wash basin, saying that he was tethered like a dog. He explained to his counselor that he never had a friend, only a pet dog, and that he was like his dog. (During his stay in our program, he often barked, much to the annoyance of staff and other patients, but could never explain his reasons for doing so.) He displayed other bizarre behavior, talking concretely about having penile erections which disturbed him, describing voices he would hear of people who were watching him, and occasionally scratching his arms.

While Nick was incarcerated, his parents—particularly his mother—had refused to have any further contact with him. Mother explained that they had tried everything to help him but could no longer tolerate his disturbed behavior or entertain any hope of his eventual reintegration into the family in an acceptable manner. Nick, however, continued to hope that he could establish a relationship with his mother and stepfather that would permit his return home following parole and met with his caseworker at the prison to develop such a plan. When the counselor called mother and learned that there was no possibility of Nick's returning home, he began thinking about a parole plan that would involve placement in a psychiatric facility. He met Nick by chance at the prison, and when asked if he had talked with mother, told Nick that he would discuss it the following day during their regularly scheduled session. About three hours later, Nick was found lying face down on the floor, his neck tied in a sheet suspended from the wash basin.

One can speculate that Nick's suicide derived from his recurrent sense of being different and unwanted, and that in some way he recognized or believed that he was again to be regarded as unacceptable and expendable by his family. In the nine years since his discharge from our program, Nick's delinquency had persisted, but what initially appeared to be a hyperactive, impulsive adolescent turned out to be a seriously psychotic and depressed young man.

CASE EXAMPLE 3

Selma, a fifteen-year-old black girl, was referred to the program by the juvenile court. Her presenting problems included occasional truancy and misdemeanors, a moderate amount of promiscuity and prostitution, and frequent running away. Selma's delinquent behavior appeared to be closely connected with escalating disruption within her home environment. Her natural father deserted the family and left them financially destitute when Selma was two years of age. He was succeeded by a number of men who remained with her mother just long enough for Selma to attach and then suffer the pain of their abandonment. A potentially stable father figure was presented when mother remarried during Selma's latency, but the closeness which Selma might have experienced in this relationship took a destructive turn when stepfather sexually molested her at age nine. Mother tried to support her daughter by pressing charges, but they were dismissed due to insufficient corroboration. From this point on, the mother-daughter relationship became openly conflictual. Selma started stealing from mother, displayed her precocious sexualization at school, and soon began running away from home. She was often found in the company of older men, from whom she sought both physical closeness and material favors, and on one occasion reported that she had been raped. By age fifteen she was soliciting for prostitution and was placed on probation.

During the course of her hospitalization, Selma alternated between anger and depression. She both stated and displayed her conviction that people were withholding and untrustworthy, and that nurturant supplies could be obtained only through oblique means. She repeatedly stated that she felt used and cheated, engaged in minor episodes of delinquency, and sought a sexual relationship with a male patient. She presented many somatic complaints, experienced painful dysmenorrhea, and appeared accident prone to the point of repeatedly injuring herself during unit activities. These were especially noticeable when her therapist was on vacation. As she neared termination, she displayed a great deal of aggressive acting out in an attempt to "make everyone as mad at me as I am at myself so I won't be discharged." As she left the unit, she warned that one day staff would read of her death in the newspapers. Plans had been made for her to continue in therapy as an outpatient, but she kept only one appointment, during which she announced that she had married.

Selma was interviewed almost two years after discharge. She looked haggard and gaunt during the interview but seemed comforted and replenished by the contact with the program. She felt very positive about the treatment program, talked fondly about a number of the staff members, but stated that she continued to have serious personal and interpersonal problems. She had been unable to maintain a stable job or residence, had been arrested for shop-lifting and for being in a car that had been used to commit a robbery, and for a time had used heroin. She had separated from her husband, who had physically abused her, had been involved in several unsatisfactory heterosexual relationships, and was deeply concerned about the extent to which she had established self-destructive patterns in her choice of mates. She was pregnant at the time of the interview and had decided to keep the baby and try to be a good mother. She did think she would be better off in ten years than she was at the time of that interview, but seemed to view this prediction as contingent on pursuing further treatment. Therapy was again offered to her and an appointment was arranged, but she neither kept the appointment nor responded to a follow-up letter.

About eight years after discharge, at age twenty-four, Selma was found raped and strangled in an alley near her home. She had been on her way to the store but had never returned. No one was arrested for this crime. She had been living in Chicago with yet another man who was physically abusive to her and addicted to drugs. He was the father of the two youngest of her three children; the father of her first child was a known gang member who was in prison for burglary. She had neither continued her education nor worked at all since discharge and was being supported through public aid. At the time of her death, she was addicted to both alcohol and heroin and was in a methadone maintenance program. She had received no treatment of an intensive nature, though she had been in a supportive group in conjunction with the drug therapy program. She was not prostituting at the time of her death. Her mother advised us that Selma would frequently talk about her stay in our hospital as being the "happiest times of her life" because she had received so much help in the program.

The specific details of Selma's rape and murder are unknown, but the outcome is not entirely surprising given her history of acting-out rage at her mother through self-destructive activity, provoking and/or seeking abusive men in an attempt to master the original sexual abuse, and, as seen in her prostitution and drug addiction, a constant fascination with a chaotic and risk-ridden milieu. These self-destructive propensities made it impossible for Selma to accept treatment when offered; even though she recognized how she had benefited from treatment, she had hinted at her eventual murder.

CASE EXAMPLE 4

Bart was almost fifteen when admitted to the program. He was a black youth who was referred by his probation officer because of frequent truancy, runaways, and breaking and entering. He was a boy who had a knack for getting caught in his delinquency and had been placed in the detention center five times in the eighteen months preceding his admission.

Bart was born with serious congenital defects. The lower third of his right arm was missing, as were two fingers on his left hand. His left leg was also seriously deformed, and was amputated at age two to be fitted with a prosthesis. Throughout his early childhood, Bart underwent surgery on his leg and arm five times.

Mother initially was horrified at Bart's condition and refused to see him for several days after his birth. Her family urged her strongly to give the baby up, but when she could bear to look at him, his eyes seemed to be saying to her, "Love me, mommy, and take care of me," and so she resolved to keep the baby and "love him as much as I could." Though mother stated that she and other family members tried to treat Bart as a normal child, she also was aware of having particular difficulty setting limits on him in sympathy for his handicaps. Moreover, mother reported that Bart was frequently manipulative around the handicaps in order to win special favors. While she was highly susceptible to these manipulations, mother also developed a conviction that she could not trust her son, "just like I could not trust his father"—a heroin addict who had spent most of the last twenty years in jail for drug-related crimes. When father was home, he refused to have much to do with Bart because of his delinquent behavior. An older brother, whom Bart reportedly idealized, also had a history of delinquency and drug addiction.

Bart had been involved in mischief at school from early years, often clowning and otherwise showing off in the classroom in an attempt to make light of his physical handicaps. His delinquent peer formation began after he was transferred into a mainstream school and, by his own report, was directly related to the fact that the other boys teased him and convinced him that he had to prove himself in this manner in order to win their favor.

During his six months on our unit, Bart displayed a continuing inability to establish meaningful interpersonal relationships or to assess his own behavior. He adopted a stance of grandiose and immature bravado, tried both to entertain and to manipulate others with his deformities, and was both actively and passively aggressive in testing limits and threatening violence to others. The overanxious and provocative behavior, through which he desperately tried to become a member of the patient group, barely masked a profound depression and fear of abandonment. He often waited and hoped for a visit from his parents, who never came, even on his birthday. He was extremely needy, demanding, and intensely lonely, yet he continually found fault with others and threatened to elope from the unit. He reported several dreams of killing people, being killed in very brutal, mutilating scenes, and demonstrated an obsessive terror of death.

After Bart had spent six months on our unit, we recommended that he remain with us in order to receive long-term treatment. However, this would have necessitated a change of therapists, which he was unable to tolerate. He eloped from the unit just prior to his therapist's departure and was discharged against medical advice when he failed to return.

Bart was interviewed a year and a half following discharge, when he was sixteen. He had been placed in a youth correctional program five months earlier, following his arrest for truancy, burglary, and car theft. He apparently was quite moved by the interview and expressed a good deal of anger and hostility. However, he also expressed positive feelings about the treatment program, based on the fact that staff "were kind to me and tried to help me." Bart felt the need for further therapy; he felt very pessimistic and uncertain about his future. He stated that in ten years he hoped to be "living."

Three years and four months after discharge, when he was eighteen years of age, Bart was shot by an emotionally unstable security guard who had previously killed two policemen but had not been imprisoned because he was deemed "mentally handicapped" and incompetent to stand trial. Working as an armed guard in an apartment building, he said that Bart was trying to enter the building illegally. He later changed his story to say that the gun discharged accidentally.

Bart's death may have been provoked by the same immature bravado, manipulative behavior, and aggressive limit testing he showed on the unit. There, we speculated, it served to mask his depression. With the disturbed security guard, it may simply have misfired and provoked an inordinate response, or it may have fulfilled the very demands of Bart's deep depression and his suicidal wishes.

CASE EXAMPLE 5

Sheldon, a white youth, was fifteen when admitted to the program. He had been referred by his high school social worker because he was incorrigible at home, chronically truant, and a frequent runaway. He had also been arrested for stealing a car and presented a history of serious drug abuse. He frequently smoked marijuana, took barbiturates, experimented with heroin, and had used LSD at least thirty to forty times. He had been picked up by the police for selling drugs at school.

At the time of his admission, and for the majority of his stay in the program, Sheldon displayed an extremely negative self-presentation which reportedly was of long standing. He was disheveled in his dress, careless of his personal hygiene, obese, and afflicted with considerable facial acne. He soiled himself until a year prior to his admission. He made himself yet more unattractive to others through obnoxious, malicious, and aggressive behavior. Though highly reactive to slights both large and small, Sheldon would continually provoke others to dislike and tease him; when they did so, he would retaliate with assaultive behavior. It was not hard to credit his parents' statement that Sheldon had never had a close friend of either sex.

It also was not hard to understand the deep disappointment with which Sheldon's parents regarded him or the difficulty which they had always experienced in relating to him in a nurturant fashion. There was a striking polarity in the parents' self-presentation as compared to that of the son whom they had adopted at age eight weeks. Both mother and father were immaculately groomed, rigidly moral, and uniformly cheerful to the point of being saccharine. They described their marriage as being "unusually wonderful" and initially denied any bitterness or shame toward their son, declaring instead that they had never minded doing their "duty" toward this alien creature. The social worker who conducted the marital and family therapy had a strong conviction that much of Sheldon's acting out was motivated by a desperate desire to elicit some emotional response from his affectively restricted parents. This conviction was borne out during the six-month course of treatment, which uncovered a deep well of depression in both parents, and served to reduce the extent to which marital conflict was denied, displaced, and acted out through their son. As the relationship with his parents improved, Sheldon achieved greater comfort and appropriateness in his peer relationships. He began to recognize the ways in which his combativeness precipitated scapegoating and, with the support of staff, was able to gain some impulse control, curtail his self-destructive behavior, and acquire some basic social skills. At the time of his discharge, however, he was still regarded as having severe ego deficits.

Sheldon appeared to have maintained some positive self-regard when seen for a follow-up interview approximately a year after his discharge. He dressed neatly, articulated clearly, and seemed generally more socially appropriate. He had dropped out of school but was working and had begun to date. He had been living at home with his parents, though their relationship continued to be strained. His use of drugs had abated considerably, and he had been arrested only once since discharge, for hitchhiking. While he regarded himself more positively, he felt negative about the treatment program. He wished the staff had been more personable and that the unit had not been locked. He would have preferred more and better food. He stated that his therapist had been very important to him, but he felt no desire to continue treatment. He had goals for the future, particularly to move away from his family, and he hoped that he would eventually marry and own a service station.

Sheldon died in an automobile accident eight years after discharge. The car in which he was a passenger was hit on an expressway ramp by another car that was entering the highway in the wrong direction; he was thrown from the car and killed instantly. Sheldon had "straightened out" according to his parents, and had been doing "beautifully" for about a year, working in apartment renovation.

The details of Sheldon's death offer no indication for any psychological or psychopathological factors within Sheldon's own personality or personality adjustment that could be deemed responsible for having caused or contributed to his violent death; it seems to have been truly an accident.

Discussion

These case reports can indicate only the more striking aspects of the desperate struggles against both rage and despair which marked the pathology of these five youths. When placed side by side, however, these brief biographies highlight the great extent to which their histories were loaded with a number of factors identified in the literature as being highly correlated with suicide and other forms of violent death among adolescents. Two of our subjects (Selma and Nick) were sexually abused by stepfather and father, respectively. Three subjects (Selma, Nick, and Bart) had lost their father at an early age, and in all cases the father was absent emotionally if not physically. Additionally, in two instances (Nick and Bart) the son was used by the mother in an attempt to replace the lost father. Four of these youths (Fran, Selma, Nick, and Bart) were subjected to chronic and severe parental discord. In Sheldon's case, the parents' facade of marital bliss was maintained only at the expense of the boy's depression. In three instances (Fran, Bart, and Sheldon) the child was regarded as expendable by the parents, as evidenced either by their being treated as a burden or by not being visited at any time during their hospitalization. We know that Nick was also subsequently viewed as expendable. All of our subjects showed difficulties related to sexuality, expressed either through promiscuity (Fran and Selma), perverse homosexual ideation (Nick), inappropriate sexualization of relationships with staff members (Bart), or lack of heterosexual interest (Sheldon). All had very disturbed peer relations and had been absent from school for nonacademic reasons. Four of these youths—Fran being the exception—had threatened or made suicide attempts either prior to or during their stay in our program.

While only Nick committed overt suicide, the weight of these factors in the case histories and our understanding of the dynamic struggles of these youths strongly compel the inference that at least three of the other four deaths were the result of suicidally equivalent behavior.

After reviewing the case reports, the research data which had been collected on these five subjects were studied independently to generate hypotheses which might help to account for the violent nature of their deaths. A number of variables included in previous research studies of the patient population (see Offer et al. 1979) were examined in order to compare these patients with the entire group of fifty-six delinquents who participated in the study. Fran had to be eliminated from this aspect of the study because her stay was not long enough and data collection was too incomplete for her to be included in the final sample. All variables were standardized (t-scores) over the entire delinquent sample in order to facilitate comparisons and readily detect patients with extreme scores on any of the measures. It was found that all four subjects differed from the rest of the sample on a single variable: amount of poorly modulated response to color cards on the Rorschach. Clinically, this elevation would suggest deficiencies in cognitive controls, leading to difficulties in responding to affective stimuli in a reflective manner. All four patients who died violent deaths were in the extreme 16 percent of all delinquent patients studied. Furthermore, all four were in the younger half of the sample at the time of admission to the program, that is, around fifteen years of age or less. This would suggest a tendency to be more seriously disturbed and to have shown problems earlier in life.

Since the investigators examining the research data were blind to the identity of the four target patients, an attempt was made to predict who these patients might have been based upon the research data and manner of death prior to actually identifying them. Two of the four were more alike in having low IQs and low spatial skills, which suggested some kind of cognitive impairment which might interfere with their judgment. It was correctly predicted that these would be Bart and Selma, both of whom had placed themselves in dangerous situations. One subject was very different from the other three. He was seen to be very impulsive on the psychological testing, showed a great deal of impulsivity and destructiveness on behavioral measures, and had been institutionalized longer than the rest. This was correctly predicted to be Nick, the subject who hanged himself. One of these subjects turned out to be very similar to the rest of the adolescent population in the sample, except that he was viewed on Teachers' Ratings to be socially insensitive and not at all motivated; this subject was correctly predicted to have been Sheldon, the patient who died an accidental death.

In addition to the research data, historical material from the delinquent sample was reviewed using a measure developed by Gunderson, Kolb, and Austin (1981) in order to assess these data for indices of borderline pathology. These ratings pointed definitely to Fran, Selma, Nick, and Bart as showing significant borderline pathology, particularly in the areas of impulsive behavior, poor interpersonal relationships, and depressive affect.

Sheldon showed no evidence of borderline pathology, and none of the five subjects demonstrated signs of psychosis.

Conclusions

It has been amply demonstrated that violent death by murder, suicide, or accident is a serious mental health problem for adolescents and young adults. We believe this present study also indicates that the population of behaviorally disordered and delinquent adolescents may be at particular risk for violent death. Many of these people continue to live unhappy, deviant lives, and, for some, the seriousness of their psychiatric disabilities becomes even more apparent as they grow older.

When working with behaviorally disordered adolescents, it is necessary to confront directly the destructiveness and hostility toward others that are expressed in much of their behavior. We would underscore here that it is equally necessary to search and treat the depressive, self-destructive components of their lives or their need to master despair by engaging in risk-taking behaviors. If this is not done, we run the risk that such serious pathology will be repressed, avoided, split off, or diffused by the patient. Alternatively, the staff and/or therapist may experience the emergence of such pathology as treatment failure and may suppress, deny, or avoid the implications of such behaviors out of their own narcissistic vulnerability.

For many behaviorally disordered adolescents, the subsequent ten years are not happy ones, and many of them do not live out that decade. For some, their deaths are intimately intertwined with their own psychopathology. Self-destructive tendencies, whether or not presented as overtly or classically suicidal in nature, must be carefully delineated in the course of both initial and ongoing treatment. To fail in this regard is to abandon these youth just as surely as many of their significant others may have done and to render ourselves even less capable of understanding the extent to which they are at risk of violent death.

NOTES

1. From the Adolescent Program and Tri-Agency Adolescent Services, Illinois State Psychiatric Institute, Chicago, Illinois.

2. We wish to express our thanks to Daniel Offer, Eric Ostrov, and Jaime Trujillo for their work in both the original study and the follow-up study of the subjects.

REFERENCES

Beck, A. T.; Resnick, H. L. P.; and Lettieri, D. J. 1974. *The Prediction of Suicide*. Bowie, Md.: Charles.
Bigras, J.; Gauthier, Y.; Bouchard, C.; and Tasse, Y. 1966. Suicide attempts in adolescent girls: a preliminary study. *Canadian Psychiatric Association Journal* 11:275–282.
Caine, E. 1978. Two contemporary tragedies: adolescent suicide/ adolescent alcoholism. *Journal of the National Association of Private Psychiatric Hospitals* 9(3): 26–31.
Conger, J. J.; Gaskill, H. S.; Glad, D. D.; Hassel, L.; Rainey, R. V.; Sawrey, W. L; and Turrell, E. S. 1959. Psychological and psychopathological factors in motor vehicle accidents. *Journal of the American Medical Association* 169:1581–1587.
Eisen, P. 1976. The infantile roots of adolescent violence. *American Journal of Psychoanalysis* 36(3): 211–218.
Eisenthal, S. 1967. Suicide and aggression. *Psychological Reports* 21:745–751.
Finch, S. M., and Poznanski, E. O. 1971. *Adolescent Suicide*. Springfield, Ill.: Thomas.
Freud, S. 1901. The psychopathology of everyday life. *Standard Edition* 6:1–279. London: Hogarth, 1960.
Freud, S. 1920. Beyond the pleasure principle. *Standard Edition* 18:3–64. London: Hogarth, 1955.
Glaser, K. 1965. Attempted suicide in children and adolescents: psychodynamic observations. *American Journal of Psychotherapy* 19:220–227.
Gould, R. 1965. Suicide problems in children and adolescents. *American Journal of Psychotherapy* 19:228–246.
Gunderson, J. G.; Kolb, J. E.; and Austin, V. 1981. The diagnostic interview for borderline patients. *American Journal of Psychiatry* 138(7): 896–903.
Harbin, H. T. 1977. Episodic dyscontrol and family dynamics. *American Journal of Psychiatry* 134:1113–1116.
Hollinger, P. 1977. Suicide in adolescents. *American Journal of Psychiatry* 134(12): 1433–1434.
Hollinger, P. 1978. Adolescent suicide: an epidemiological study of recent trends. *American Journal of Psychiatry* 135(6): 754–756.

Hollinger, P. 1979. Violent deaths among the young: recent trends in suicide, homicide, and accidents. *American Journal of Psychiatry* 136(9): 1144–1147.

Hollinger, P. 1980. Violent deaths as a leading cause of mortality: an epidemiological study of suicide, homicide, and accidents. *American Journal of Psychiatry* 137(4): 472–476.

Jacobs, J.; and Teicher, J. D. 1967. Broken homes and social isolation in attempted suicides of adolescents. *International Journal of Social Psychiatry* 13(2): 139–149.

Jalali, B; Jalali, M.; Crocetti, G.; and Turner, F. 1981. Adolescents and drug use: toward a more comprehensive approach. *American Journal of Orthopsychiatry* 51(1): 120–130.

Kaufman, I.; Peck, A. L; and Tagiuri, C. K. 1954. The family constellation and overt incestuous relations between father and daughter. *American Journal of Orthopsychiatry* 24:266–277.

Kovacs, M., and Beck, A. T. 1977. The wish to die and the wish to live in attempted suicides. *Journal of Clinical Psychology* 33(2): 361–365.

Lester, D. 1967. Suicide as an aggressive act. *Journal of Psychology* 66:47–50.

Lewis, D. O.; Shanok, S. S.; Balla, D. A.; and Bard, B. 1980. Psychiatric correlates of severe reading disabilities in an incarcerated delinquent population. *Journal of the American Academy of Child Psychiatry* 19:611–622.

Lewis, D. O.; Shanok, S. S.; Pincus, J. H.; and Glaser, G. H. 1979. Violent juvenile delinquents: psychiatric, neurological, psychological and abuse factors. *Journal of the American Academy of Child Psychiatry* 18:307–319.

Litman, R. E. 1967. Sigmund Freud on suicide. In E. S. Schneidman, ed. *Essays on Self Destruction*. New York: Science House.

Litman, R. E.; Curphey, T.; Schneidman, E. S.; Farberow, N. L.; and Tabachnick, N. E. 1963. Investigations of equivocal suicide. *Journal of the American Medical Association* 184:924–929.

McCandless, F. D. 1968. Suicide and the communication of rage: a cross-cultural study. *American Journal of Psychiatry* 125:197–205.

MacDonald, J. M. 1964. Suicide and homicide by automobile. *American Journal of Psychiatry* 121:366–370.

MacDonald, J. M. 1967. Homicidal threats. *American Journal of Psychiatry* 127:475–482.

Margolin, N. L., and Teicher, J. D. 1968. Thirteen adolescent male suicide attempts: dynamic considerations. *Journal of the American Academy of Child Psychiatry* 7:296–315.

Marohn, R. C. 1974. Trauma and the delinquent. *Adolescent Psychiatry* 3:354–361.

Marohn, R. C. 1977. The "juvenile imposter": some thoughts on narcissism and the delinquent. *Adolescent Psychiatry* 5:186–212.

Marohn, R. C. 1980. The psychiatric response to delinquency. In M. Sugar, ed. *Responding to Adolescent Needs*. New York: Spectrum.

Marohn, R. C.; Dalle-Molle, D.; McCarter, E.; and Linn, D. 1980. *Juvenile Delinquents: Psychodynamic Assessment and Hospital Treatment*. New York: Brunner/Mazel.

Marohn, R. C.; Dalle-Molle, D.; Offer, D.; and Ostrov, E. 1973. A hospital riot: its determinants and implications for treatment. *American Journal of Psychiatry* 130:631–636.

Marohn, R. C.; Offer, D.; and Ostrov, E. 1971. Juvenile delinquents view their impulsivity. *American Journal of Psychiatry* 128:418–423.

Marohn, R. C.; Offer, D.; Ostrov, E.; and Trujillo, J. 1979. Four psychodynamic types of hospitalized juvenile delinquents. *Adolescent Psychiatry* 7:466–483.

Menninger, K. A. 1935. Purposive accidents as an expression of self-destructive tendencies. *International Journal of Psycho-Analysis* 17:6–16.

Menninger, K. A. 1938. *Man against Himself*. New York: Harcourt Brace.

Neuringer, C. 1975. Problems in predicting adolescent suicidal behavior. *Psychiatric Opinion* 12(6): 27–31.

Offer, D.; Marohn, R. C.; and Ostrov, E. 1975. Violence among hospitalized delinquents. *Archives of General Psychiatry* 32:1180–1186.

Offer, D.; Marohn, R. C.; and Ostrov, E. 1979. *The Psychological World of the Juvenile Delinquent*. New York: Basic.

Ostrov, E.; Offer, D.; and Marohn, R. C. 1976. Hostility and impulsivity in normal and delinquent Rorschach responses. *Mental Health in Children* 2:479–492.

Otto, U. 1964. Changes in the behavior of children and adolescents preceding suicidal attempts. *Acta Psychiatrica Scandinavica* 40:386–400.

Porterfield, A. L. 1960. Traffic fatalities, suicide and homicide. *American Sociological Review* 25:897–901.

Rabin, P. L., and Swenson, B. R. 1981. Teenage suicide attempts and parental divorce. *New England Journal of Medicine* 304:1048.

Rosen, A. 1954. Detection of suicidal patients: an example of some limitations in the prediction of infrequent events. *Journal of Consulting Psychology* 18:397–403.

Rosenbaum, M., and Richman, J. 1970. Suicide: the role of hostility and death wishes from the family and significant others. *American Journal of Psychiatry* 126:1652–1655.

Sabbath, J. C. 1969. The suicidal adolescent: the expendable child. *Journal of the American Academy of Child Psychiatry* 8(2): 272–285.

Schneer, H. I.; Kay, P.; and Brozovsky, M. 1961. Events and conscious ideation leading to suicidal behavior in adolescents. *Psychiatric Quarterly* 35:507–515.

Schrut, A. 1964. Suicidal adolescents and children. *Journal of the American Medical Association* 188:1103–1107.

Schrut, A. 1968. Some typical patterns in the behavior and background of adolescent girls who attempt suicide. *American Journal of Psychiatry* 125(1): 69–74.

Selzer, M. L., and Payne, C. E. 1962. Automobile accidents, suicide and unconscious motivation. *American Journal of Psychiatry* 119:237–240.

Shaffer, D. 1974. Suicide in children and early adolescents. *Journal of Child Psychology, Psychiatry, and Allied Disciplines* 15:275–291.

Shaffer, J. W.; Schmidt, C. W.; Zlotowitz, H. I.; and Fisher, R. S. 1977. Social adjustment profiles of female drivers involved in fatal and nonfatal accidents. *American Journal of Psychiatry* 134(7): 801–804.

Spellacy, F. 1977. Neuropsychological differences between violent and nonviolent adolescents. *Journal of Clinical Psychology* 33(4): 966–969.

Stanley, E. J., and Barter, J. T. 1970. Adolescent suicidal behavior. *American Journal of Orthopsychiatry* 40(1): 87–96.

Tabachnick, N. 1975. Subintentioned self destruction in teenagers. *Psychiatric Opinion* 12(6): 21–26.

Tabachnick, N.; Litman, R. E.; Osman, M.; Jones, W. L.; Cohn, J.; Kasper, A.; and Moffat, J. 1966. Comparative psychiatric study of accidental and suicidal death. *Archives of General Psychiatry* 14:60–68.

Teicher, J. D., and Jacobs, J. 1966. Adolescents who attempt suicide: preliminary findings. *American Journal of Psychiatry* 122:1248–1257.

Tillman, W., and Hobbs, G. 1949. The accident-prone automobile driver. *American Journal of Psychiatry* 106:321–331.

Weinstein, E. A., and Lyerly, O. G. 1969. Symbolic aspects of presidential assassinations. *Psychiatry* 32:1–11.

Wolfgang, M. 1959. Suicide by means of victim-precipitated homicide. *Journal of Clinical and Experimental Psychology* 20:335–349.

13 ADOLESCENCE: PSYCHOLOGY OF THE SELF AND SELFOBJECTS

ERNEST S. WOLF

There is general agreement among psychoanalytic theoreticians and clinicians that adolescence, however it is defined or subdivided, is a transitional period between childhood and adulthood. Through an integration of basic psychoanalytic principles and theories with a growing body of clinical data derived from analytic work with adolescents, with attention to data from cognitive psychology, cultural anthropological studies, and the historical context in which generational change occurs, it is also assumed that a causal relationship exists between the pubertal changes brought about by biological maturation and the psychological, social, and behavioral manifestations studied by psychoanalysts. In this view of adolescence, cultural, social, and historical factors appear as modifiers of a basically biological process.

Freud himself saw the child's psychosexual development as basically genetically determined and relatively independent of the impinging environment. The causal hypothesis, together with the close relationship between physiological changes and psychological changes, led to the conclusion that in childhood the Oedipus complex must be a universal phenomenon and that the psychosocial changes of adolescence are similarly universal accompaniments of the biology of the changing adolescent body. To be sure, the environment is not ignored, but it assumes a secondary importance in Freud's conceptualization. Relationships to objects are significant in that they may affect the vicissitudes of drive and defense. Society's values, morals, and ideals become important in that they enter into the formation of the superego.

Freud paid little attention to puberty and adolescence (the term "adolescence" occurs only six times in the index to the *Standard Edition,* with all six references pertaining to *The Interpretation of Dreams).* Post-Freudian psychoanalysts have stressed puberty and adolescence as an important phase in psychological development. Anna Freud (1958) has called particular attention to the role of sexual maturation in the instinctual resurgence of libido. The influx of newly mobilized libido causes psychological turmoil that needs to be calmed by the defense mechanisms available to the ego, especially those of asceticism and intellectualization.

The Freudian conceptualization elegantly and efficiently organized the data obtained from the psychoanalytic situation. Psychoanalytic theories of instinctual conflict and defense have greatly advanced the science of psychology and the practice of psychiatry and psychotherapy; psychoanalysis has had an immeasurably enriching and stimulating impact on all the sciences and arts of man. However, the limitations of what is basically a biopsychological view of man have become increasingly apparent. Post-Freudian psychoanalytic theory—not psychoanalytic method or data—became unnecessarily narrow and quasi-biological by making instincts and their vicissitudes the center of the conceptualization.

Although the advent of ego psychology and the adaptive point of view apparently freed psychoanalysis from this reduction to a psychology of instinctual fates, in fact, ego psychology is a facade that hides but does not really do away with an obsolete, nineteenth-century biologism at the base of classical theory. This was in keeping also with nineteenth-century positivism and the natural science model which the great physiologist von Helmholtz had introduced into the medical science of that century. Only now, under the pressure of contemporary data from infant-mother observations, can one observe the beginning of a shift from nineteenth-century psychoenergetics to twentieth-century interactionism, as is represented by the work of Mahler (Mahler, Pine, and Bergman 1975).

The data of psychoanalysis and, particularly, adolescence must be seen in a different framework, one without the traditional metapsychology of drives and defenses, of id, ego, and superego. Kohut organized the data of psychoanalysis in a different framework—a conceptualization of experiential states. This latter theory takes the place of traditional metapsychology and is usually referred to as the psychology of the self.

Kohut puts the self into the center of the theory. Self psychology is a psychology of the vicissitudes of the self—its emergence and development, cohesion, boundaries, structure, functions, and disorders. The initial impetus for the emergence of self psychology from classical psychoanalysis did not arise from theoretical considerations but from clinical stalemates which forced Kohut to reconsider his theory-laden interpretations and to recognize transference constellations that did not fit into the classical conceptualizations. At the time, Kohut (1971) designated these newly discovered transferences as narcissistic, and he attempted in his conceptualization to stay within the Freudian model. But then he recognized the usefulness of a conceptual shift to a model in which the self was the center of the theoretical structure. Today we designate these narcissistic transferences as selfobject transferences.

The essence of this model of self psychology is a view of man that recognizes that psychological man cannot exist in a psychological vacuum. By "psychological man" I mean a human being, a person who is aware of being a human being, with wishes, desires, fears, expectations, ambitions, and ideals; that is, he is aware of having an inner life. In short, psychological man is a man with a self. Psychological man can exist only in a psychological environment which makes the emergence and maintenance of the self possible. Physiological man can exist only in a physiological environment that sustains him. Without appropriate nourishment, oxygen, temperature, pressure, moisture, and so forth, physiological man would undoubtedly die. However, physiological man is not yet psychological man, as anyone can testify who has seen or experienced the human organism when it is attached for a prolonged period of time to the wires and tubes of a life-sustaining machine. To become psychological man, the organism must also be connected to an appropriate psychological ambience that supplies a self-sustaining psychological experience.

I use the word "experience" deliberately to emphasize the subjective aspect of the theory of self psychology. The self that does not experience itself as a self is not a cohesive self but is merely a fragmented existence. Thus, impairment of a self-sustaining psychological environment inexorably leads to some loss of self, some more or less fragmented state, as demonstrated by the frequency of transient psychotic episodes in intensive care units when there is insufficient psychological support of the patients by the staff. Another example: in orphanages, initially healthy infants may not survive, even with perfectly adequate physiological care, in the absence of personal care from a dedicated nurse. At the other end of the life cycle, the deprivation in

173

psychological sustenance sometimes brought about by retirement often results in a collapse of self which is soon followed by physical death.

These are dramatic examples of the self in extremis. However, self psychology did not emerge from the contemplation of extreme conditions but from the everyday experiences of ordinary analysands in the psychoanalytic situation. Here one can observe the usually transient self-fragmentation that occurs when a self-sustaining extraanalytic relationship is lost or when the selfobject transference relationship to the analyst is seriously disrupted. The ups and downs of a fluctuating self-state, as a precariously put-together self moves through the vicissitudes of a day in the now sustaining, now depriving selfobject ambience of everyday life, have not escaped the attention of sensitive artists. Virginia Woolf's (1925) *Mrs. Dalloway* paints a vivid picture of one fragile lady's painful experience of her self through one long, ordinary day.

These examples should illustrate that psychological man cannot exist in a psychological vacuum but only in a psychological environment that makes the emergence and maintenance of the self possible. Self psychology has investigated this relationship between psychological man and his need-sustaining psychological environment. Since the very emergence of the self-experience depends on the presence and appropriate functioning of certain objects in the psychological environment, these objects have been designated as selfobjects. In fact, if the selfobject functions appropriately, the sustained but psychologically unsophisticated self usually is not conscious of being sustained; the self is merely aware of an experience of joyful wholeness. The selfobject function ordinarily is a silent one that manifests only in the cohesion of the sustained self, analogous to the organism's silent need for oxygen. Awareness ordinarily means awareness of an unsatisfied need, either a psychological need that manifests by symptoms of fragmentation or a physiological need that announces itself, for example, by shortness of breath. It took thousands of years for science to discover that the oxygen content of the surrounding air was needed to sustain physiological life. It has taken even longer for scientific investigation to discern the self-sustaining selfobject function in the psychological ambience.

Since there can be no self-experience without the sustaining selfobject function, the selfobject becomes part of the experienced self. Thus one arrives at the seeming paradox that the selfobject, as a psychological function, is experienced both inside and outside the self at the same time (as is true for the oxygen breathed). The selfobject, strictly speaking, is not an object but a psychological function performed by an object for the self. And what is the self? It is an abstraction, usually cohesive and enduring, with a past, a present, and a future, knowable only in its manifestations as an experience but not knowable in its essence, and thus defying precise definition—at least until now. Since our interest focuses on the vicissitudes of self-experience, the vicissitudes of the relationship between the self and its selfobjects, perhaps the most fitting name for our field of study is not self psychology but selfobject psychology. Yet the gain in precision in such a name change may not be worth the loss of elegance.

It was in the psychoanalytic situation that Kohut initially became aware of his analysands' needs for selfobjects. These needs were manifest in the analysands' expectations of the analyst. Kohut, in recognizing that these expectations originated as repetitions of archaic residues of early child-parent relationships, designated these clinical phenomena as transferences and described two major varieties of these transferences: the mirror transferences and the idealizing transferences. Since we are mainly concerned with theoretical and developmental issues, particularly as they relate to adolescence, it is sufficient to mention that the clinical phenomenology of selfobject transferences and countertransferences has been discussed extensively elsewhere (Kohut 1968, 1971, 1977; Wolf 1976, 1979, 1982).

Development of the Self

The discovery and investigation of selfobject transferences allowed Kohut to study the development of the self and to delineate the major components of its structure. He theorized that the neonate is born preadapted to thrive in a certain physical environment which contains the necessary elements of nourishment and a certain psychological environment which makes available the selfobject functions needed for the emergence and maintenance of the self. At birth, no self can be said to exist, but parents already think of their baby as a person and address him as such in their total attitude as well as in their speech. This parental disposition to respond to the baby as a self, by making available responsive selfobject functions, is necessary not only for the infant's healthy development but also for its very survival. Many children grow into psychologically crippled individuals, but the survivors are recognizably human persons in their psychological being. Each has a personality, even when he does not reach the level of a cohesive self.

In recent years, studies of mothers and their babies have clearly demonstrated that a dialogue begins almost immediately after birth and that the neonate from the very beginning is an active participant in this dialogue which shapes the emerging self. Sometime during the second year of life the self is constituted as a cohesive entity that can be conceptualized as a psychological structure. For this structure Kohut has used the term "bipolar self," which refers to the observation that enduring memories of the mirroring selfobject function cluster together, forming the self's pole of grandiosity and ambition, while the analogous residues of idealizing selfobject functions cluster into the self's pole of values and ideals. Once the self has consolidated as a particular constellation of ambitions and ideals together with its given talents and learned skills, it remains a unique combination of its constituent parts, setting out on a uniquely determined course of life toward its goal of fulfillment.

The development of the self can be viewed somewhat narrowly as the development of the self's selfobject needs or as the development of the relationship of the self to its selfobjects (Wolf 1980a, 1980b). The need for selfobjects—by which I mean the needed self-sustaining functions carried by the selfobject—never disappears during the self's life. However, the intensity and form of the needed mirroring and idealizable selfobject ambience change in an age-appropriate manner. With increasing solidity of the self, the need for the immediacy and closeness of the surrounding selfobject milieu becomes less fervent; therefore, demands on the human carrier of the selfobject function become less peremptory. The connection to the parental selfobject, for example, becomes less intimate and gradually diffuses to include others, such as siblings, peers, teachers, and friends, all of whom can become carriers of the selfobject function. More and more, the maturing self is embedded in a network of selfobject relationships.

It is important to point out, however, that the development of the selfobject relation, while central in human psychology, does not by any means exhaust the potential for psychological development; other areas of psychological development are proceeding at the same time. We must differentiate especially between the development of social relationships and that of selfobject relations. Children and adolescents have social needs for companions, playmates, friendships, teachers, and so on. The interpersonal relationships that characterize the social scene perform important functions and services to the self. They are not needed for the maintenance of the self as a structure, that is, they are not carriers of the selfobject function to any discernible degree merely by virtue of their social usefulness. Some of these social relationships may at times take on selfobject functions, that is, for some reason they draw upon themselves the expectations that the self has for needed selfobjects. For example, I have observed in adolescents that the frequency, intensity, and emotionality often associated with being taught a skill by an expert teacher may result in the interpersonal relationship to the teacher, as teacher, gradually becoming submerged in the vicissitudes of a selfobject tie, often to the dismay of both student and teacher, who may not easily understand their own so-called irrational reaction to one another.

Thus all types of interpersonal relationships may become drawn into the selfobject matrix. When this happens in heterosexual dating relationships, people speak about love and often they marry. Securing the selfobject tie is a more potent motivation for marriage than either sex or economic gain.

What of the role of sexuality? Freud's discovery of infantile sexuality and the stages of its development will always remain a landmark in the history of psychoanalysis. However, clinical experience led Kohut to a reconceptualization of the role of sexuality in psychological development. Self psychology recognizes in sexuality an important factor, at times even the most important factor, affecting the self in both its development and its maturity. But unlike Freud, Kohut no longer sees sexuality as the central motivator of behavior. Instead, the motivators are the maintenance of the self's cohesion and self-expression experienced as self-esteem. The success and failure of sexual desires have a deeply felt meaning for the self and influence its cohesion as well as its self-esteem. Thus the child will normally arrive at the oedipal phase, and, with appropriate selfobject responsiveness, the oedipal phase will be traversed—perhaps with some tension but mostly with joyfully assertive and lustily sensuous attachment to the parent of the opposite gender, provided the ambience in the family allows it. If, however, the selfobject responses are faulty, for example, overly stimulating, seductive, or overly suppressive and counteraggressive, then the normal oedipal phase will be distorted into a pathological Oedipus complex that leads to the familiar phenomena of neurotic sex and neurotic aggression.

The Self and Adolescent Process

In addition to social relations and sexuality, other developmental areas impinge on the developing self in its matrix of selfobjects, for example, cognition (see Piaget 1969). Cognition deserves a special place, particularly in our reconsideration of adolescence, because at age twelve to fourteen the shift from concrete to formal operations takes place. This newfound capacity to combine propositions, to isolate variables in order to confirm or dispose of hypotheses, and to carry out these operations with symbols rather than only with objects or concrete events has a great impact on the adolescent self.

In a personal communication from the Adolescent and Family Development Project at the Harvard Medical School, Noam reported that the shift to formal operations depends on the facilitating support of the psychological ambience created for the youngster by parents and teachers. Not all fourteen-year-olds make this final step into maturity; a great number remain stalled at a level of concrete operations in spite of the capacity for further development. The realization of the cognitive developmental potential depends on the psychological ambience. This observation is analogous to the point of view presented here about oedipal and adolescent sexuality, namely, that the potential for sexual maturity depends on the facilitating selfobject ambience.

These observations, as well as the data on the adolescence of analysands, lead to a reconsideration of the adolescent process. It seems that the radically new insights into the surrounding world and its associated selfobject milieu, made possible by the leap in cognitive capacity, more than pressure from maturing sexual capacities, force the self into a restructuring of itself—the restructuring that we call the adolescent process.

Encouraged by Kohut's brief comments on adolescent sexual activity in the service of primarily narcissistic purposes (Kohut 1971), Gedo, Terman, and I outlined the transformations of self-structure during adolescence in a first attempt to apply self psychology to the adolescent process (Wolf, Gedo, and Terman 1972). At that time, we proposed the transformation of the self as the major task of the adolescent phase of development. We had noted how the age-appropriate deidealization of parental selfobjects entailed a greatly increased vulnerability of the self. The fragile or even fragmented self of the adolescent may temporarily strengthen itself by the intensification of special peer relationships, for example, by the formation of "secret societies" with one's best friends. In many cases, it is the larger peer group that performs the same self-sustaining selfobject function by devotion to shared ideals or by sharing an admired group idol as an idealized selfobject. We also noted that, with the rebuilding of the more permanent value system, the now strengthened self can discard the peer group relationship.

My analytic experience during the almost ten years since the publication of that paper has confirmed the essential correctness of our view. However, in 1972 we did not realize that the need for selfobjects was lifelong and continuous. We thought the adolescent's need for the selfobject function would eventually diminish, allowing not only peer group but all selfobject relations to be discarded. We were still influenced by the model of an ego striving for independence, self-sufficiency, and autonomy. Since then I have recognized the enduring nature of the self's selfobject needs. The self's goals are not autonomy and independence but cohesiveness in its striving for integration into a reciprocally responsive matrix of selfobject relationships. The self discards the peer group's function as a selfobject not out of a decreased selfobject need but because the maturation of its cognitive capacity allows the construction of symbolic selfobjects. The maturing adolescent is now capable of formal operations. He can construct hypotheses and test them. He can create his own philosophy of life—a whole system of values, ideals, and ethics becomes his needed idealized selfobject. He can set sail along the path of the life plan determined by the constitution of his individual self. This same greatly increased cognitive capacity is also a major contributor to the deidealization of the archaic idealized parental imago. The adolescent can no longer hide from himself the inevitable discrepancies between who he has imagined his parents to be and who the parents really are. For the first time, he can look at and also see through his admired selfobjects; there is no escaping a severe, perhaps traumatic, disappointment.

But what of pubescence and sexual maturation, which have usually been thought to be pivotal in the psychosocial upheaval and turmoil of adolescence? To find oneself in a rapidly changing body and to be exposed suddenly to unpredictable moods, strange feelings, and passions is indeed a formidable challenge to the self's cohesion and integrity. However, it is my impression, based on work with adolescents as well as from the analysis of adults with a retrospective view on their adolescent years, that it is not the intensity of physiological upheaval leading to puberty but the quality of empathic responsiveness and understanding that the youngster receives from the self-supporting, selfobject ambience that is of decisive importance in making the adolescent passage into adulthood either smooth or filled with turmoil.

If we take developmental psychology seriously, we cannot escape the observation that development does not come to an end when maturity is reached. There are average expectations from the surrounding selfobject ambience at each developmental level. Thus, parents need their youngsters as selfobjects, perhaps as much as children need parents. Usually these reciprocal expectations are in phase with each other, but sometimes supervening social conditions produce a clash of out-of-phase, conflicting expectations. Usually we talk about parents' failure to provide the self-sustaining ambience for their children, but the reverse failure also occurs, and not infrequently. For example, the parents' capacity to respond to the adolescent's needs diminishes, phase appropriately, as the need to idealize their offspring is increasing. In our culture, the trauma of selfobject deprivation as a result of being left by the youngster's departure for college, for example, is quickly overcome, at least by the parent. It is not so easy for either when, in an apparent regression of the normal progress of development, the youngster, for various economic or social reasons, returns to live at home. There are other examples, but these will suffice to call attention to a neglected area of research in selfobject psychology.

Conclusions

Adolescence has come to an end when the young adult has chosen, and has chosen well, the vocation, the companions, the milieu, and the paths and ideals which will be available to function as selfobjects in supporting the self's cohesion as it strives to express itself in the fulfillment of its life plan. In our contemporary open society, the multiplication of available options makes the adolescent's task of choosing more difficult and more time consuming.

I hope I have persuaded the reader to consider the self-concept in the center of psychological theorizing. The failure of anthropologists to confirm the universality of the Oedipus complex, the absence of a definite phase of adolescence as reported by some historians, and the escape from the adolescent turmoil (required by traditional psychoanalytic theories) observed in studies of normal adolescents displace the biological core of the drive and defense concept of traditional psychoanalytical theory.

Theories are not true or false but approximations that more or less comprehensively make sense out of data. Whether in the long run the theory of self psychology will have turned out to be superior—that is, to be a more useful, more encompassing, more significant tool in making sense out of the psychology of being human—remains to be seen. That question will be answered empirically over the coming decades.

REFERENCES

Freud, A. 1958. Adolescence. *Psychoanalytic Study of the Child* 13:255–278.
Kohut, H. 1968. The psychoanalytic treatment of narcissistic personality disorders. *Psychoanalytic Study of the Child* 23:86–113.
Kohut, H. 1971. *The Analysis of the Self.* New York: International Universities Press.
Kohut, H. 1977. *The Restoration of the Self.* New York: International Universities Press.
Mahler, M. S.; Pine, F.; and Bergman, A. 1975. *The Psychological Birth of the Human Infant: Symbiosis and Individuation.* New York: Basic.
Piaget, J. 1969. The intellectual development of the adolescent. In G. Caplan and S. Lebovici, eds. *Adolescence: Psychosocial Perspectives.* New York: Basic.
Wolf, E. 1976. Ambience and abstinence. *Annual of Psychoanalysis* 4:101–115.
Wolf, E. 1979. Transference and countertransference in the analysis of disorders of the self. *Contemporary Psychoanalysis* 15:577–594.
Wolf, E. 1980a. On the developmental line of selfobjects. In A. Goldberg, ed. *Advances in Self Psychology.* New York: International Universities Press.
Wolf, E. 1980b. Tomorrow's self: Heinz Kohut's contribution to adolescent psychiatry. *Adolescent Psychiatry* 8:41–50.
Wolf, E. 1982. Empathy and countertransference. In A. Goldberg, ed. *The Future of Psychoanalysis.* New York: International Universities Press.
Wolf, E.; Gedo, J.; and Terman, D. 1972. On the adolescent process as a transformation of the self. *Journal of Youth and Adolescence* 1:257–272.
Woolf, V. 1925. *Mrs. Dalloway.* London: Hogarth.

14 CONTINUITIES AND TRANSFORMATIONS BETWEEN INFANCY AND ADOLESCENCE

JOSEPH D. LICHTENBERG

Since Freud's original formulations, psychoanalytic researchers have been applying patterns of development from early childhood to later stages. Examples of this are Winnicott's (1951) observation of the infant's use of cuddlies and transitional objects; Mahler, Pine, and Bergman's (1975) observation of a developmental phase of separation-individuation and rapprochement crisis; and Kohut's (1971) hypothesis about self-cohesion. In many instances, where analogies have been noted between early childhood developments and events of later stages, differences in the organizational tasks have been minimized or ignored. While no careful observer would claim that adolescence is simply childhood recapitulated, continuities—properly noted—have often been described without counterbalancing statements about transformations[1] that exist between infancy and adolescence as well as those that occur within each.

The most obvious example of a continuity is that the infant is born a human being and continues to be that particular unique being through the permutations of childhood and adolescence. The most striking examples of transformation are apparent when we consider the different tasks and organizational principles of each stage. In infancy the organizational principles are those involving the transformation of a multipotential neonate with biological-neurophysiological-behavioral patterns into a child capable of functioning at a symbolic level of awareness. In adolescence, the organizational principles are those involving the transformation of a fully integrated personality, adapted to the patterns of childhood, into one adapted to the requirements of adult life.

It is a matter of individual judgment among researchers how much emphasis to place on continuities and how much weight to give to differences in the organizational principles involved. When we note how frequently children with mostly serene infancies pass through adolescence relatively productively, and how often children with stormy infancies have turbulent adolescent experiences, we are struck by the continuities—or, at least, the compulsion to repeat. But when we recognize that one adolescent with a relatively serene infancy is relatively colorless and mundane and another is exploratory and creative, we are aware that for a given person in a period such as adolescence, one or another personality facet may be heightened by virtue of the specific organizational potentialities of the phase. In similar fashion we tend to generalize in the case of an adolescent disturbance in order to connect it with a disturbance in infancy; that is, we say this person had a disturbed childhood so it is not unexpected that he has had a stormy adolescence. But the forms of disturbance, when we become specific, are usually not easily predictable. Will one difficult toddler become a problem drug user or another hold his school progress together while getting into violent battles with his family? Continuities in these instances should interest us less than transformations.

To make a discussion of this inexhaustible subject more manageable I shall discuss both infancy and adolescence under five headings: eating, sleeping, and eliminating; socializing; play and work; sexuality; and thrills and risks. These headings do not refer to distinct entities. In the discussion of eating, sleeping, and eliminating the emphasis is on biophysiological regulation, but eating is a social event and sometimes a sensual experience. The section on socializing emphasizes interactive behavior; play and work deal with perceptual-cognitive developments; sexuality deals with regulation of bodily sensation coordinated with gender identity; and the thrills and risks section examines a unique, affectively charged, behavioral pattern.

Eating, Sleeping, and Eliminating

Example 1: Susan was a baby who was easily fed, and for whom a pattern of longer night sleep was easily established and elimination caused no problem. She ate the foods added to her diet but showed a preference for milk. At about ten months, the time her mother chose for her weaning, she evidenced distress, and her mother discontinued the effort. Three months later, after a difficult period of anticipation, her mother separated from her parents, who returned to Europe. That night Susan vomited her milk and refused the next bottle and the next with clear aversion. She readily ate the remainder of her diet but remained averse to milk throughout childhood.

As an adolescent she ate a wide variety of foods and was generally willing to try new tastes. She remained unwilling to drink milk, even with the peer pressure of camp life. As a camp counselor, however, she began to drink milk with mild interest and it became an occasional beverage. During adolescence, by general observation, no evidence of any remnants of problems based on her sudden (traumatic?) weaning were discernible—either with respect to eating or problems with separating.

Example 2: Kate's parents had problems with obesity to the extent that no morsel of food was eaten in the household without anxiety or argument. Kate's eating patterns as an infant and young child were mildly erratic but appeared well within a normal pattern. As a late adolescent she entered analysis for other problems. During adolescence she had established a pattern of wanting to eat only the "junk" foods of her peer group, rejecting any effort on the part of others to expand her restricted range. A problem with overweight soon developed, and it became evident that Kate lacked awareness and attunement to her state of hunger and satiety. Weight and body form had taken on many symbolic meanings in the areas of socialization and sexuality, but these overlay the basic problem of her inability to regulate her food intake on the basis of inner cues. The external situation had so colored her feeding experience since infancy that what had become internalized were signs signaling yes or no, allowed or forbidden. These were, however, without linkage to her own inner physiological state.

Example 3: Vincent entered analysis as an adult with an assortment of generalized complaints, one of which was a reluctance to get up in the morning resulting in frequent lateness. This pattern had begun in adolescence when he went to college at sixteen. This was his first time away from home, and he began to stay awake in the dorm as late at night as he could find company. This problem with sleep, which persisted in his adult life, had begun in his early adolescence. There it took the form of a struggle over masturbation and the fear of eternal damnation. When Vincent had been a little boy, his father had had to arise very early to work a factory shift. He would take the half-asleep, half-awake Vincent and put him in bed with his mother—providing, he thought, companionship for both. There had been no known prior sleep problem in infancy, nor did any overt problem arise in latency. In analysis, Vincent's difficulty with sexual overstimulation was worked through, and the sleep difficulty abated without requiring much analytic focus.

The organizational principle that underlies the infant's pattern of eating, sleeping, and eliminating is the mutual influence of his caregiver's regulatory efforts and the infant's predispositional tendencies. The neonate's functional capacities can be organized into five temporally sequential behavior states: alert wakefulness, quiescent wakefulness, REM sleep, non-REM sleep, and crying. The time-circumscribed intense domination of behavior that results from hunger is an event occurring during the state of active alertness and is as well a causal factor in bringing this state about. During elimination, especially of the bowel, a shift of active alertness occurs from an external stimulus to an internal one. Sleep, too, exerts a powerful pull on the infant and is a powerful stimulus for the caretaker to coordinate her efforts with the baby's impelling need for this change of state. The success or failure of the mother's attempt to coordinate her feeding procedures and scheduling with the neonate's needs is decisive in the initial and subsequent regulation of the infant's states within the diurnal cycle. Looking at the first year as a whole, the organizing of the infant's states, and the advancing coordination within states, begins with the caretaker's molding of a biologically primed activity and moves on to early instances of learned actions (toy cuddling before sleep, thumb sucking to stave off hunger while waiting for a feeding). Learned actions pass rapidly to complex discriminations (helping mother on the diaper table) and then to behaviors that convey a quality of choice and intentionality. (For a more detailed account of these findings and their sources see Lichtenberg [1981a, 1981b]).

During the second year, the toddler who develops a clear-cut sense of self as director of his intentions does so within the context of being his mother's (and family's) child. He has been regulated for better or for worse—as the particular infant of his parents especially in respect to his physiologically based patterns. The regulation may be more or less agreeable, or more or less averse, but it operates as a given. In contrast the adolescent begins to challenge this given, not to destroy this essentially indestructible base but to operate preferentially with respect to the details of the patterns of eating, eliminating, and sleeping habits. To do so he joins an outside family of self-regulators—his peers in their fads. The significant feature is not to establish a new fixed pattern of eating, sleeping, and eliminating—this pattern is often short-lived—but to exercise a choice to be different, to experience a sense of self-regulating in the direction of greater flexibility, if possible. Thus Susan's choice to reexperiment with milk was a kind of rebellion against her childhood pattern but in the interest of exercising a self-regulated choice. In her case the basic regulatory success had continuity, the trauma seemed to have become dissipated within the preadolescent development, and the choice to reexperience milk was a normal adolescent transformation in the interest of flexibility. Kate's regulatory failure in infancy had a crippling continuity in adolescence. It acquired a complex overlay of symbolic meanings, but no transformation of these meanings—either in her adolescent efforts with peer-group copying or analytic working through—sufficed to undo the continuity of the problem itself. It required a hyperattentive retraining. Vincent's sleep problem did not have its base in an early regulatory failure; or stated differently, the regulatory functional potential for sleep was intact (continuous). His sleep disturbance was based on the continuity of oedipal period overstimulation. Its permutations were a product of the particular transformation of adolescent sexuality.

Socializing

Example 1: Stanley was sixteen when his mother brought him for treatment because of her concern about his relatively solitary life. His friendships seemed strained and superficial, his relationship to his therapist, while formally correct, was quite distant. A very bright student, especially in math, he had a reputation for attention-getting odd behavior such as setting off the fire alarms in the school with a remote control device. Because of his distancing proclivities, a schizophrenic process was feared, but none was found on testing. The parents both seemed socially warm and caring. Stanley's mother described him as having been a model child to look after—noting that he had met all his milestones of development ahead of schedule. She had kept a record and her husband had taken home movies from the time of Stanley's birth. The puzzled therapist availed himself of this rare opportunity, and to his astonishment he observed in one of the first scenes that Stanley was being fed by his mother while he lay on his back on a diapering table and his mother sat a full arm's length away. The therapist realized that one quality that marked the proper but joyless interaction was Stanley's neither seeking nor responding with pleasure to eye contact.

Example 2: Ginny had been a trial to her mother since birth. Where her older brother had molded comfortably into their mother's arms for feeding or presleep cradling, Ginny wiggled and kicked to free herself—only to cry if let go. On the diapering table, her brother had been playful, with runs of eye contact and synchronous kicks and coos, while Ginny maneuvered herself physically into positions that so interfered with the process that little of this loving exchange was possible. Ginny's father filled in as best he could and often had greater success than Ginny's mother—his greater physical strength seeming to provide a more secure holding environment. This general pattern continued throughout childhood. It was as though mother, father, and brother were going in one direction, with Ginny taking off in another.

During adolescence Ginny went through a series of transformations. First she competed with her brother by outdoing him in fields where she was more talented. Then abruptly she changed direction. She turned against accomplishing, became involved with a psychopathic boy, and became a rather heavy user of drugs. A suicide attempt followed, and Ginny seemed appreciative of the family's efforts to care for her, structuring her return to school. She chose then a path of endeavor, different from her parents and her brother, that while erratic was not oppositional in principle but more self-determined.

The neonate is born biologically primed for social contact. His hearing is especially keen in the auditory range of the female voice. The fixation point of his visual gaze is about eight inches—the distance to his mother's face when he is held in a feeding position. Thus social contact is initiated when even as a very young infant (seven to ten days) he will interrupt his feeding to roll his eyes up to initiate a sequence in which the mother will respond to his heightened alertness, speaking to him in a rhythmical tone. His arms will move in a rhythm synchronous to her speech. The number of such looking, talking, moving runs will be determined by a mutual signal reading. His facial expression, when examined with slow-motion photography, reveals an unexpected capacity to imitate his mother's emotive expressions. By four weeks, the cues from the baby are often sufficiently clear that the mother can sense the infant's readiness to prolong the state of playful interactive attentiveness; by three months, contact runs have the quality of conversational games.

Communications having more formal characteristics develop at about five months, at a time when the infant undergoes a general expansion of his whole state of alertness. This transformation of heightened attentiveness is associated with neurophysiological maturation and reorganization. Communications in both the behavior and affective sense are two ways from the beginning—positive meaning more and negative meaning an averse turning off or protest. In the social interaction these are not adventitious but commonly represent responses to violations of the expected response patterns (Beebe and Stern 1977; Call 1980).

Thus the infant perceives and reacts behaviorally in increasingly complex ways within an affectively toned, social interactional matrix of himself and his family. However, only with the maturation of many capacities, beginning after the end of the first year, does a child develop the ability to create an image of the self and of others perceived as having continuity not determined by the behavioral interaction itself (self- and object permanence). By a series of transformations in the second year, social communication moves from signal information exchange to the use of language as a part of a symbolic exchange. It is during the second half of the second year that the toddler is able to give firm representation to what I consider to be the basic unit of social experience—consisting of self, object, and an exchange between them (interpersonal or intrapsychic); of perceptual cognitive elements; and of affective coloration in a context of space and time.

Stanley's infancy was deprived of an essential beginning for optimal social interactional development. There was reason to believe that he received enough contact to stabilize a sense of self, but one with a severe deficit in emotional color and range. Thus when as an adolescent he reached out for peer contact, he did so in ways so awkward that he precluded success. He ended up more guarding himself from hurt and embarrassment than succeeding in using the peer relationship to gain the flexible range of emotions he had failed to develop in early childhood.

For Ginny, as for Stanley, the continuity between infancy and adolescence was striking. Her neonatal motor restlessness had become an oppositional tendency she associated with her sense of self. This persisted during adolescence when the potential transformations of that period offered serious dangers, not in the form of the psychopathic experimentation but in drug usage. The altered state of consciousness this produced was a toxic state deleterious to any potential resolution. Fortunately it allowed the family to fulfill a rescuing function, and this initiated a sufficient change in the interaction to permit a forward move. Because of the potential for a mature adaptation, chosen on her own terms, Ginny was able to be her own "independent" self—constructively oppositional in the sense that she chose to be outside the family's social pattern but with their support and approval.

Play and Work

Example 1: What had seemed a slight awkwardness in Hannah in her infancy was recognizable as a small motor coordination deficit when she was a small child. This restricted the pleasurable range of play of this good-natured child. She was able to swim and perform large muscle tasks with average competence, and so this was encouraged. Her handwriting was poor, and in school she evidenced some learning disabilities in math and written testing. With her parents' help, plus tutoring, she worked on all of these limitations without loss of her cheerful, optimistic outlook. In adolescence she made an early career decision to become a teacher of small children and to work especially with children with learning disabilities—an identification, in a general way, with her parents' profession as well as to their approach to her.

Example 2: Harold, as infant and toddler, was a child to whom play accomplishments came very easily. Endowed with excellent coordination, he could tie shoes before his older brother could. But Harold also evidenced a pattern in childhood in which he would become intensely involved in some activity until he mastered it with praiseworthy skill, only then to lose all interest and abandon it—to his parents' dismay. This continued in adolescence with hobbies but on a larger scale. Work in a more formal sense seemed to interest Harold more. He enjoyed the independence earning money gave him, and he planned and worked quite seriously—not so much for the intrinsic pleasure of the work but for the rewards earning brought him in the adult world.

Play in the form of response to stimuli begins very early in the life of the neonate. If a toy is dangled on a string in an area ten or twelve inches in the midline, everything about the baby changes. His eyes fix on it, his pupils dilate. His whole body goes into immediate motion. His fingers, toes, and mouth point toward the object. At a slightly older age, he will instantly swing his arm toward the object, his fingers contracting to a grasping position. He may miss making contact with it, only to try again, coming closer. When he finally hits it, he will react with excitement. It is noteworthy that this response to an inanimate object is different from the response to the mother. Brazelton and Als (1979) claim that as early as four weeks of age, they can tell from looking at a toe or a finger whether the infant was in an interaction with an object (more jerky movements) or a parent (more smooth movements), and even which parent (mother softer, father more excited). Thus the infant would seem to be biologically primed to respond to two different forms of play, human interactive play and play with inanimate stimuli.

Studies of sensorimotor learning indicate the lawful nature of the developing child's play-work. Experimental studies (Broucek 1979; Papousek and Papousek 1975) have added an understanding of the affective component. Four-month-old infants exposed to patterned flashing lights react with interest and then with habituation. When the infant learns that by turning his head thirty degrees he can activate the light show, he will do so with delight. It was noted that after a while his interest was far less in watching and far more in doing—in enjoying his competence and efficacy. During the second year of life, a major transformation occurs in play when it becomes the area for the work of symbolically representing and resolving problem situations. This constitutes a lifelong connection between work and play. In adolescence the severing of this connection is often more symbolic than actual, especially if the flexibility to work at play and play at work can persist. Competence pleasure can serve as a guide to both.

Hannah's play experience as a child delineated for her a problem in competence. This introduced a relatively early working-at-the-problem context to her play. The nature of infancy did not permit the same solution that she could arrive at in adolescence. Her identification with helpers, derived from rescue fantasies of early adolescence, provided the solution to her work choice and need for competence. For Harold there seemed to be a surfeit of competence pleasure, but his responsiveness to the specific challenge of the stimuli lacked holding power. The modality of adult life—earning money, achieving position, and power—supplied the needed motivation. Thus for Harold this final transformation of adolescence into adult life provided the steadying he needed.

Sexuality

Example 1: Phil entered treatment as a young adult because he could not make up his mind about what he wanted to do. He spent most of his time at home playing his clarinet and daydreaming. Despite a very high intelligence potential, he had had a mediocre school record, including college. Gradually he revealed that he never dated, had never had any sexual contact with a girl, but was very involved in a voyeuristic perversion. Phil's infancy had been normal, his toddler period strained by attacks from his undisciplined older sister. This promoted a fearfulness and passivity for which he attempted to compensate by an exhibitionistic proclivity. This was taken as natural in his family—his parents went about nude in the home, being what they thought of as modern, free, sexually uninhibited people. The level of sexual overexcitement was accordingly intense, and Phil remembers displaying himself to his two younger sisters, encouraging the youngest to kiss his penis. In early adolescence, he had an inguinal hernia repair which was followed by a reversal from exhibitionism to shyness and reticence. The prior trend remained in his fantasies, which had a strong narcissistic quality. His voyeurism began with his sisters, who were willing accomplices, and then extended to strangers.

The powerful effect of sensual pleasure—to establish conceptual connectedness among erotogenic zones and between each erotogenic zone and other nonsensual experiences—is by now a psychoanalytic truism. What infant research has added is the recognition that gender differentiation has been established, based on a combination of biological differences and environmental selective responses. By the middle of the second year, there is an upsurge of genital sensation and fondling. Recent evidence suggests that how the toddler's autoerotic play is responded to will color the degree of embarrassment-shame responses (Amsterdam and Levitt 1980; Kleeman 1975).

Boy-girl differences can be observed in the older toddler exposed to a baby. Girls will coo and fuss over the baby, while boys will demonstrate no such ecstatic response. Boys at this stage are more apt to prance about as gorillas or supermen (Parens 1979). All this, it should be noted, is prior to and independent of anxiety reactions to genital differences and the attendant body danger misinterpretations.

Little more need be said about development in the oedipal period. What I should like to emphasize is that gender identity, which is already well established before the oedipal period, is quite distinct from sexual object choice. And sexual object choice is only begun in the oedipal period; it is primarily a task of adolescence. In examining pathological situations such as Phil's, we have become so accustomed to the oedipal experience and the oedipal love object casting a shadow over the adolescent choice that we have lost sight of the flexibility available to the more normal (less fixated) adolescent. While the love objects both chosen and rejected will bear an associative connection to the oedipal love object, the linkage may be relatively insignificant.

The adolescent is not a preschool child to whom mother and father mean everything. Mother's hair, blended with father's pensiveness, and a will possessed by neither may attract an adolescent, but the sensual experience that will constitute love is not a repeat or a continuity but a transformation. It is one made possible by a restructuring of values—prohibitions appropriate to a six-year-old must be restructured. It is more accurate to say that in adolescence the restructuring of values continues because, contrary to the usual concept of latency, sexuality continues its powerful hold over the symbolic process in the elementary school child. It may be overshadowed by the cognitive advances and general physical development of this period, but the idea of the latency child is more a Victorian illusion than an observable fact. In adolescence, however, the presence of adult genitalia and the excitement of postpubertal sensations, buttressed by curiosity, must be responded to. Thus I believe clinical examples, such as Phil's, may have confused the issue about the adolescent transformation of oedipal preferences into highly flexible (not necessarily successful) sexual object choices.

Another question that is unanswered is, To what degree does the intensity of sexual urgency constitute a continuity or a transformation? For one adolescent, the power of the urgency for erotic outlet may be so intense as to assume a central focus—either to seek gratification or to be defended against. Another adolescent may rather easily fit the intensity of his or her sensual desires into the ordinary patterns of his other life tasks and choices. What we do not know is whether these intensities—strong, moderate, or mild—reflect continuities from prior childhood experiences or whether puberty and its physiological maturations constitute an independent factor. If it is an independent factor, then the pattern of transformations of sexual seeking in adolescence itself must be given greater weight in our conceptualizations.

Thrills and Risks

Example 1: As a baby, Jerry was famous as the redheaded daredevil. He was extremely motor active, and when he saw something he wanted he went after it in headlong fashion. As a ten-month-old, he almost leaped out of the window of a moving car in pursuit of a dog. As a two-and-one-half-year-old, he disappeared from the family group on the beach. He was found several blocks away walking in the road toward home to get a favorite toy that had been left behind. Consequences such as falls seemed to have no effect on his risk taking. He would climb or jump or run headlong toward whatever attracted him or occurred to him to want. His family essentially gave up on warnings, concentrating instead on preventing him from hurting himself. As a teenager, Jerry was a popular boy and excellent student. He was relatively conventional in his approach to risk taking. He often cited risks to others in his peer group, an indication of the possibility of a reaction formation to his early proclivities. However, there did not seem to be a compulsive or phobic need to avoid going along with the group or occasionally to take the lead.

Example 2: Professor G entered analysis in his early forties because he feared the failure of his second marriage. He had two paradoxical symptoms: first, he reacted with violent alarm if any member of his family exposed him- or herself to the slightest danger; second, he was unusually prone to involve himself in situations of excitement and risk. These involved creating social scenes, having sexual escapades, and speculating with investments. Because of his thrill seeking, his friends often compared him with an adolescent. Professor G thought that ironic since as a teenager he had been inhibited, studious, and conventional and had considered himself physically, sexually, and socially backward. His principal memory of his adolescence was of hating his home, where he felt confined and stifled, and loving the occasions when he could escape to the street and play ball with

193

his friends. In respect to his actual family, his teenage years had been his most stable. Shortly after his birth, his mother was diagnosed as having a brittle form of diabetes. There were frequent periodic panics in the home during his mother's diabetic crises—and very serious concerns for her life. She was hospitalized recurrently, and he was looked after by worried but sympathetic relatives. His father, whose work also involved danger and deception, was in and out of his life during these early years. Finally the mother's condition stabilized, but the slightest complaint on her part could, even in his adult years, trigger his alarm or violent rage. His pleasure and thrill seeking and his risking of exposure were modeled on his identification with his father, although he was unaware of the connection.

Jerry's example illustrates the premise that risk taking in infancy is not thrill seeking but stimulus seeking. Children like Jerry are neurophysiologically primed for this behavioral response; researchers sometimes speak of them as being wired that way. When neurophysiological maturation is complete—a rather slow process—these children can and often do develop workable controls based on appropriate upper-level symbolic reasoning. It is the quality of the interrelationship with their family members, often signified in their reputation as wild, that they may have to work out in later stages.

In saying that the risk taking of the infant's spontaneous behavior is to respond to stimuli and not to seek thrills, I do not mean to imply that thrill seeking and risk taking are not important experiences of this phase of life. The age-appropriate experience of thrills and risks is, I believe, a facet of normal caretaker-child regulation. A mother learns how her infant responds to exciting conversational games and to regulate the outer limits. Motion excitement can provide an enormously pleasurable sense of thrill and risk or a highly dystonic experience. Each father must learn how much his baby or toddler likes to be held high in the air or tossed free for a second and allowed a momentary sense of falling—then to be caught with shared glee. Parents must observe at what age the child responds favorably to a particular exposure, such as to the water's edge of a brook, splashing in a baby pool, to games of chase and "gotchya," or to witch and monster scares. Of course, unpleasurable excitements will occur in any child's life—a narrow escape from an automobile accident, a loud family argument, the anguish or hushed anticipation of death or a birth. All of this underlies the special nature of thrills and risks. Almost anything can be considered one or both—a trip on a trolley, a cable car ride up a mountain, a fight, a sexual experience, or being sadistic or masochistic. When these are experienced as a thrill, what they have in common is a special accentuated sense of self. As an adolescent patient stated, "You know you are for sure alive when chills run up and down your spine." It is therefore a part of the regulatory challenge to a parent to see that the child has exposure to thrills in which the self is enhanced, the risks are controlled, and the interrelationship is positive. A prototype is the sense of being in father's strong, safe arms when thrown in the air and caught, or when jumping from not too high a place, or being pushed on a swing higher and higher—but not too high.

In adolescence, unlike infancy, thrills and risks are actively sought for their own sake. This is primarily for their self-enhancing effect, although they may serve other functions as well. In addition, the adolescent attempts to bring this experience under a degree of self-regulation. He will now choose the form of his thrill seeking—the risks or challenges he will or will not take. And he will choose whose "arms" he will trust to hold him—a speaker against nuclear power, a diet cultist, or a political leader. The thrilling quality of these idealizations serves the purpose of increasing the intensity of self-experience, either primarily or from the radiated glory of the leader (parent replacement). Both sexual pursuits and power operations are transformed from the more intrinsic pleasures of sensuality, companionship, and competence pleasure into sources of thrills and risks that stimulate a sense of self-expansiveness.

All of this activity in adolescence—the egging of one another on toward daring exploits or risk taking—I regard as normal in itself. An attempt at regulation may succeed or fail, but if the attempt is aimed at achieving self-regulation, success or failure does not in itself determine the adaptedness. In the case of Professor G, there was a serious defect in the regulation of spine-chilling thrills because of the dramatic shifts in his mother's physical states. His adult choice of profession, research into body chemistry and physiology (not of diabetes), had some relevance to an attempt at control and mastery. His adolescence itself served more like a latency period. This was indeed useful to him because he was ill prepared to handle thrills and risks that a more normal teenager could take in stride. Because of this developmental lag, he was able to use his excellent mind productively in school with a minimum of interference. This left him, however, with an unresolved, almost addictive, attraction to thrill seeking and little experience in setting limits. This surfaced first with alarm reactions to his children and then became more intense as he approached what he regarded as a mid-life crisis. It is significant that in his analysis he regarded the analyst as offering him a positive "arm" to catch him as he hurtled through the air. This was, I believe, a special type of idealizing transference, one not frequently described in the literature.

Conclusions

Many continuities between infancy and adolescence can be demonstrated for both normal and pathological development. Accomplishments in socializing and in play and work; regulatory skills with respect to eating, sleeping, and eliminating; regulatory achievements in seeking and enjoying sensual pleasure; and thrills and risks will persist. Alternatively, disturbances in socializing, play and work, and especially basic regulations remain in need of later resolution. But when an adolescent resolves a disturbance that has persisted from an earlier period, he does so under entirely different circumstances than existed in that earlier phase. While he also has to accommodate to often rapid changes in bodily sensation, he does so with a fully formed body schema. While he also experiences the pressure of assertiveness and a tendency toward reactive aggression, he has a fully formed set of controls and defense mechanisms.

On the other hand, while the infant is buttressed as much as possible from the exigencies of social and political unrest, the adolescent must come into contact with them. Society may provide him a relatively quiet period in which to swallow goldfish, or a terrible period of war, or the temptation to go underground (with or without consciousness-altering drugs). When the adolescent works to achieve goals and values that will adapt him to the adult world, he builds on those internalized from childhood. But if he must make drastic changes, he is equipped with the capacity for symbolic logic through the twin modalities of primary and secondary process thinking. It is this accomplishment, the capacity for a symbolic level of cognition, that represents one of the major transformations in infancy and does not have to be recapitulated in adolescence. Nor does a cohesive self have to be formed; rather, an established cohesive sense of self must be expanded in its range and skills—bodily, socially, and with respect to self-esteem, self-expansiveness, and the idealization of others. As anyone who works with adolescents knows, these are indeed transformations enough for one epoch.

196

NOTE

1. *Transformation* is used here to refer to any changes by which a function is more or less irreversibly affected. Thus transformations include physical maturational changes and psychological differentiations, integrations, organizings, and reorganizings. The term is used for changes occurring both during a specific phase of development and between different phases. It refers to an alteration of a function that is adaptive (and relatively irreversible) and to an alteration of a function that is maladaptive (and at least sometimes relatively reversible). This definition is purposefully broad in order to suggest an organizing principle having general applicability.

REFERENCES

Amsterdam, B., and Levitt, M. 1980. Consciousness of self and painful self-consciousness. *Psychoanalytic Study of the Child* 35:67–84.

Beebe, B., and Stern, D. 1977. Engagement-disengagement and early object experiences. In M. Freedman and S. Grand, eds. *Communicative Structures and Psychic Structures*. New York: Plenum.

Brazelton, T. B., and Als, H. 1979. Four early stages in the development of mother-infant interaction. *Psychoanalytic Study of the Child* 34:349–371.

Broucek, F. 1979. Efficacy in infancy: a review of some experimental studies and their possible implications for clinical theory. *International Journal of Psycho-Analysis* 60:311–316.

Call, J. 1980. Some prelinguistic aspects of language development. *Journal of the American Psychoanalytic Association* 28:259–290.

Kleeman, J. 1975. Genital self-stimulation in infant and toddler girls. In I. Marcus and J. Francis, eds. *Masturbation: From Infancy to Senescence*. New York: International Universities Press.

Kohut, H. 1971. *The Analysis of the Self*. New York: International Universities Press.

Lichtenberg, J. D. 1981a. Implications for psychoanalytic theory of research on the neonate. *International Review of Psycho-Analysis* 8:35–52.

Lichtenberg, J. D. 1981b. Reflections on the first year of life. *Psychoanalytic Inquiry* 1:695–729.

Mahler, M.; Pine, F.; and Bergman, A. 1975. *The Psychological Birth of the Human Infant*. New York: Basic.

Papousek, H., and Papousek, M. 1975. Cognitive aspects of preverbal social interaction between human infant and adults. Ciba Foundation Symposium. *Parent-Infant Interaction*. New York: Associated Scientific Publishers.

Parens, H. 1979. *The Development of Aggression in Early Childhood*. New York: Aronson.

Winnicott, D. 1951. Transitional objects and transitional phenomena. In *Collected Papers*. London: Tavistock, 1958.

15 THE REVISION OF OBJECT REPRESENTATIONS IN ADOLESCENT MALES

MARY C. LAMIA

The primary love object for the boy remains the same throughout the phases of his development. With cognitive and emotional growth, his internal representation of his mother is subject to change. These changes take place through the processes of introjection, identification, and projection (cf. Jacobson 1964; Sterba 1947). In adolescence, an increase in instinctual drives reviving the Oedipus complex, the need to disengage from preoedipal object ties, and corresponding ego and superego reactions have a significant impact on the development of the boy's object representations.

Modifications in the psychic structure during adolescence have been, since Freud, discussed by Blos (1962), Deutsch (1967), Erikson (1968), A. Freud (1966), Jacobson (1961), and others. However, psychoanalytic literature gives insufficient attention to the revision of self- and object representations in adolescence, the relationship between the adolescent's self-representations and object representations, and the manifestations of these representations in conscious and unconscious attitudes toward the opposite sex.

Detailed accounts of the development of self- and object representations stop short of a discussion of these processes in adolescents (see Jacobson 1954; Klein 1948; Kohut 1966). Jacobson (1954) points out that "the adolescent reactivation of early infantile conflicts finds again expression in the youngster's confusion about himself and the world. The vicissitudes of self- and object representations during this stage are rather complicated and would deserve special studies" (p. 125).

The adolescent male's unconscious representations of women are necessarily a component of his sexual life. However, studies of adolescent sexuality, such as those concerned with the development of sexual identity (Deutsch 1967; Greenacre 1975), sexual attitudes and behavior (Offer and Offer 1975, 1977), and the relationship between narcissism and sexual activities (Kohut 1971), are not illuminating with regard to the adolescent's unconscious representations of the opposite sex.

While lecturing to groups of adolescent males on the topic of female sexuality, it appeared that the kinds of questions they asked about women presented particular patterns that warranted theoretical explanation. In light of psychoanalytic theory, a content analysis of questions asked by adolescent males about female sexuality is reported and discussed in this chapter.

Method

Data were obtained from 281 adolescent males who were asked to write anonymously two questions they would like answered about female sexuality.[1] The students ranged in age from sixteen to eighteen. Their average age was 16.8.

The adolescents were students in human sexuality classes at a middle-class, urban, Catholic high school for boys. They had received instruction in human sexual anatomy by a male teacher prior to filling out the questionnaire. They were told that a selected number of their questions would be answered by a female psychologist.

Results

The adolescents wrote 550 responses (questions) averaging nearly two questions per adolescent. The content of their responses fell into fourteen categories outlined in table 1. The categories were derived from manifest content of the adolescents' responses. Categories 1 (strength of the female sexual drive) and 5 (quality of the female sexual response) both contain quantitative and qualitative elements. Responses pertaining to how much females wanted or enjoyed sex were grouped under the category "strength of the female sexual drive." In contrast, "quality of the female sexual response" is related to the female's physiological arousal.

TABLE 1

QUESTIONS ON FEMALE SEXUALITY

Response Category	Frequency	Percent
1. Strength of the female sexual drive	201	36.5
2. How a male can arouse a female	57	10.4
3. Female emotions	56	10.2
4. Women's roles	53	9.6
5. Quality of the female sexual response	52	9.5
6. What the female looks for (at) in the male	45	8.2
7. Premarital sex	21	3.8
8. Menstruation	12	2.2
9. Female anatomy	12	2.2
10. Birth control	10	1.8
11. Oral sex	10	1.8
12. Pregnancy......................................	10	1.8
13. Female sexual fantasies	5	.9
14. Other	6	1.1

NOTE.—These response categories were offered by respondents ($N = 550$) who were asked to "Write two questions that you would like answered about female sexuality."

In terms of the distribution of responses, the categories fall into three major groups. The first group is category 1, which accounted for 36.5 percent of the responses. Group 2 consists of categories 2 through 6, ranging from 8.2 percent to 10.4 percent of the response. Group 3 is composed of categories receiving less than 4 percent of the response.

Discussion

Questions about the strength of the female sexual drive were asked most frequently by the adolescents (36.5 percent). They wondered how much females wanted or enjoyed sex. Typical inquiries were: "Why are males more interested in sex than females?" "Is the female's sex drive as strong as the male's?" and "Is sex gratifying to a woman?" Overall they saw women as having less sexual interest and enjoyment than men. At the same time, women who liked sex were seen as deviant. For example, "Is there such a thing as a nymphomaniac or is that just a female with the same sexual desires as a normal male?" or "Why do some girls enjoy sexual activities?" Women who wanted sex were also seen as having ulterior motives: "Does a woman have sex for pleasure or just so she won't lose her boyfriend?" Some adolescents wondered about the purpose of sex and separated the sex drive from the reproductive drive: "Do women still want to have intercourse even if they don't want to get pregnant?"

From the point of view of drive theory, this category of questions seems to demonstrate the interrelationship between drive strength and mobility and ego and superego activity. Questions about the strength of the drive seem to differentiate self from object, male from female. The mobility of the drive also seems to contribute to this division of representations. What we may be seeing in this category of questions is a process in the male's formation of a stable self-image by defining the sexuality of the female as different from his own—an attempt of the ego to define the self in terms of what females are or are not.

These representations of women as different from men can also be viewed as a consequence of the decathexis of the boy's early identification with his mother. This early identification creates a crisis for the boy in puberty when the conflict of bisexuality presses for final resolution and the boy is confronted with the problem of sexual identity (Blos 1962). According to Blos, the bisexual position is resolved in adolescence as sex-alien tendencies that threaten to disrupt the unity of the ego are conceded to the other sex. The sex-inappropriate component acquires ego syntonicity by becoming the property of the love object, which in turn is cathected with object libido.

Distortions of female sexuality can also be seen as manifestations of defensive activity in relation to the emergence of oedipal themes evoked by an increase in drive energy at puberty. The images of women held by these adolescents were frequently divided into those who do enjoy sex and those who do not. Lichtenberg and Slap (1973) present evidence for a defense of splitting of representations which separates currents of strong feelings and urges that would arouse castration anxiety and guilt if experienced simultaneously toward an object.

In Freud's (1905) discussion of the transformations of puberty, he claims that a normal sexual life is only assured when an exact convergence of the affectionate current and the sensual current are together directed toward the sexual object and the sexual aim. He was pessimistic about the ability of most men to fuse the currents of affection and sensuality properly. The man's respect for a woman acts as a restriction on his sexual activity, and the delay between sexual maturity and activity results in the need for men to debase their sexual object. This male debasement of the sexual object is comparable to the condition of forbiddenness in the erotic life of women (Freud 1912).

Although some might argue that only in previous times did the adolescent male make a direct division between "good (respected) girls" and "bad (sexually active) girls," Deutsch (1967) believes that "in our time, the young male makes this differentiation less consciously, and even protests upon being confronted with it" (p. 26).

The second most frequently asked question had to do with how a male can arouse a female (10.4 percent). Typical questions in this category were: "What turns women on?" and "What are the places on a woman's body that she likes to have touched?" Many of the adolescents' questions reflected the notion that the female must be made interested in sex. For example, they asked: "How do you get a female in the mood to make love?" and "What makes women want to have sex?"

Questions about the emotions of females were also prevalent in the adolescents' responses (10.2 percent). The males wanted to know what women are all about. For example, "How do you understand females?" "Why are women so unpredictable?" "How can you tell if a girl loves you?" "Describe the emotional life of a female (in general)," and "Why do most girls tease the guys into something that they know they won't do, but they act like they will?"

It appears that the adolescent male's attempt to cope with his own anxiety about sexuality leads to distorted notions about females and interferes with his understanding of the female psyche and female sexuality. Even Freud was aware of his limited understanding of women. In his *Three Essays on the Theory of Sexuality* (1905), he states that the sexuality of women "is still veiled in an impenetrable obscurity" (p. 151). And in 1926, he wrote that "we know less about the sexual life of little girls than of boys. But we need not feel ashamed of this distinction; after all, the sexual life of adult women is a 'dark continent' for psychology" (p. 212). Freud's own struggle with his unconscious representations of women is suggested by his choice of terms. Although he has been criticized for being sexist, it appears that Freud's difficulty in understanding the female psyche was not simply a result of conscious sexism. It might benefit women to understand that sexism is not merely a product of culture. Sexism has its roots in the unconscious foundations of beliefs on which male development is based.

Questions concerning the roles of women included 9.6 percent of the total responses. Prevalent in these questions was anxiety about powerful or dominating women and the changing roles in society. The adolescents asked: "What are women trying to prove in women's lib?

They know they can't do a man's job so why continue?" "Do you think women are becoming too powerful now?" "Do you think in days to come that sex roles will change?" "How do you feel about the female being the aggressor in sex?"

The questions asked by the adolescents reflect issues of power and competition with women. They may be viewed as narcissistic concerns related to the active, producing, threatening preoedipal mother. The boy's normal fear, envy, and rivalry with the mother have been related to the preoedipal wish to be pregnant and bear children like mother (Van der Leeuw 1958). On the other hand, Anna Freud (1966) asserts that the discovery of the difference between the sexes may strengthen the boy's defenses against his own feminine wishes and identifications and may "give rise to the pitying contempt for the castrated female" (p. 192).

We can also turn to the revival of oepidal themes in adolescence to explain the manifest content of questions concerning the roles of women. The view of women as active or powerful increases castration anxiety and fear of dependency in men. Freud (1918) believed that the influence of the castration complex on the opinion in which women are held "underlies the narcissistic rejection of women by men, which is so mixed up with despising them" (p. 199). This is seen in man's fear of passivity or of the active woman. This devaluating and defensively belittling attitude toward women conceived during the phallic phase often persists as a lifelong contemptuous attitude toward the female sex (Blos 1962).

The adolescents showed curiosity about the quality of the female sexual response (9.5 percent). The majority of responses in this category were variations on the themes illustrated in the following examples: "What does a woman feel during sexual intercourse?" "What does the female orgasm feel like?" "Why do women make noise while having sex?" "Is sex painful for the female?" The concept of multiple orgasm was expressed with both awe and fear: "Can a woman have a lot of continuous orgasms?" "Can a female get knocked unconscious by having several orgasms in a row?"

Here again is the adolescents' need to separate male from female sexuality. We also get a glimpse of aggressive, destructive fantasies that may be the result of envy and fear of the preoedipal mother or may represent versions of externalization, namely, concern about their own intense sexual interest and fear of the strength of their own sexual and aggressive impulses.

Another concern of the adolescents involved what the female looks for (at) in a male (8.2 percent). They were curious about what attracts a female to a male and how important a man's physical attributes are to women. Anxiety about appearance and penis size was obvious in their questions: "Does a woman only want good looks in a man?" "What is the first thing a girl looks at when a guy enters a room?" "Does the size of the man's penis make a difference?" Narcissistic issues are evident in their concerns, as are oepidal issues of competition and rivalry.

Less frequently, issues about premarital sex (3.8 percent), menstruation (2.2 percent), female anatomy (2.2 percent), birth control (1.8 percent), oral sex (1.8 percent), pregnancy (1.8 percent), and female sexual fantasies (0.9 percent) were subjects of inquiry for the adolescents. Questions in these areas, which were sometimes unusual, included: "Is premarital sex right or wrong?" "Why is the female such a bitch at that time of the month?" "If a female has sex frequently, like a prostitute, can her vagina get stretched out of shape or worn out?" "Do women want to use birth control?" "Why won't most women submit to having oral sex?" "Why is the woman the one who can get pregnant?" and "Describe a woman's sexual fantasies (if any)."

Although the adolescents showed less frequent manifest concern about these issues, such matters may be more subject to repression and a higher degree of defense may be involved.

Conclusions

Questions about female sexuality asked by 281 adolescent males were reported and discussed in light of psychoanalytic theory. Alternative explanations for patterns of questions asked by the adolescents were offered.

A cross-sectional view of the adolescent poses limitations in specifying antecedent conditions and predicting future development. However, it brings to our attention certain aspects of adolescents' functioning that are worthy of speculation and further study.

The population on which this study was based calls for further exploration into the effects of religious beliefs and the impact of schools segregated by sex on the development of object representations.

Longitudinal studies and clinical data from the treatment of male patients might determine what aspects of the object representations of adolescent males are phase specific and what aspects represent processes on the way toward firm establishment in the adult.

Finally, we can observe in the content of the male adolescents' questions the existence of double standards and sexist attitudes. It appears that attitudes toward sex roles, child rearing, and sexual stereotypes can be altered on a conscious intellectual level but are destined to persist in the unconscious. Anatomical differences between the sexes, and the child's reaction to these differences, will remain despite cultural revolution, social influences, and parental attitudes. The early perception of gender differences leads, in boys and girls, to different mental representations of self and object (Blos 1980). Jacobson (1964) believes that the universal unconscious fixation in men and women to the fantasy of female castration discloses our limited ability to form realistic object representations.

1. Data were collected between 1976 and 1978.

REFERENCES

Blos, P. 1962. *On Adolescence*. New York: Free Press.
Blos, P. 1980. Modifications in the traditional psychoanalytic theory of female adolescent development. *Adolescent Psychiatry* 8:8–24.
Deutsch, H. 1967. *Selected Problems of Adolescence*. New York: International Universities Press.
Erikson, E. 1968. *Identity: Youth and Crisis*. New York: Norton.
Freud, A. 1936. *The Ego and the Mechanisms of Defense*. New York: International Universities Press.
Freud, A. 1966. *Normality and Pathology in Childhood: Assessments of Development*. New York: International Universities Press.
Freud, S. 1905. Three essays on the theory of sexuality. *Standard Edition* 7:125–243. London: Hogarth, 1953.
Freud, S. 1912. On the universal tendency to debasement in the sphere of love. *Standard Edition* 11:179–190. London: Hogarth, 1953.
Freud, S. 1918. The taboo of virginity. *Standard Edition* 11:193–208. London: Hogarth, 1953.
Freud, S. 1926. The question of lay analysis. *Standard Edition* 20:183–258. London: Hogarth, 1953.
Greenacre, P. 1975. Differences between male and female adolescent sexual development as seen from longitudinal studies. *Adolescent Psychiatry* 4:105–120.

Jacobson, E. 1954. The self and the object world. *Psychoanalytic Study of the Child* 9:75–127.

Jacobson, E. 1961. Adolescent moods and the remodeling of psychic structure in adolescence. *Psychoanalytic Study of the Child* 16:164–184.

Jacobson, E. 1964. *The Self and the Object World.* New York: International Universities Press.

Klein, M. 1948. *Contributions to Psychoanalysis, 1921–1945.* London: Hogarth.

Kohut, H. 1966. Forms and transformations of narcissism. *Journal of the American Psychoanalytic Association* 14:243–272.

Kohut, H. 1971. *The Analysis of the Self.* New York: International Universities Press.

Lichtenberg, J., and Slap, J. 1973. Notes on the concept of splitting and the defense mechanism of the splitting of representations. *Journal of the American Psychoanalytic Association* 21:772–787.

Offer, D., and Offer, J. 1975. *From Teenage to Young Manhood.* New York: Basic.

Offer, J., and Offer, D. 1977. Sexuality in adolescent males. *Adolescent Psychiatry* 5:96–107.

Sterba, R. 1947. *Introduction to the Psychoanalytic Theory of the Libido.* New York: Nervous and Mental Diseases Monographs.

Van der Leeuw, J. 1958. On the preoedipal phase of the male. *International Journal of Psycho-Analysis* 34:112–115.

16 ANTICIPATION AND EXPERIMENTATION: THE SEXUAL CONCERNS OF MID ADOLESCENCE

ADRIAN SONDHEIMER

Adolescents are exposed to opportunities for learning in various settings, including the home, among peers, at work, and in school. Although the majority of youths in this country complete part or all of high school, many unfortunately suffer through the experience owing to inadequate planning on the part of those responsible for their education (Buxton and Sondheimer 1979; Friedenberg 1965).

Mental health professionals are frequently utilized as consultants to school systems as educators seek the benefit of their expertise. General principles underlying approaches to the consultative enterprise have been thoroughly elaborated by Caplan (1970). The school environment clearly presents an ideal opportunity for consultation to enhance and improve the students' didactic experience. Decades ago Anna Freud (1930) described benefits that would ultimately accrue to students as teachers learned from mental health professionals about psychological issues of childhood growth and development. In the intervening years others (Berlin 1962; Forman and Hetznecker 1972; Kandler 1979) have outlined and broadened approaches available for the consultant to the education system. These include traditional individual case consultation, discussions with teachers and administrators, the utilization of audiovisual aids, and meetings occurring between the consultant and groups of students, at times specifically in the classroom setting.

Education about sexual matters has relatively recently been legitimized as an appropriate area of concentrated instruction within the school system. As Calderone (1966) points out, this new mandate corresponds with sex education becoming distinct, for the first time, from reproductive education. Coincident with this change, the mid 1960s produced a spurt of articles and activities concerning this new area of instruction (Peltz 1968). Thus the White House Conference on Children and Youth (1960) recommended that family life courses be made integral parts of elementary through high school curricula, and the National Association of Independent Schools, in 1966, offered similar proposals. Mental health personnel were encouraged to contribute their expertise by consulting in the creation of sound, school-based sex education formats. But all has not been smooth sailing for the sex education movement; it has aroused considerable antagonism, even among professionals (Anchell 1969).

Of course, learning about sex has been a human enterprise for millennia, but misconceptions and fears about the subject, as well as the development of troubling consequences resulting from experimentation, have also arisen repeatedly. Masters and Johnson (1970) suggest that 50 percent of the adult population suffers from various forms of sexual dysfunction. Statistics (National Center for Health Statistics 1977; U.S. Department of Health, Education, and Welfare 1973) continue to describe the explosive growth in the number of teenage pregnancies, as well as the increased perinatal risks associated with these births. Skeptical questions have also been raised about changes in sexual mores that seem to have occurred among adolescents in the past fifteen years (Blaine 1968; Josselyn 1974), although a prevailing sentiment appears to regard with approval the increased openness about sexuality stemming from these new currents.

Various studies indicate that changes have also occurred recently in the origin of initial sex information for adolescents. Whereas parents and written material once seemed to have primacy, a shift to peers as the major source appears to have taken place (Dickinson 1978; Thornburg 1978). Unfortunately a great deal of the information shared in such a manner is grossly inaccurate (Reichelt and Werley 1976). Not that the situation existing a generation earlier was superior. In that era, when discussion of sexual issues was largely discouraged, the youths had to rely for their instruction on the older generation or on the prevalent sex education literature. At best, their parents were poorly informed and the literature was woefully lacking, in both its substantive content and its potentially alienating tone (Rubinstein, Watson, and Rubinstein 1979).

It is likely that the shift from parents and books to peers as informational sources is due to the adolescent's greater awareness of the paucity of his elders' knowledge coupled with the increase in his opportunities for sexual encounters, both verbal and experiential. Offer (1969) has described the importance and the magnitude of peer group communication and value sharing for adolescents. Others have strongly suggested capitalizing on these phenomena as a means of imparting accurate information in subject areas in which the voicing of common concerns is beneficial. These features, characteristic of adolescent development, lend themselves naturally to sex education in the group setting. The teaching exercises can be approached in varied fashion. The context may be that of classroom or rap center, adult educators or peer counseling might be emphasized, and family participation is occasionally pursued (Brandenburg 1976; Reichelt and Werley 1975; Rosenberg and Rosenberg 1976; Zuckerman, Tushup, and Finner 1976). Whatever the environment, the authors stress the importance of group sharing, which has even been deemed "therapeutic" (Seiden 1976).

The desire on the part of adolescents for an adult "sex educator" emerges consistently (Calderone 1970; Thornburg 1978). Repeatedly the authors and the data emphasize the need for an individual who is both knowledgeable about and comfortable with the material, and who will not fall easy prey to interpersonal errors that can rapidly alienate the adolescent (Jensen and Robbins 1975). The psychiatrist has been suggested as the professional most appropriate for this task in the school setting (Finch 1968; Peltz 1968) as he presumably would be best able to marshal information derived from physiological, neurological, developmental, and psychological perspectives.

Efforts have been made (Lief 1965; Wabrek and Lief 1972) to educate physicians in sexual matters and to train them to teach others. Nevertheless, there exists a meager amount of data in the general psychiatric literature describing the sexual concerns of various populations grouped by age. Noteworthy exceptions include the contributions of Sorensen (1973), who utilized self-administered questionnaires and personal interviews to describe sexual issues relevant to adolescents, and Werner (1975), who similarly solicited inquiries through the mail from college-age youth. Gordon (1973, 1978) has written extensively and appealingly on the subject for both adult and adolescent audiences.

This chapter represents an attempt to focus on sexual issues of concern to mid adolescents, and it is based on consultative work performed in the school setting. The open-ended study seeks to determine the specific sexual concerns, how they are expressed, the issues that may lurk beneath the surface, the effect group discussion may have on the members, and those approaches by an educator that might prove most beneficial.

Methodology

Sex education sessions, spread out over two and one-half years, took place in a single public high school situated in a large northeastern city. The particular school differs from the majority in that admission is open to students living throughout the city, rather than limited to those of the local community. Thus the student body is composed of a mix of ethnic, religious, racial, and socioeconomic backgrounds. The institution's admission requirements necessitate passing an entrance examination which emphasizes the potential for above-average academic achievement.

As part of the health education curriculum for high school juniors (average age, sixteen years), each class received one forty-minute session for this sex education exercise. Twenty-five to thirty students, with an essentially equal number of males and females, attended on each occasion.

The presentation began with a brief verbal description of changes in physical characteristics and emotions that are characteristic of the onset of adolescence. This introduction was followed by two minutes of desensitization, in which "four-letter" expressions for parts of the body and descriptions of sexual activities were solicited from the students, after which additional slang terms were provided by the author. This technique, which may seem more shocking in print than in the actual practice, provided relatively rapid relaxation of the students' anxieties and subsequently permitted considerably more openness and exchange of material than might otherwise have been expected, given the brief time available for the exercise.

I subsequently described the use of such expressions as a product of individuals' anxieties about sexual matters. The hope was expressed that the students could inquire about sexual issues of concern to them in a setting in which they now felt more comfortable. To that end the students were asked to write their questions on paper without identifying themselves. These were subsequently collected, and all questions, without exception, were read aloud. Appropriate responses were attempted and classroom discussion solicited.

Results

Previous studies (Rubinstein et al. 1979; Werner 1975) have compartmentalized the sexual concerns of junior high school and college students, respectively, into categories suitable for investigation. The older students' questions were divided into two major subcategories: anatomy and physiology, and sexual activity. The latter was further subdivided into the categories of sexual intercourse, oral and anal; petting; masturbation; and homosexuality. A review of the inquiries submitted by the high school population of this study suggested the need for other groupings in addition to several mentioned above.

The students participating in the sessions numbered 541, and questions were received from 507. Table 1 lists the categories in order of decreasing frequency. Though a question may pertain to more than one category, it was placed in that group which described the dominant theme of the inquiry.

TABLE 1
FREQUENCIES OF QUESTION CATEGORIES

	N in Each Category	% of Total
Normality/abnormality:	90	16.7
Male-female sharing of experience	38	7.0
Friendship versus sex	29	5.4
Fantasies	23	4.3
Psychological issues	89	16.5
Moral/ethical/social:	82	15.2
General issues	47	8.7
Authority/psychiatrist as arbiter	35	6.5
Masturbation	59	10.9
Anatomy and physiology	50	9.2
Pregnancy and contraception	47	8.7
Homosexuality	43	7.9
Sexual practices	28	5.2
Adolescent whimsy	18	3.3
No question asked	34	6.3

MORAL/ETHICAL/SOCIAL

GENERAL ISSUES

What part does religion play in these new moral values and sexual liberation? What should I do or think about this, follow my friends no matter what, or follow my own mind?

Is premarital sex wrong?

Is the morality of today more open than in our parents' day, or is it just used as a cover-up to hide what our parents might have done?

A good many of the questions raised by the students serve as entrees to a wide-ranging discussion of the issues rather than mandate specific limited responses. Questions in the moral sphere are indicative of one of the major developmental tasks of adolescence, that is, the need to deal with conflicts arising between new information and old training and experience, between the comfort and familiarity of home and the stresses brought about by options formerly unavailable. The recently acquired capacity for sexual potency and the vastly increased importance of the peer group as a source of support and enhanced self-esteem are major phenomena that foster greater awareness of different modes of behavior.

Adolescents struggle with these matters in often poignant fashion, and they are often not as clear about their stands on the issues as occasional declarative statements and even overt behaviors might indicate. They also often function as potent hypocrisy detectors, subjecting much of their elders' moral guidance to incisive scrutiny.

AUTHORITY: PSYCHIATRIST AS ARBITER

Why does one feel so secretive about sex, so prohibited, if it is a thing of nature (in your opinion please!)?

What is your definition of being a man?

How slow should a boy go with introducing sex to a girl?

213

Are sexual feelings and attitudes reflective upon a person's personality, that is, reflective upon the need for a psychiatrist to help him through a problem or defect in his personality?

The importance of adult role models to adolescents cannot be overemphasized. The elders are utilized not as individuals who provide answers but as persons who have undergone the anxieties of that earlier developmental stage and who are subsequently able to share the results of their experiences combined with factual knowledge. The youths are seeking neither externally imposed restrictions on their behavior nor license but, rather, support and encouragement as they explore their sexual feelings and those of their partners. Reassurance derived from an elder authority is a major component in the educative process. The knowledge of anatomy and physiologic processes, combined with an awareness of the anxieties attendant on the variety of life's problems, may suggest the psychiatrist to the students as an individual with appealing qualifications and allow him to be heard when others may not.

NORMALITY VERSUS ABNORMALITY

FRIENDSHIP VERSUS SEX

I consider myself asexual or neuter—is true neutrality really possible?

If a person doesn't feel any strong sexual feelings at our age, will that person develop them later?

Is it okay for a couple who are just friends to have physical contact with each other?

The onset of adolescence generally corresponds with the start of puberty, which brings about changes in both physical characteristics and emotions. The rates of change in both spheres do not necessarily correlate, however, and the youths frequently indulge in surreptitiously comparing themselves with each other. Unable to avoid these issues as they are bombarded by sexually stimulating material in the media, they are also often required to address sex-oriented, sensibly presented educational material. As wide-ranging differences in degrees and rates of emotional maturation and development exist among adolescents, they limit acknowledgment of their sexual feelings to a pace with which they feel comfortable. Some move hesitantly and deliberately, others act with greater rapidity, at times impulsively. Reassurance, coupled with information about the ranges of normal development, is of paramount importance. Discussion of the various kinds of relationships into which adolescents enter, some of which may include sexual thoughts and/or shared physical experiences, is equally essential.

MALE-FEMALE SHARING OF EXPERIENCE

Do girls feel the same way as the boys feel? For example, would girls want to touch a guy's penis like guys would want to feel up a girl?

If you express your sexual feelings, how are you to make sure you are not classified as a C.T. (cockteaser)?

Do girls have as much a sex drive as boys?

Considerable anxiety develops concerning the other gender's perceptions as the opposite sex takes on much greater importance for most adolescents than existed previously. Looks, dress, feelings, reputation, and the handling of sexual opportunities are major matters, as are culturally sanctioned stereotypes which often foster fuzzy notions of male-female differences regarding the urgency of their respective sexual desires.

The adolescent confronting these issues often mistrusts his own responses, and the new underlying question rapidly becomes "Am I normal?" The opportunity for the sexes to discuss their anxieties and self-doubts allows them to discover the similarity of concerns that they share as well as the differences. It also permits the individual to compare himself with others of the same sex, and this provides him with the means to evaluate his standing on the normality continuum.

FANTASIES

What kind of sexual fantasies do people have?

When, if at all, does fantasizing become excessive?

The adolescent spends much time in learning, in both the academic setting and his surrounding environment. Though physically capable, he is not yet emotionally equipped to engage adult responsibilities or relationships, and he needs time to learn in these areas as well. Much preparatory work occurs through fantasy, and the most exciting and stimulating ones generally involve sexual depictions. But fantasies are private and they can be experienced as very powerful, to the extent that they may often arouse concern and even fear. The assertion that such activity is common, frequent, and indeed necessary for emotional growth dispels a good deal of trepidation; the notion that "excessive" implies a major disruption of the individual's functioning is reassuring for the vast majority.

PSYCHOLOGICAL ISSUES

If a girl feels she would like to have intimate relations with someone, but she has been brought up to believe that it is wrong, how should she go about making a decision, without feeling guilty either way?

How do you accept and cope with rejection?

How does one explain frigidity?

Is a girl still a virgin if she uses a tampon? If she masturbates?

Should you always be honest in a relationship? What about the games?

What is the proper age for teenagers, or adults, to begin having intercourse?

Finding a partner?

Approximately one-fifth of the submitted questions fall into the category of psychological issues. Adding to their number, the queries slotted into the sphere of morals and ethics indicate that one-third of the questions essentially reside in the region of personal philosophic concerns. These results strongly imply that many adolescents are struggling with choices involving the creation of moral values. All the youths are dealing with feelings engendered on the intrapsychic level, and some are better prepared to address the issues maturely than others. Duplicity versus

216

honesty, appropriateness of timing, and the loneliness of being alone are examples of lifelong concerns, but they are felt with particular intensity during the mid-adolescent years. Virginity is generally lost and first intercourse consummated during adolescence or young adulthood, and these issues in particular are best approached by emphasizing the value of mature consideration and decision making. Guilt, sadness, and fear are unavoidable emotions intimately intertwined with interpersonal and sexual behavior. An acknowledgment of that truth allows for subsequent intrapsychic contemplation and emotional development.

ANATOMY AND PHYSIOLOGY

Why are wet dreams necessary?

What is an orgasm?

Can a person contract VD any way other than intercourse?

Can a man run out of sperm and still have an erection and orgasm?

Shifting from the area of feelings and psychological issues to the sphere of biologic and morphologic concerns necessitates the availability of concrete, factual knowledge. Ignorance of the correct response is best admitted openly, instead of perpetuating mis- or half information. Penile and breast size; doubts about potency; the physical components of sexual arousal; venereal disease; and the absence or presence of the hymen and its susceptibility to penetration by tampon, finger, or penis are prevalent concerns. Though a few students may have been previously exposed to sex education courses, much inaccurate information and "old wives' tales" nevertheless circulate freely. It is most prudent to assume a considerable lack of basic knowledge and, therefore, to start at the beginning. More sophisticated information, as well as a discussion of thoughts stimulated by these subjects, should only be introduced after the knowledge of fundamentals is conveyed and assimilated.

MASTURBATION

Does masturbation really take you away from the real world and cause people to live in a fantasy land (I read this). P.S. How can you stop?

What is the difference in the normal age of termination of masturbation for males and females?

Can a guy tell if a woman masturbates by having sexual intercourse with her?

Is massive masturbation wrong when it doesn't seem to bother you?

Masturbation is closely related to fantasy as self-stimulation rarely occurs without the formation of mental images. Fantasy invariably depicts individuals acquiescing to the demands and requests of the director of the scenario, and the process dispenses with the otherwise necessary requirement of first obtaining consent. The resort to masturbatory activity is a normal developmental step which permits an individual to experience the pleasure of mounting sexual excitement and release while the tempo remains totally under his control. For the adolescent it serves as an opportunity to discover those images and physical sensations he finds most enjoyable. Though the maneuver is generally indulged in isolation it does entail true risk. Discovery may occur when a family member unexpectedly barges into a room, the undetected disposal of semen may prove difficult, and excessive indulgence can lead to painfully chafed skin.

The realization of such a new, powerful, and easily accessible experience is also frequently perceived as frightening. Aside from the superstitious warning of the development of "hand warts and brain rot," such fears commonly have a vague foundation and are generally related to the intensity of desire over which the adolescent feels he has little control. Disturbing images may occasionally intrude as well. The fantasies accompanying the self-involved practice of masturbation also raise the issue of eventual intimacy, that is, involvement with others, a phenomenon the adolescent may prefer to defer for the more distant future. In addition, a sensation so pleasurable which must be practiced on the sly frequently arouses feelings of shame, to which many adolescents respond with the plea of "When will it end?" A discussion of the prevalence of masturbation in normal development, male-female differences in incidence, its subsequent incorporation into mutual sexual encounters, and its continued accessibility as an opportunity for pleasurable release helps allay many of the concerns.

218

PREGNANCY AND CONTRACEPTION

Can a girl become pregnant the first time she has intercourse?

When is the safest time to have sex without birth control?

How long before intercourse must the Pill be taken to guarantee proper contraception?

Is it true that a girl can't get pregnant if she has sex about a week or ten days before her period?

What's the safest abortion method?

More than half of all teenagers in the United States engage in sexual intercourse during their junior and senior years of high school (Zelnik, Kim, and Kantner 1979). The extent to which a great many of these same adolescents are ignorant of the physiologic principles underlying the menstrual cycle, of perineal anatomy, and of the processes resulting in pregnancy is particularly striking.

Sexual intercourse is best described as a potentially pleasurable enterprise that often involves emotional sharing but which demands responsibility. It naturally follows that acknowledgment and discussion are required of the common reluctance among adolescents to deal with the subject of contraceptive approaches. Explanations for this disinclination include complaints about "lack of naturalness," the interference of contraceptives with the subconscious desire for impregnation, the acknowledgment via the use of such devices that one is actually engaging in sexual activity, and/or the powerful wish to deny massively the potential for conception. It becomes necessary, therefore, to focus on the practical implications of pregnancy and youthful motherhood, situations which the majority of students claim to be eager to avoid. It is also of considerable importance for the students to learn that a "Pill" on the day of intercourse, a double dose of pills the day after, and the state of previous virginity are all ineffective impediments to determined spermatozoa.

SEXUAL PRACTICES

Can anal intercourse create pregnancy?

How safe is giving blow jobs?

Why do some young, intelligent women want to be beaten before intercourse?

Does it hurt a guy to squeeze his balls?

The comparison of relatively sophisticated questions with those suggesting hesitation about private thoughts and solitary practices indicates the wide range of experience that exists among youngsters of essentially identical age. Just as students appreciate learning from each other of the concerns they share with regard to fantasies and emotions, so, too, they welcome the communal discussion of sexual practices that some have experienced but about which all are aware. This beneficial effect of the group setting was well illustrated by a male student who immediately flung himself across his desk and let out a banshee scream of disbelief in response to the "genital compression" query. The tumultuous laughter that instantly followed increased further with the educator's comment that the questioner had gotten the most authentic and accurate reply possible.

As the varieties of sexual activity are discussed, emphasis should be placed on the desirability of their being acceptable to both partners. Factual knowledge, however, requires dissemination as well. For example, a description of fellatio includes the comment that while spermatozoa, and not germs, are most commonly admitted into the mouth, it is the placement of teeth that generally requires the most caution.

HOMOSEXUALITY

Is homosexuality considered to be a disease, a natural phenomenon, a product of society, or what, by the so-called experts?

What is the reason for young kids fooling around with their own sex?

What do you do if you are approached by a homosexual and you don't want to be a part of it?

The wish to be emotionally close with members of one's sex remains present throughout life. Same-sex touching and exploration, as part of

220

normative development, occasionally occur during late latency or early adolescence. With the arrival of the mid-adolescent years, such activity is generally considered far less acceptable in both the social and intrapsychic contexts. The expression of less explicit remnants of this desire, however, remains culturally permissible in North American society. Females are thus allowed to hug each other in greeting and to cuddle when one or both are upset, while males may clap each other on the back in signs of approbation.

It appears that a relatively small proportion of the total population, approximately 4 percent (Kinsey, Pomeroy, and Martin 1948), is predominately homosexual in orientation, and those who describe themselves as bisexual do not add greatly to the numbers. During the past decade we have witnessed a greater awareness of the difficulties faced by this minority group, as well as the raising of a broader debate among psychiatrists and other professionals concerning questions of etiology. As "homosexuality as mental illness" becomes a less acceptable doctrine, normalcy and deviance become more a determination of the individual's capacity to function in society rather than simply a measure of the statistical prevalence of his sexual orientation. This hesitant shift in attitude and approach among mental health experts is mirrored by the perplexity of younger people, some of whom have not necessarily brought their own sexual identities to complete resolution. Consequently it is not surprising to find that the individual who states that "being exposed to them (homosexuals) as real people has changed my attitudes a lot" might well be the friend of another adolescent who declares, "If I was ever approached by one, I'd probably shit in my pants."

ADOLESCENT WHIMSY

Is a curved penis common? . . . how common? . . . how curved?

Is Miss J (the health education teacher) wearing a bra?

Is it strange if you don't particularly like the taste of a female's genitals? Could it be that particular female just doesn't wash herself or what?

Have you ever jerked off into a vacuum cleaner hose?

The need to test oneself against adults is a major component of adolescent development. The verbalization of outrageous suggestions, or at least of notions that depart from accepted convention, is one such method. When presented in humorous form the edges soften, the mood becomes more relaxed, and the underlying serious intent can be addressed in an atmosphere of reduced tension. Adolescent humor thus differs from that of the child's naive concreteness in that awareness of hidden content, intent, and possible outcomes is often quite conscious.

The nature of sexual subject matter provokes the development of considerable anxiety. Physiologic dissimilarities, hesitation about diverse sexual practices, varieties of maturbatory approaches, and the need for personal hygiene are therefore more easily considered after the laughter dies down. The immediate blushing of the youthful Miss J, a well-liked teacher, was noted by those who were teasing her in a challenging but affectionate manner. The students obtained a graphic illustration that sexual awareness and concerns remain even after the end of adolescence.

For this expert pedagogue, the following question was perhaps the most difficult one posed: "Are you crazy, or do you enjoy doing these dumb lectures?" This marvelous opportunity to spur cognitive development to a higher level of abstraction was not to be lost, however, as it was immediately pointed out that a consultant is eminently capable of being "crazy or dumb" simultaneously.

Conclusions

It was not the intent of this study to measure objectively the amount of knowledge gained from the exercises; rather, the aim is to provide insight into the sexual concerns and misconceptions of adolescents. One may reasonably conclude from the questions posed by the students that increasing the availability of improved and more extensive sex education courses, as part of preventive health services, seems strongly indicated in order to correct significant deficiencies in adolescents' knowledge of basic sexual material. Other studies (Garrard, Vaitkus, Held, and Chilgren 1976; Reichelt and Werley 1976; Rosenberg and Rosenberg 1976; Zuckerman et al. 1976) indicate that information derived from sex education courses is retained to a considerable degree, and it is reasonable to assume that similar learning occurs in the context of the approach described in this chapter.

Two potential drawbacks to the acquisition of this information may nevertheless have occurred. A brief period of only one session was available for each class, and it is likely that the quantity of knowledge obtained was consequently limited. It is also possible that the presence of the health education teacher during the session represented a hindrance to the freedom of verbal expression. However, the frankness with which questions were asked and the candidness of the subsequent discussion suggest that such was not the case. In all likelihood the anonymity of the questioners' identities was the primary protection the students required. In addition they were simultaneously aware of, and interested in, implicitly advising their teacher about those issues they deemed particularly important.

It seems evident that this approach works well in the mixed-sex group setting. Perhaps the major finding to emerge is that the student's greatest desire, irrespective of gender, is to unearth the sexual thoughts and interests of his classmates, and his major concern is self-measurement against peers. Awareness derived from the discussion of similarities and ranges of normalcy provides considerable reassurance, probably the adolescent's greatest need.

This work was performed in a setting in which the students shared the features of common chronologic age and above-average academic interest. The finding of a considerable similarity of sexual concerns suggests that the issues categorized above are the ones most prominent in the mid-adolescent years. By contrast the ethnic, racial, socioeconomic, religious, and geographic factors impinging on the students were considerably disparate. The influence of these heterogeneous elements probably contributes to the wide range of sexual experience and emotional maturity suggested by the questions. It is interesting to note that a relatively low percentage (14 percent) of the inquiries was devoted to issues of pregnancy, contraception, and heterosexual practices. This finding may in part be explained by the delay exercised in these matters by students with high academic aspirations and may not be typical for this age group.

As emphasized elsewhere (Jensen and Robbins 1975; Peltz 1968), these educative procedures operate most effectively when a leader communicates with sensitivity and a sense of humor, and encourages discussion as well. Didactic lectures, by way of contrast, patently alienate students. The consultant psychiatrist who combines information derived from training with these desirable approaches will perform this function well. The mental health expert should be prepared, moreover, for the occasional presence of disturbed individuals. One student, who described himself as "hetero-, homo-, and bi-sexual" asked, "What proof could someone use to convict someone of a sexual crime?" Such a query stands out as bizarrely different from the rest, and it presents an opportunity for the leader to amplify on issues of mental health and disturbance for all the students, with suggestions about the indications for, and availability of, psychological assistance.

Approximately one-third to one-half of the questions were concerned with what can broadly be described as psychosocial issues. This impressively large number suggests that adolescents, given the opportunity, can articulate issues well, are not necessarily too negativistic or embarrassed to do so, and will even share their philosophical concerns and personal worries with adults. For this exchange to occur, however, they require a supportive atmosphere that encourages such expression.

Given this impressive degree of openness, it is striking that the question, "How come I feel for only one girl and no others?" was one of only two inquiries of more than five hundred denoting the issue of love. Perhaps this poor numerical representation was due to the brief duration of the class; if more time had been available, this issue as well as other new ones might have received increased attention. The likelier explanation, however, was provided in question form by the other student who asked, "Do you think that until you get to a specific age an adolescent doesn't know what love is?" Adolescents are certainly capable of loving, but in the sexual context the mid adolescent, having outgrown the naive romantic visions of earlier years, generally remains too self-involved to undertake the mature responsibility of deeply caring for another peer. In contrast, questions of college-age and adult students solicited in similar exercises reflect a considerable shift to concerns about relationships and mutual caring. Such a change in emphasis indicates the strong influence of developmental issues on sexual concerns.

Finally, the perplexity underlying seemingly innocuous questions must be emphasized. Adolescents become increasingly aware of the insubstantiality of easy answers and of the need to acknowledge discomfiting emotions such as apprehension, doubt, and guilt. Some questions demand simple educative responses, but many require examination on a deeper level. The identifying markers for the one and for the other are often difficult to locate. Nevertheless, the struggle with complexity and the delight in a myriad of possibilities often help to stimulate adolescents to further exploration and growth. These factors can well be utilized by consultants in their efforts to aid adolescents as they strive to achieve a more comprehensive and comfortable sense of their sexuality.

REFERENCES

Anchell, M. 1969. The psychological effects of sex education in public schools. *Child and Family* 8(1): 81–84.

Berlin, I. 1962. Mental health consultation in schools as a means of communicating mental health principles. *Journal of the American Academy of Child Psychiatry* 1(4): 671–679.

Blaine, G. 1968. Sex among teenagers. *Medical Aspects of Human Sexuality* 2(9): 6–11.

Brandenburg, J. 1976. Peer counseling for sex related concerns: a case study of a service in a college medical setting. *Journal of the American College Health Association* 24(5): 294–300.

Buxton, M., and Sondheimer, A. 1979. Who's in control? School violence and its impact on adolescent development. *Journal of Current Adolescent Medicine* 1(4): 11–16.

Calderone, M. 1966. Sex and the adolescent. *Clinical Pediatrics* 5(3): 171–174.

Calderone, M. 1970. Sex education and the physician. *Postgraduate Medicine* 47(2): 100–104.

Caplan, G. 1970. *The Theory and Practice of Mental Health Consultation*. New York: Basic.

Dickinson, G. 1978. Adolescent sex information sources: 1964–1974. *Adolescence* 13(52): 653–658.

Finch, S. 1968. The physician's role in sex education. *Medical Aspects of Human Sexuality* 2(1): 37–40.

Forman, M., and Hetznecker, W. 1972. Varieties and vagaries of school consultation. *Journal of the American Academy of Child Psychiatry* 11(4): 694–704.

Freud, A. 1930. The relation between psychoanalysis and education. *The Writings of Anna Freud* 1:121–133. New York: International Universities Press, 1974.

Friedenberg, E. Z. 1965. *Coming of Age in America*. New York: Random House.

Garrard, J.; Vaitkus, A.; Held, J.; and Chilgren, R. 1976. Follow-up effects of a medical school course in human sexuality. *Archives of Sexual Behaviour* 5(4): 331–340.

Gordon, S. 1973. *The Sexual Adolescent*. Charlottesville, N.C.: Ed-U-Press.

Gordon, S. 1978. *Facts about Sex for Today's Youth*. Charlottesville, N.C.: Ed-U-Press.

Jensen, G., and Robbins, M. 1975. Ten reasons why "sex talks" with

225

adolescents go wrong. *Medical Aspects of Human Sexuality* 9(7): 10–23.

Josselyn, I. 1974. Implications of current sexual patterns: an hypothesis. *Adolescent Psychiatry* 3:103–117.

Kandler, H. 1979. Comprehensive mental health consultation in high schools. *Adolescent Psychiatry* 7:85–111.

Kinsey, A.; Pomeroy, W.; and Martin, C. 1948. *Sexual Behavior in the Human Male*. Philadelphia: Saunders.

Lief, H. 1965. Sex education of medical students and doctors. *Pacific Medicine and Surgery* 73(1A): 52–58.

Masters, W., and Johnson, V. 1970. *Human Sexual Inadequacy*. Boston: Little, Brown.

National Center for Health Statistics. 1977. *Teenage Childbearing: United States 1966–1975*. Monthly Vital Statistics Report: Natality Statistics vol. 26, no. 5, suppl. DHEW publication no. (HRA) 77-1120. Washington, D.C.: Government Printing Office.

Offer, D. 1969. *The Psychological World of the Teenager*. New York: Basic.

Peltz, W. 1968. Sex education programs in schools. *American Journal of Psychiatry* 125(2): 206–213.

Reichelt, P., and Werley, H. 1975. A sex information program for sexually active teenagers. *Journal of School Health* 45(2): 100–107.

Reichelt, P., and Werley, H. 1976. Sex knowledge of teenagers and the effect of an educational rap session. *Journal of Research and Development in Education* 10(1): 13–22.

Rosenberg, P., and Rosenberg, L. 1976. Sex education for adolescents and their families. *Journal of Sex and Marital Therapy* 2(1): 53–67.

Rubinstein, J.; Watson, F.; and Rubinstein, H. 1979. An analysis of sex education books for adolescents by means of adolescents' sexual interests. *Adolescence* 12(47): 293–311.

Seiden, A. 1976. Sex roles, sexuality, and the adolescent peer group. *Adolescent Psychiatry* 4:211–225.

Sorensen, R. 1973. *Adolescent Sexuality in Contemporary America*. New York: World.

Thornburg, H. 1978. Adolescent sources of initial sex information. *Psychiatric Annals* 8(8): 70–77.

U.S. Department of Health, Education, and Welfare. 1973. *The Women and Their Pregnancies: The Collaborative Perinatal Study of the National Institute of Neurological Diseases and Stroke*. DHEW publication no. (NIH) 73-379. Washington, D.C.: Government Printing Office.

Wabrek, A., and Lief, H. 1972. Medical school involvement in sex counseling for college students. *Journal of Medical Educaton* 47(9): 740–741.

Werner, A. 1975. Sex questions asked by college students. *Medical Aspects of Human Sexuality* 9(5): 32–61.

Zelnik, M.; Kim, Y.; and Kantner, J. 1979. Probabilities of intercourse and contraception among U.S. teenage women, 1971 and 1976. *Family Planning Perspectives* 11(3): 177–183.

Zuckerman, M.; Tushup, R.; and Finner, S. 1976. Sexual attitudes and experience: attitude and personality correlates and changes produced by a course in sexuality. *Journal of Consulting and Clinical Psychology* 44(1): 7–19.

17 MORAL NIHILISM: DEVELOPMENTAL ARREST AS A SEQUELA TO COMBAT STRESS

HELENE COOPER JACKSON

The Vietnam conflict was unique in American history. Even more than ten years later, veterans were experiencing significantly more psychological and social problems than their peers who did not go to war (Egendorf 1981). Clinical observations indicate that Vietnam combat veterans who suffer from posttraumatic stress disorder[1] present a severity of disorganization in their internal and external lives that is inconsistent with their relatively benign, premorbid personalities. Although all combat inflicts psychic injury, the enormous stress, which Lifton (1976) called a "combat situation of absurdity and evil," forced many soldiers to move precipitously from an age-appropriate phase of idealism to a nihilistic position of meaninglessness. Superego restraints were lost; terror and violence were sanctioned by authorities and/or peers. The disparity between the adolescent's inner life and the reality of the chaotic and irrational combat world in which he found himself was so great that he was unable to integrate the experience either cognitively or morally. Expansion and growth were inhibited. In addition, the "homecomer" (Schuetz 1944–1945) found that society's values had changed; the veteran's efforts were denigrated. Thus the experience became dysfunctional for the development of an integrated ego ideal and superego, the psychic agencies to which moral development is attributed and which, under normal conditions, become consolidated during late adolescence.

The difficulties this group of Vietnam veterans experiences may, in part, be related to being fixed in an adolescent phase of moral development strikingly similar to nihilism. Like the nihilist described by Wein (n.d.), the Vietnam veteran abrogates his own vitality, often

228

HELENE COOPER JACKSON

feeling "dead to himself and dead to other people." Although his life continues, he feels it is over and done with.

Moral Nihilism

The philosophy of nihilism developed in Russia in the nineteenth century among those who believed that their society's statements of values and ideals were hypocritical or false. Although nihilism became popular after its first appearance in Turgenev's (1862) novel, *Fathers and Sons*, Nietzsche was the only major philosopher to make extensive use of the term. As the concept spread, it lost its anarchistic and revolutionary flavor and is currently used "to denote a mood of despair over the emptiness or triviality of human existence" (Edwards 1967).

Many Vietnam soldiers, during combat or following their return home, experienced traumatic disillusionment with the military establishment, with the policies that were carried out in Vietnam, and with their society's values and attitudes toward its returning "heroes." Like the nihilist who "will dissociate himself from conventions, behave as a stranger who belongs nowhere, [and] be imbued with the feeling that nothing matters" (Wein, n.d.), these veterans are estranged from themselves and the world. A Vietnam veteran says, "I am driven. I can't stop. Underneath there is nothingness, a void, no meaning, just black death. I died back there. I feel nothing."

Theories of Moral Development

Morality is usually defined as an evaluation or means of evaluating human conduct. Most believe that "morality is a device of social control, an indispensable primary way in which societies have always prevented the breakdown of social order and their own eventual self-destruction" (Holt 1980).

According to Freud (1933), the source of moral development is in the initial parent-child relationships which are characterized by obedience to authority. He attributed the development of moral judgment to two agencies of the mind—the superego and ego ideal. Derived from instinctual attachments and defenses, the superego develops through identification with the parent of the same sex. The ego ideal is formed in a continuous attempt to recapture the narcissistic perfection of the original primary dyad and proceeds in the context of relationships throughout life. As disappointments are survived, expectations are re-

229

ordered. The vicissitudes of ego ideal development move from hallucinatory wish fulfillment to the relinquishment of the "grandiose, heroic, inflated self-image to an ideal which can function as a guide to reasonable aims and goals in terms of object choice, career and role in society" (Ritvo 1971).

Focusing on the development of cognitive judgment, Piaget (1948) investigated the moral development of the child within the context of rules. He traced the progression in young children from heteronomous morality (dependence on the external environment) to autonomous morality. Relatively autonomous morality arises from the development of the self through the process of being able to take the roles or attitudes of others in ongoing interactions with peers. This stimulates moral development instead of producing any one particular value system.

Piaget (1948) postulates two developmental lines of morality: the morality of constraint and the morality of cooperation. The morality of constraint evolves from the unilateral relations between the child as inferior and the adult as superior. From this perspective, justice is reduced to demands of authority; intentions and motives have no bearing on judgment. The morality of cooperation, on the other hand, is created out of reciprocal relationships among peers and is based on mutual respect.

While Piaget believed that a high level of cognitive development is necessary for adult development to proceed, it is by itself insufficient. That is, a high level of cognition does not necessarily yield a high level of moral reasoning. On the other hand, the stage of logical development clearly limits the moral stage attainable. Flavell (1963) writes that cognitive development and moral development are ongoing, interactive, organizing processes formed in the "spontaneous give and take, [and] in the interplay [of thought and action] which take place in peer interactions." Both depend on the ability of the organism to assimilate new material to its own existing stage structure or schema. Through conflict and its resolution, the individual moves from stage to stage via the processes of assimilation, accommodation, and equilibration. Conflict arises when one perceives a discrepancy between existing organization and that which is to be assimilated. In other words, the person can only assimilate that for which past experiences have prepared it. There must be a preexisting system of meanings, an organization sufficiently advanced and flexible enough to admit and then assimilate the new stimulus.

Building on the work of Piaget and Freud, Gilligan and Kohlberg

(1973) use the drama and conflict of adolescence to trace moral development as it moves through various levels. Each represents successive degrees of internalization of moral sanctions and an increasingly complex and differentiated internal reordering of the previous level of moral reasoning. The levels correspond to Piaget's phases of concrete operational thinking and formal operational thought. Data collected from moral dilemma interviews with male adolescents led the authors to postulate an invariant, hierarchical stage and sequence theory of moral development that moves from an individual, egocentric focus (preconventional) through a societal focus (conventional), culminating in a focus on universal principles (postconventional) that transcend any particular culture. This process occurs within the principles of justice and reason and is based on the logic of equality and reciprocity.

Kohlberg's and Piaget's hierarchical models place priority on the value of equality and reciprocity and on the use of rationality to determine moral choices. Kohlberg's preconventional level of moral reasoning is characterized by a lack of awareness or appreciation of conventional or societal rules. What is "right" is limited to following concrete rules or orders blindly from a self-serving orientation of obedience to authority. Rules and expectations are experienced as external to the self. Kohlberg's conventional level moves beyond the egocentric position to a concern for the approval, opinions, and well-being of others. The concept of "right" is seen as conformity to the rules, roles, and expectations of a small group or of society. The postconventional level in Kohlberg's scheme is characterized by a perspective that defines values and principles that exist prior to the organization of society. Thus "right" is viewed in terms of general or universal human rights, values, or principles that society should uphold. The postconventional person has differentiated himself from convention and defines values in terms of self-constructed, reflective principles which he has developed by logical thought (Kohlberg and Gilligan 1971).

Each stage, then, contains maxims or principles that may be seen as analogous to Freud's stage paradigm of the individual's movement from "id-bound" child to law-abiding citizen and, ultimately, to the well-analyzed adult who questions the rules instead of following them blindly—an adult who resolves moral issues through rational means.

Theories of Adolescence

The term "adolescence" refers, in the male, to a period between childhood and adulthood from ages fourteen to twenty-five. The defini-

231

tion is, literally, "becoming an adult." Gilligan (1968) writes that the "convergence of developmental themes in late adolescence around questions of morality, together with the intellectual capacity of the adolescent mind to think about moral questions in a new way, points to adolescence as a critical time for moral development in the human life cycle."

While the universality of major psychic turmoil as a necessary phase of normal adolescence has been challenged (Masterson 1968; Offer 1969), the traditional view of adolescence has been that it is a period of psychic instability and vulnerability (Blos 1962; Erikson 1956, 1958; A. Freud 1958). Blos (1979) writes that the ability to progress to adulthood is predicated on the capacity to regress in the service of development. What Blos describes as "regression" is similar to what Kohlberg calls "transition" and Erikson (1958, 1968, 1970) labels "moratorium."

Kohlberg's phase of "transition" was originally labeled "retrogression." This was perceived as a period in which the adolescent reverted to what appeared to be earlier, more primitive cognitive and moral structures in order to give meaning to the world. This stage is now seen, as is Blos's concept of regression and Erikson's moratorium, as a normative phase of adolescent development in which "moral relativism and nihilism [are a] transitional attitude in the move from conventional to principled morality" (Gilligan and Kohlberg 1973). When regression was first observed, it was feared that fixation at this point in development might result in the "moral defiance of a Nietzsche or a Raskolnikov [or an] asocial, amoral, hedonism." Although these fears proved to be unfounded for Kohlberg's sample of college males, they were, unfortunately, accurate predictions for many of the adolescents who fought in Vietnam.

According to Erikson (1968), the moratorium is a "period of delay, a time in which to test the rock bottom of some truth before committing the powers of the body and mind to a segment of the existing [or coming] order." Erikson (1958) believes this phase is "built into the schedule of human development" and that a mishap at this time may result in an arrest at the "rock bottom and deplete the energy available for [the adolescent's] reemergence." He writes, "It is probable that in all historical periods some, not necessarily the least gifted, young people do not survive their moratorium; they seek death or oblivion, or die in spirit." This phenomenon of late adolescence is usually followed by a period of consolidation in which the disparity between two moral systems is integrated into an awareness that there is no single version of the truth.

All three concepts are analogous to a nihilistic position that is characterized by the disillusionment caused by the contradiction between the reality of the world and the adolescent's ideals. These contradictions often lead the adolescent to feel isolated and disconnected from his sense of self and the world. He feels that his truth is fractured, that the world holds no meaning. He recognizes that his system of beliefs and values is no longer valid. His task is to combine his vision of the ideal with the irrationality of the world around him, to which he has become exquisitively sensitive. When this phase is prolonged long beyond its age-appropriate time, it becomes pathological.

Clinical Data

The four Vietnam veterans whose interviews are reported here are part of a larger group of sixteen combat veterans who participated in a project on the impact of combat stress on adolescent moral development.[2] At the time of enlistment, the four men were chronologically in mid adolescence, between the ages of eighteen and nineteen. During the study they ranged in age from twenty-nine to thirty-four years. Their retrospective reports suggest that they were at a phase prior to moral nihilism, that is, the time when cognitive development has not yet "lost its innocence [or] knowledge, its naive objectivity" (Gilligan 1968). The clinical data suggest that this phase of idealism strongly influenced their decision to enlist. Adolescent idealism is dramatically illustrated by the following excerpts.

I wanted to go. It was the right thing to do, to stop Communist aggression in the world so everybody can be free. I believed in my country. I felt the most honorable thing I could do was to die for my country.

I was Mr. Patriotic, and I believed in what our country was doing. So I went over there with this incredible sense of patriotism.

We were just proud of the uniform itself, showing it off. We were going somewhere and proud to be Americans. I believed what I read in the history books.

All expressed an innocence, a singular view of the world, a naiveté that is characteristic of a normal, idealistic phase of adolescence. All had a strong belief in God.

233

I was brought up, "Don't hurt anybody," you know the difference between right and wrong, how to be a good Christian.

You know, I was an altar boy. I was going to be a priest.

I was brought up a Protestant in the Baptist church. You have all these morals.

I believed in God. He was the one thing I had left. When I lost him, I lost everything. Nothing was left. Life had no meaning anymore.

The last statement suggests a link between nihilism and a loss of belief in God. This veteran chose to "face nothingness" rather than to submit to a faith that to him had become what Erikson (1958) calls a "cant of pious words."

The loosening of infantile object ties and the increased capacity for heterosexual relationships are closely tied to the structural development of the ego ideal. Veterans retrospectively describe their attempts to deal with these adolescent tasks.

I knew when I went to board the Air Force plane that if I'd looked back at my mother I wouldn't have been able to go.

I wanted to get out of the house. I didn't like my parents at the time. They were domineering. I needed to feel independent, so from the time I was fifteen, I had a job, had my own money, and helped the family.

I guess it was pride, a certain glamour, the John Wayne macho stuff.

Adolescence is a period of significant internal and external pressure in which optimal development can occur only with support from many sources. Esman (1977) writes, "In an ordered society, with clear structure and functioning institutions, the developmental support offered will keep the adolescent's psychic vulnerability within the limits necessary for his survival." According to Erikson (1970), the adolescent needs a stage on which he can interact freely and safely with individuals and the social community.

The process of deidealization is the "most painful subjective experience within the adolescent psychic restructuring" (Blos 1979). Historically the military has provided adolescents with a structured community within which they could safely accomplish their tasks. Unfortunately, rather than facilitate a recapitulation, by which the tasks of adolescence might be accomplished, Vietnam became a "horror show" in the theater of the absurd.

It's like in phases. At the time I thought I knew it was for real. When you first go in, it's a game. Then all of a sudden the game starts taking you around the board. And it stops being a game all of a sudden. You reach each phase on the board and it's increasingly becoming more real and more obvious it's not a game, it's really final.

The first time I got shot at I jumped up and looked around. I thought to myself, "That's funny, what's going on?" One of the guys who knew pulled me back down and I jumped up again. I couldn't believe it. He pulled me down again. I really didn't expect it. It was real!

The absurdity of it. Waste. Waste of life. It really stunk. It was lousy. A general once said, talking about the boys in Vietnam, he said, "They may be nineteen years old but they're going on forty-two." And damn! We grew up awful fast.

The encounter with death undermined the adolescent's magical sense of omnipotence and vulnerability "by means of its terrible inner lesson that death is real, that one will oneself die" (Lifton 1979).

For some, nihilism was experienced early. The following quotation is a graphic example of Nietzsche's imperative that "disillusionment is a necessity before a way could be cleared for new avenues of thought" (Breisach 1962). This insight has clearly been long recognized by the military.

In the Marine Corps, from the beginning, they really broke you down. And then built you right back up into a machine. They build you into one unit, one machine.

These young men experienced a precipitous broken connection in the developmental process toward mature adult functioning. They were forced to give up the old morality in a situation where no universal ethics prevailed.

When I first went, it was all good. You've got to do it to stop communism. Then it became confusing. You didn't really understand what was happening.

It was a sad and depressive awakening to reality. There's a difference between what you want to believe and what you see.

For some, questioning the reality and rightness of the war came when they returned home.

This girl came up to me, this beautiful girl. I'll never forget her. She had a big smile, and just came right up to me and she said, "Did you just come back from Vietnam?" I said, "Yes," proudly, you know. She asked me, "Did you kill any babies?" and then she spit on me! And I was like nineteen years old, and we were home. And I said this doesn't make sense.

There is a shocked awareness of the disparity between the ideal and the irrationality of the world. Forced into a nihilistic position by a situation he cannot comprehend, the veteran is unable to integrate the contradiction. It is generally accepted that a crisis may offer an opportunity for growth, development, and a capacity for more mature and complex psychic structuring. Or, it may be so traumatic that it seriously arrests development. Disillusionment persists.

Well, everything that I had believed in ended up being a big bunch of bullshit as far as I'm concerned.

Despair persists.

Lost, lost, it's gone. Never get it back again. No. You can't get it back. It's gone, it's past.

The adolescent ideals and illusions were destroyed, leaving a vacuum into which no meaning of life can develop.

I decided the whole thing was useless and meaningless. A lot of things happened that I can't find any justification in my heart and that I'll never find any justification for.

The inability to give meaning to the Vietnam experience has left many veterans in the nihilistic position of moral despair, skepticism, meaningless, and isolation, sometimes leading to self-destructive behavior.

About a year ago, I guess, I took an overdose of medication and stuff. I just didn't give a shit, you know. I felt that was the answer, just to get out.

According to Arendt (1977), the capacity for moral response depends on the "activity of thinking [and is] among the conditions that make men abstain from evil-doing." The nihilistic experience in Vietnam was out of phase with the adolescent's stage of development. In Piaget's terms, the soldier was too overwhelmed to use the processes of accommodation and assimilation for testing more complex and adequate structures of thought which would enable him to make sense of his experience. Some of these young men did not even discern the moral problem; the disparity was too great. Unable to abstain from "evil-doing," some took refuge in drugs and alcohol.

I never really thought. You didn't have time to think about it over there. And the times you could sit back and relax for three or four days, everyone would sit down and smoke dope and get juiced. I used to just want to forget.

When asked how he would describe what happened when he saw innocent civilians killed, one veteran said,

At the time, no feeling whatsoever. No, you don't feel anything at all. I had no feelings.

Another replied,

I just sat there numb, dumbfounded. I still feel numb.

According to Lifton (1976), numbing expresses a "situation of meaninglessness and unfulfilled life," of broken connections. Meant to ward off anxiety, unfortunately, it also wards off autonomy and self-understanding. In his expression of numbness, the veteran presents a defensive posture in which "being dead, one cannot die and one cannot kill" (Laing 1965).

Some would ward off the anxiety of the combat situation with disintegration and a return to an earlier primitive stage of functioning.

> After you see someone hung up by the balls, you want to reciprocate.

> At the time when I hit the seven that I got, I was saying to myself, "This one's for that one. This one's for that one, this one's for that one."

> Killing women and children. Pay them back. Revenge for the guys that had been killed. That makes it right.

They were fixed in a nihilistic situation of self-preservation and a nihilistic process of self-destruction (Wein, n.d.). In attitude, some regressed to a hedonistic position, like the child who unabashedly delights in torture.

> At the time it was fun. I really enjoyed it.

> There was no conflict at the time. That kind of makes you sick.

> It was a good feeling. A feeling of power. The thrill had that kind of power.

When asked if those feelings were reminiscent of another time, one veteran replied,

> No, because before, as a child, it wasn't real. It was like pretend. It was fun. You played games, it wasn't real. No.

They were in the midst of a "counterfeit [moral] universe" in which perverse "inner corruption [situationally reinforced] became the price of survival" (Lifton 1976).

> It was kill or be killed. It was easy to kill.

238

Arrest in Adolescent Development

These four veterans seemed to fall within a preservice, normal range of adolescent development. There were no signs of gross psychopathology prior to enlistment, that is, no reports of serious delinquency, psychiatric history, suicide attempts, drug or alcohol abuse, or police records. None had a service psychiatric history.

The striking feature of this clinical material is that these men have not made gains in moral development in the decade since their combat experience. As a result of the size and selected nature of the sample (the men are all enlistees and patients at the Mental Hygiene Unit), these veterans are not representative of the general population of Vietnam veterans who suffer from the residual stress of combat trauma. However, this study suggests that the inability to integrate the combat experience has led to an arrest in adolescent development. For these men, the apparent arrest or stasis in the phase of moral nihilism, by its very duration, has become pathological. Unable to progress or to find new meanings that transcend the old, the connection remains broken between self and others.

I don't know. I just seem to have lost all the drive out of my life. I've lost something. It's been taken away. It's awfully hard to find something to replace it with.

Unable to renegotiate old relationships the veteran remains in limbo, frozen and numb, in a pervasive mood of despair, hopelessness, and alienation.

I can't function in my family or in society. I just haven't come to a conclusion of the whole damn war. As much as I try to figure it out, I still can't understand it.

They are stuck in an "egocentric isolation of a perpetual adolescence" (Gilligan and Kohlberg 1973).

I was young and immature when I went in. I'm still young and immature, as far as I'm concerned.

Therapeutic Implications

Therapeutic interventions must be designed to assist these men in the resumption of the developmental thrust that was precipitously and traumatically aborted by their combat experience and subsequent homecoming. They have severed connections with their past values and ideals. An imbalance between the aggressive and libidinal drives is evidenced by defensive passivity, outbursts of rage, and an inability to effect satisfying relationships. Often they have difficulty in maintaining even a tenuous connection with their therapists. They may require extensive outreach, something many therapists find difficult to respond to or to provide. As a result, dealing with countertransference becomes difficult (Haley 1974).

I have found group therapy to be particularly well suited to facilitate the thrust of development and the accomplishment of the tasks that have been disrupted. As an external superego and ego ideal, the group protects the veteran's ego in this vulnerable period. It serves as a surrogate family as well as a societal displacement. It establishes a clearly structured community of interest where members may begin to reconstruct and reorganize their experiences, past and present, in a different, more complex way. The group provides a milieu in which peer relationships can stimulate the veteran's capacity to think about moral questions in a new way. In a benign, supportive atmosphere, the veteran begins to perceive a discrepancy between his own and other members' perceptions, between his perceptions and the new environment. He becomes a "treater" as well as "treated," active rather than passive. Heroic, inflated ideals are given up for more reasonable aims and goals. Members begin to develop the capacity to renegotiate relationships, moving from a position of mistrust, inferiority, powerlessness, and narcissistic rage to one of reciprocity, collaboration, responsibility, and caring—from a morality of constraint to a morality of cooperation.

Conclusions

These veterans present a difficult and challenging therapeutic task. The concept of moral nihilism as a prolonged phase of normal adolescent development provides a different and useful basis for observation and a possible explanation for the apparent inconsistency between the relatively benign premorbid personalities and the severity of disorganization this group of veterans present. The image of the Vietnam veteran as the prototype of the moral nihilist forces one to reexamine one's view of these patients. As different moral judgments determine different moral actions, a new definition of the problems of some Vietnam veterans may lead to new perceptions and perhaps more effective treatment strategies.

NOTES

1. According to DSM III, diagnostic criteria for posttraumatic stress disorder are existence of a recognizable stressor that would evoke significant symptoms in almost anyone, accompanied by reexperiencing of the trauma, numbing of responsiveness or reduced involvement with the external world, and feelings of detachment. Symptom picture is marked by diffuse anxiety, intrusive recollections of trauma, nightmares, and headaches.

2. This research project was conducted in partial fulfillment of the requirements for the doctoral program, Smith College School for Social Work. All participants were patients at the Veteran's Administration Outpatient Clinic, Mental Hygiene Unit, Boston, at the time of the interviews. They were selected and referred by staff members.

REFERENCES

Arendt, H. 1977. *The Life of the Mind: Thinking.* New York: Harcourt Brace Jovanovich.

Blos, P. 1962. *On Adolescence.* New York: Free Press.

Blos, P. 1979. *The Adolescent Passage.* New York: International Universities Press.

Breisach, E. 1962. *Introduction to Modern Existentialism.* New York: Grove.

Edwards, P. 1967. *The Encyclopedia of Philosophy.* New York: Free Press.

Egendorf, A. 1981. *Legacies of Vietnam: Comparative Adjustment of Veterans and Their Peers.* New York: Center for Policy Research.

Erikson, E. H. 1956. The problem of ego identity. *Journal of the American Psychoanalytic Association* 4:56–121.

Erikson, E. H. 1958. *Young Man Luther.* New York: Norton.

Erikson, E. H. 1968. *Identity, Youth and Crisis.* New York: Norton.

Erikson, E. H. 1970. Reflections on the dissent of contemporary youth. *International Journal of Psycho-Analysis* 5:11–22.

Esman, A. 1977. Changing values: their implications for adolescent development and psychoanalytic ideas. *Adolescent Psychiatry* 5:18–34.

Flavell, J. H. 1963. *The Developmental Psychology of Jean Piaget.* New York: Van Nostrand.

Freud, A. 1958. Adolescence. *Psychoanalytic Study of the Child* 13:255–278.

Freud, S. 1933. The dissection of the psychical personality. *Standard Edition* 22:57–80. London: Hogarth, 1964.

Gilligan, C. 1968. Moral development in the college years. In A. Chickering, ed. *The Modern American College.* San Francisco: Jossey-Bass.

Gilligan, C., and Kohlberg, L. 1973. From adolescence to adulthood: the rediscovery of reality in a post-conventional world. Paper presented to Jean Piaget Society, Philadelphia, June.

Haley, S. 1974. When the patient reports atrocities. *Archives of General Psychiatry* 30:191–196.

Holt, R. R. 1980. Psychoanalysis and ethics: Freud's impact on modern morality. *Hastings Report* (April), pp. 38–45.

Kohlberg, L., and Gilligan, C. 1971. The adolescent as a philosopher: the discovery of the self in a postconventional world. *Daedalus* (Fall), pp. 1051–1085.

Laing, R. D. 1965. *The Divided Self.* London: Penguin.

Lifton, R. J. 1976. *The Life of the Self.* New York: Simon & Schuster.

Lifton, R. J. 1979. *The Broken Connection.* New York: Simon & Schuster.

Masterson, J. 1968. The psychiatric significance of adolescent turmoil. In A. Esman, ed. *Psychology of Adolescence.* New York: International Universities Press, 1975.

Offer, D. 1969. Adolescent turmoil. In A. Esman, ed. *Psychology of Adolescence.* New York: International Universities Press, 1975.

Piaget, J. 1948. *The Moral Judgment of the Child.* New York: Free Press.

Ritvo, J. 1971. Late adolescence: developmental and clinical considerations. *Psychoanalytic Study of the Child* 26:241–263.

Schuetz, A. 1944–1945. The homecomer. *American Journal of Sociology* 50:369–376.

Turgenev, I. 1862. *Fathers and Sons.* New York: Washington Square, 1962.

Wein, H. n.d. Discussion of nihilism. *Universitas* 6(2): 173–182.

PART III

PSYCHOPATHOLOGICAL ASPECTS OF ADOLESCENT DEVELOPMENT:

AFFECTIVE DISORDERS IN CHILDREN AND ADOLESCENTS

18 CHILDREN AND ADOLESCENTS AT RISK FOR MANIC-DEPRESSIVE ILLNESS: INTRODUCTION AND OVERVIEW

CLARICE J. KESTENBAUM

During the past twenty-five years, research efforts focusing on individuals with a high probability of becoming schizophrenic in adult life have vastly increased (Erlenmeyer-Kimling, Cornblatt, and Fleiss 1979). Risk research, however, has only recently begun to address the issue of vulnerability to affective disorders. Despite epidemiological data indicating that a first episode of bipolar illness in adolescence is not uncommon (Loranger and Levine 1978; Perris 1966; Winokur, Clayton, and Reich 1969), it had long been believed that manic-depressive illness similar to the adult disorder did not occur in childhood. In recent years single-case reports have begun to appear in the literature. Feinstein and Wolpert (1973) reported the case of a three-year-old girl whose intermittent impulsivity, distractibility, hyperactivity, and destructive activity warranted, in their opinion, the diagnosis of manic-depressive illness. McKnew, Cytryn, and White (1974) described a hypomanic eight-year-old who exhibited jocularity, grandiosity, rage attacks, and inappropriate behavior. These case reports are uncommon, however, and as Carlson and Strober (1978) noted, true mania in childhood is extremely rare and probably masked by developmental issues.

The literature concerned with descriptions of the childhood precursors of adult bipolar illness is equally sparse. Retrospective accounts of some individuals who later developed bipolar illness indicate that their premorbid functioning was normal or often superior. Cohen, Baker, Cohen, Fromm-Reichman, and Weigert (1954) found from in-

245

tensive psychotherapy with adult manic-depressives that in childhood many were highly functioning, extroverted, ambitious, and sociable (despite superficial relationships characterized by clinging dependence). What, then, are the indications that a child might be vulnerable to a manic-depressive disorder in adult life? That the illness should develop in adult life without recognizable precursors in childhood seems as improbable as Athena's springing fully formed from the brow of Zeus.

The following five chapters constitute a careful examination of many of the features so troublesome to investigators in the field of affective disorders; namely, the contribution of genetic predisposition and the role of environmental stress, clinical and psychological assessment, therapeutic interventions, and possible underlying neurophysiological mechanisms.

Before discussing the childhood disturbance, either the illness or the prodromal state, I would like to review some basic assumptions about bipolar adult illness.

Mania and melancholia have been well documented from antiquity to the present day. Kraepelin (1921) in 1896 classified manic-depressive psychosis as a unitary form of mental illness distinct from schizophrenia, with periodic and circular manifestations. In 1921 he described the classical mood changes and stated that the various forms of manic-depressive illness arose from their individual temperamental predispositions: manic, depressive, cyclothymic, and irritable. These were, he concluded, lifelong dispositions manifested by intermittent mood disturbances. Episodic periods of illness, however, could occur. The depressive form was usually predominant, but on termination of the episode the patient would return to his premorbid temperamental state. Kraepelin believed that the illness had hereditary roots and that there was a continuum between affective temperaments and full-blown affective disorders.

Present-day (1980) DSM III diagnostic criteria for bipolar disorder include one or more distinct periods with a predominantly elevated, expansive, or irritable mood of at least one week's duration, manifested by some of the following symptoms: increase in activity; pressured speech; flight of ideas or racing thoughts; grandiosity, often delusional; decreased need for sleep; distractibility; and reckless activities such as foolish business investments, buying sprees, and sexual indiscretions. There may be psychotic features such as delusions and hallucinations. Shopsin (1979) describes the manic patient as euphoric, unconcerned, carefree, and devoid of problems. Affects are exhibited without any concern for reality or the feelings of others. Mood is often expansive, and some patients have extraordinary delusional notions about their power and importance and characteristically involve themselves in various senseless and risky enterprises. However, some gifted individuals in a more organized hypomanic state demonstrate a quick wit and a good sense of humor, unlike schizophrenics. The euphoric mood, in contrast, may be accompanied by anger and irritability. Manic patients may be provocative, contentious, and readily provoked by seemingly harmless remarks. They can react with rage to minor provocations and become verbally abusive with screaming, shouting, and even violence.

In contrast to depressed patients, manic patients are extremely self-confident, with an ego that knows no bounds; they are "on top of the world." They are seemingly selfish with an attitude of "nothing and nobody else counts." Accompanying this magical omnipotence and supreme self-esteem is an equally inordinate lack of guilt and shame. Often there is a denial of realistic danger. The patient's boundless energy, cunning, planning, scheming, and inability to forecast resulting consequences frequently lead to irresponsible enterprises and excessive spending, as well as to misdemeanors of a sexual, aggressive, and/or possessive nature. Serious criminal acts occur but are indeed rare. In contrast to the depressed phase of manic-depressive illness, patients in the manic phase have heightened libidinal drives with abounding energy and increased sexual appetite.

Accompanying the euphoric, expansive, irritable mood of manic patients is the accelerated pace of psychomotor activity. They are always active, quickly changing from one to another of their multiple enterprises. They seem to be indefatigable; they may function for days without sleep until they succumb to fatigue, sometimes becoming dangerously exhausted. Often only a few hours of sleep will suffice, after which they resume their pace in a relentless, restless agitation. They may become excessively verbose with logorrhea and flight of ideas. Except in extreme cases, the ideas usually remain sufficiently relevant to be followed without difficulty by the psychiatric examiner.

The depressive phase of the illness is more familiar to clinicians. The patient may exhibit dysphoric mood, loss of interest in all activities, loss of pleasure, poor appetite, insomnia or hypersomnia, psychomotor agitation or retardation, loss of energy, feelings of worthlessness, slowed thinking, and preoccupation with death.

Some investigators believe that there is a spectrum of affective disorders with positive family history of related behaviors. Akiskal (1981) has described cyclothymic disorders in which interpersonal problems such as repeated failures, romantic losses, episodic promiscuity, and alcohol and drug abuse mask an underlying affective disorder. He implies that this entity is similar to the borderline personality disorder as described by Gunderson and Singer (1975).

These patients are impulsive and show intense unwarranted anger and affective instability; they have difficulty being alone and frequently describe feelings of emptiness, boredom, and anhedonia. Stone (1979) has reviewed Kraepelin's list of temperamental features in manic-depression, complementary with other items relevant to this diagnostic realm. Manic items include alcoholism, ambitiousness, arrogance, boastfulness, euphoria, compulsive gambling, extroverted traits, heightened self-confidence, hypersexuality, insensitivity, intensity, lack of insight, raucous laughter, inveterate punning, stubbornness, talkativeness, teasing, and wanderlust. Several such temperamental traits obviously do not necessarily indicate the presence of a manic or even hypomanic disorder, but a premorbid history of such traits in a psychotic patient (particularly if family history is positive for affective disorder) may help to establish a diagnosis of bipolar illness.

There is little doubt that recent advances in the study of affective disorders point to a hereditary factor. Rosenthal (1970) summarized data on manic-depressive psychosis in the first degree relatives of bipolar index cases from eleven studies from 1921 to 1953 and found that the median morbidity risks were: (*a*) parents, 7.8 percent; (*b*) siblings, 8.8 percent; and (*c*) children, 11.2 percent. The important questions underlying all the studies to date are, What role does the genetic component play, and is it in and of itself sufficient for a manic-depressive breakdown to occur in later life or is a particular kind of environmental stress necessary to produce the illness (Kestenbaum 1980)?

The first chapter for the symposium, "Manic-Depressive Disorder in Children and Adolescents," by Sherman C. Feinstein, addresses the clinical aspects of bipolar illness in children. It makes the important point that the disorder may show "specific equivalent behaviors that are the precursors of the cyclothymic personality and manic-depressive states of young adulthood." He believes, furthermore, that the affective system of patients with manic-depressive illness may display a basic vulnerability which, when overstimulated, begins a discharge pattern that does not lend itself easily to autonomous emotional control. He postulates that some biological variation (probably on a genetic basis) leaves the affective system with specific vulnerability to affective stress. The case presentations of Jody, Jan, and Art are illustrative. The onset of Jody's illness was before age three, but distinct phasic disturbance was not seen until age five. The affective episodes seem to have been precipitated by loss reactions which overwhelmed the ego and resulted in a shift to affective solutions.

Jan, age ten, was described as having definite cyclic behavior. Frenzied activity, overproduction of speech, and interpersonal difficulties characterized the "manic" states. Art had a history of separation anxiety, temper tantrums, and mood swings before his psychotic breakdown in adolescence. All three children had a family history compatible with affective disorder. Since recent studies have demonstrated that there is a higher incidence of psychopathology among children of parents with affective disorders (Winokur, Clayton, and Reich 1969), the offspring are at an increased risk for developing minor depression, cyclothymia, sociopathy, and alcoholism. It would be important to discern which clinical features predate the onset of the full-blown clinical syndrome and are representative of an early expression of a bipolar diathesis in a vulnerable child, and which symptoms might be reactive to parental illness and not represent genetic vulnerability. There are, to date, few studies of bipolar offspring who were interviewed by direct questioning and not only from parental questionnaires. Where bipolar offspring were directly examined, depression was diagnosed in 25–45 percent of the children (McKnew, Cytron, Efron, Gershon, and Bunney 1979).

In 1979, I described thirteen children with a family history of bipolar manic-depressive disorder. Six of the children exhibited the following features: (1) family history positive for bipolar illness; (2) specific clinical symptomatology including temper tantrums, compulsive rituals, dysphoria, lability, obsessional preoccupation, learning disability, hyperactivity, and impulsivity; and (3) specific patterns in psychological test scores (WISC) revealing verbal achievement significantly greater than performance (Kestenbaum 1979).

The second paper, "The Offspring of Bipolar Manic-Depressives: Clinical Features," by Leo Kron, Paolo Decina, and Clarice J. Kestenbaum, addresses itself to these issues. With Susan Farber, Margaret Gargan, and Ronald Fieve we studied thirty-one children of manic-depressive parents, controlled for age, sex, and class in order to discover some corroboration of my original hypothesis. The clinical findings are particularly interesting. The experimental group was significantly differentiated from the control group with regard to depression, overactivity, overproduction of florid fantasy, and attractiveness. There was a nonsignificant trend to be more distractible, irritable, impulsive, anxious, and histrionic, and a greater tendency to demonstrate depressive equivalents, such as delinquency. Relationships tended to be disturbed. There were, moreover, positive attributes which discriminated between the two groups. The experimental group was rated as more attractive and more intelligent (probably because of high verbal ability). While only one child of the comparison group warranted a diagnosis (depression), sixteen children in the experimental group were given diagnoses by DSM III criteria.

All the cases were then reviewed by the three project psychiatrists to explore the presence of any clinical patterns of developing traits. Three broad clinical groups were recognized, into which twenty-five of the thirty-one children could be placed by unanimous consensus. These groups were identified as Extroverted, Inhibited, and Impulsive. A fourth, miscellaneous category was added. Each group contained children at various levels of functioning, the most dysfunctional group being the Impulsive one. Characteristics of children in the Extroverted and Inhibited groups resembled those frequently described in association with affective illness. As postulated, the children of manicdepressives, in a small but carefully controlled study, did show a Verbal/Performance discrepancy on the WISC-R which discriminated the experimental group from the control group. There was no relationship between this discrepancy and psychiatric diagnoses, but there was a significant association between the Verbal/Performance discrepancy and the ten children in the Extroverted group. (The mean Verbal/Performance discrepancy was 15.1 for this group versus 4.1 for the remainder of the bipolar index cases and 1.6 for the comparison group.)

Preliminary data from the small pilot project indicate that the children of bipolar manic-depressives are more symptomatic and demonstrate more psychopathology than the comparison group. No absolute premorbid picture has been defined, but several patterns seem to be worth pursuing. Certainly some symptomatic children could be reacting to the daily stress of living with an ill parent. However, a subgroup of the children of manic-depressives, including many who were asymptomatic and highly functioning, showed specific traits (triple-X) and a particular cognitive style (high verbal, lower performance). These children demonstrate a fundamental vulnerability to bipolar illness which may become manifest under stressful circumstances.

Michael Strober and Gabrielle Carlson's chapter, "Predictors of Bipolar Illness in Adolescents with Major Depression: A Follow-Up Investigation," sheds further light on the problem of differential diagnoses. The clinical importance of their findings cannot be overestimated. Carlson and Strober's (1978) original work called into question the disproportionate prevalence of schizophrenic diagnoses in young psychotic patients. Often it was not until readmission for a second psychotic break that correct manic-depressive diagnosis was finally established and appropriate pharmacological treatment instituted.

In this chapter, the effort to determine which depressed adolescent is exhibiting the first phase of a manic-depressive illness is described in detail. Sixty young adolescents, hospitalized for major depression, were studied prospectively for three to four years. Twenty percent of the cohort developed bipolar illness. Predictors were found to be: (1) rapid symptom onset, psychomotor retardation, and mood-congruent psychotic features; (2) strongly positive family history of affective disorder (often bipolar); and (3) pharmacologically induced hypomania. The implication is that bipolars are far more vulnerable than unipolars to "switches" into hypomania or mania, as Bunney (1978) has postulated.

The chapter by Donald H. McKnew, Jr., Leon Cytryn, Martine Lamour, and Alan Apter, "Fantasy in Childhood Depression and Other Forms of Child Psychopathology," explores the relationship of depressive fantasy in children to the diagnosis of clinical depression and general psychopathology. These authors have contributed much to diagnostic accuracy and nosology for affective disorders in children. Their present findings suggest that the nature of the fantasies of a small cohort of children of manic-depressive parents were not distinguishable from children with other forms of psychopathology. These findings vary somewhat from those of Kron, Decina, and Kestenbaum, who found significant differences in fantasy production of index cases as compared with controls, but other studies have corroborated their results, indicating that the presence of nightmares and morbid fantasies in children is an indication of general psychopathology and is not specific to depression.

The final chapter, "Functional Brain Asymmetry and Affective Disorders," by Harold A. Sackeim, Paolo Decina, and Sidney Malitz, is an attempt to organize the large body of information regarding lateralization in brain mechanisms subserving the regulation of mood. It also examines the evidence supporting the hypothesis of disturbance in lateralization in affective disorders, specifically characterized by right-side dysfunction. The authors review the literature on split-brain research. There seems to be greater involvement (overactivation and/or dysfunction) of the right relative to the left hemisphere in depressed states, and right-side dysfunction is reported in several studies involving bipolar probands as compared with unipolars.

The cerebral laterality studies may hold the key to the discovery of a fundamental genetic liability—the lack of some central inhibiting regulating mechanism—which may lead to a manic-depressive illness in later life. Evidence for this hypothesis may be forthcoming from further investigation of neuropsychological functions (including the study of discrepancies in cognitive functions, as with the WISC discrepancy in a subgroup of children at risk), neurophysiological data on individuals with bipolar illness, and careful clinical assessment. With such information available, the problem of intervention will be greatly simplified.

To return full circle to the paper by Feinstein: It seems highly likely that the children he describes demonstrate a genetic vulnerability to manic-depressive illness that under stress may become manifest. Bunney has conceptualized the change from depression to mania in a vulnerable adult as a "switch process" which may be brought on by bereavement or other stressful life events. The adult in the manic phase is bombarded by stimuli he cannot sort out, that is, flights of ideas, pressured speech, clang associations. When there is a breakdown of reality-testing functions, he can become delusional. The child so constitutionally prone may also exhibit similar features early in life. He can exhibit extreme silliness, hyperactivity, sleep disturbance, pressured speech, and increased magical thinking in an attempt to deny social or academic problems.

What, then, in a symptomatic child, should be the treatment of choice: psychotherapy or lithium? Ginsberg (1979) notes that "at present, whether proven or not, we assume that there are genetic, biochemical, physiological, hormonal, and psychological aspects that are relevant to mania. Our view of this condition is . . . interactional and suggests that for some a biological interaction is most efficacious; for others a psychological intervention; for most people both will be ideal."

Feinstein also recommends both supportive and intensive psychoanalytic psychotherapy in the presence of developmental defect. He believes that the affective lability of childhood may be considered a traumatic factor in early development and often results in developmental interference which may contribute to later borderline personality organization with distortions in object relationships.

Although psychotherapy is, in my opinion, a necessary component of treatment, for an individual in the manic phase insight into his condition is usually lacking and, under these circumstances, lithium has proved to be the most effective agent in facilitating a patient's acceptance of his disorder.

Children with a manic-depressive diathesis present certain particular problems for the therapist. For example, the grandiosity and inflated self-worth of these children—their narcissism—is but a thin veneer covering a host of negative feelings about themselves. Their sensitivity to the slightest criticism (and every interpretation is taken as such) causes them to construct thick walls that are difficult to penetrate. There is, moreover, a denial of problems so that the inventiveness of the most skillful therapist is strained. Finally, sensitivity to loss is often demonstrated by extreme reactions to the therapist's vacation or even an occasional session canceled due to illness.

The parents of these children are often unaware of their children's problems. They themselves may use denial as their chief defense, so that it is often difficult to convince such parents of their children's vulnerability. Children need to be made aware of their own emotional lability when under stress. One adolescent described his fear of losing control: "I feel as if I had a Cadillac engine inside all wound up to go, but my body is only a Model-T Ford. I can barely hold it down, and if I let go for a minute, it'll go off on its own and I'll never be able to stop."

On a positive note, I would like to add that young patients with an affective disorder are often among the brightest, most sensitive, and creative individuals we encounter. They are often endowed with special gifts and should be encouraged to develop them, whether in the sphere of music, art, literature, or human relationships. They are most capable of tenderness and empathy when they do not feel threatened themselves. By helping such children negotiate the difficult adolescent years (because they do need protection from the intensity of their drives as well as from the events of the external world), we are protecting them from future psychotic breakdown or at least ameliorating such breakdown as well as enhancing the quality of everyday life. Thus the rewards of at-risk research speak for themselves.

REFERENCES

Akiskal, H. S. 1981. Subaffective disorders: dysthymic, clyclothymic and bipolar II disorders in the "borderline" realm. *Psychiatric Clinics of North America* 4(1): 25–46.

Bunney, W. E. 1978. Psychopharmacology of the switch process in affective illness. In M. A. Lipton, A. DiMascio, and K. F. Killam, eds. *Psychopharmacology: A Generation of Progress.* New York: Raven.

Carlson, G. A., and Strober, M. 1978. Manic-depressive illness in early adolescence. *Journal of the American Academy of Child Psychiatry* 17(1): 138–153.

Cohen, M. D.; Baker, G.; Cohen, R. A.; Fromm-Reichman, F.; and Weigert, E. V. 1954. An intensive study of twelve cases of manic-depressive psychosis. *Psychiatry* 17:103–137.

DSM III. 1980. *Diagnostic and Statistical Manual of Mental Disorders.* 3d ed. Washington, D.C.: American Psychiatric Association.

Erlenmeyer-Kimling, L.; Cornblatt, B.; and Fleiss, J. 1979. High risk research in schizophrenia. *Psychiatric Annals* 9:38.

Feinstein, S. C., and Wolpert, E. A. 1973. Juvenile manic-depressive illness: clinical and therapeutic considerations. *Journal of the American Academy of Child Psychiatry* 12:123–136.

Ginsberg, G. L. 1979. Psychoanalytic aspects of mania. In B. Shopsin, ed. *Manic Illness.* New York: Raven.

Gunderson, J. G., and Singer, M. T. 1975. Defining borderline patients: an overview. *American Journal of Psychiatry* 132:1–10.

Kestenbaum, C. J. 1979. Children at-risk for manic-depressive illness: possible predictors. *American Journal of Psychiatry* 136:1206–1208.

Kestenbaum, C. J. 1980. Adolescents at risk for manic-depressive illness. *Adolescent Psychiatry* 8:344–366.

Kraepelin, E. 1921. Manic-depressive insanity and paranoia. In E. Wolpert, ed. *Manic Depressive Illness.* New York: International Universities Press, 1977.

Loranger, A., and Levine, P. 1978. Age of onset of bipolar affective illness. *Archives of General Psychiatry* 35:1345–1348.

McKnew, D. H.; Cytryn, L.; Efron, A. M.; Gershon, E. S.; and Bunney, W. E. 1979. Offspring of patients with affective disorders. *British Journal of Psychiatry* 134:148–152.

McKnew, D. H.; Cytryn, L.; and White, I. 1974. Clinical and biochemical correlates of hypomania in a child. *Journal of Child Psychiatry* 13:576–585.

254

Perris, C. 1966. A study of bipolar (manic-depressive) and unipolar recurrent depressive psychoses. *Acta Psychiatrica Scandinavica* (suppl. 194) 42:1–188.

Rosenthal, D. 1970. *Genetic Theory and Abnormal Behavior.* New York: McGraw-Hill.

Shopsin, B. 1979. Mania: clinical aspects, rating scales and incidence of manic-depressive illness. In B. Shopsin, ed. *Manic Illness.* New York: Raven.

Stone, M. H. 1979. A psychoanalytic approach to abnormalities of temperament. *American Journal of Psychotherapy* 32(2): 263–280.

Winokur, G.; Clayton, P. J.; and Reich, T. 1969. *Manic-Depressive Illness.* St. Louis: Mosby.

NOTE

The papers in this special section were presented in a symposium held at the 134th Annual Meeting of the American Psychiatric Association, New Orleans, May 13, 1981.

19 MANIC-DEPRESSIVE DISORDER IN CHILDREN AND ADOLESCENTS

SHERMAN C. FEINSTEIN

In adults the essential feature of bipolar affective disorders is a disturbance of mood which may assume full or partial manic or depressive symptoms. DSM III (1980) divides affective disorder into major affective disorders, other specific affective disorders (cyclothymic disorder and dysthymic disorder), and atypical affective disorders, a residual category for those reactions that do not fulfill the defined entities.

In children and adolescents bipolar affective disorder, manifesting a manic-depressive pattern, may show specific equivalent behaviors that are the precursors of the cyclothymic personality and manic-depressive illness states of adulthood. Recent findings (Feinstein 1980; Kestenbaum 1980; Youngerman and Canino 1978) suggest that the affective system of patients with manic-depressive illness may have a basic vulnerability which, when overstimulated, begins a discharge pattern that does not respond easily to autonomous emotional control. Some biological variation (probably on a genetic basis) leaves the affective system with specific vulnerability to affective stress. The typical bipolar cyclic states of adulthood, therefore, may be considered illness patterns rather than minimal criteria for diagnosis (Feinstein 1973, 1980; Feinstein and Wolpert 1973).

In Kraepelin's (1904, 1921) classical description of the disorder, manic-depressive insanity was classified a unitary form of mental illness distinct from schizophrenia with periodic and circular manifestations, including manic and depressive confusion and delirium. He also included mood changes, periodic or continuous, which seemed to stem from personal predisposition. Beyond common fundamental features,

Kraepelin noted that the clinical picture frequently changed, the prognosis was generally good, and he believed the illness had hereditary roots.

Developmental Aspects of Affective Disorders

While the normal individual is generally aware that he is subject to variations in mood, he rarely perceives that rhythmic changes affect his biological and emotional patterns daily and over a long period of time (Feinstein 1973). For the first sixteen weeks of life the infant's biological rhythms of sleep and other physiological functions normally deviate from the twenty-four-hour circadian rhythm of the adult caretakers. The maternal care provides a stimulus barrier for the still vulnerable newborn, and slowly the infant begins to exhibit activity and feeding patterns consonant with his family and the world around him.

During early childhood, from seven to eighteen months of age, phenomena of mood are of great importance. Most children demonstrate major periods of exhilaration or relative elation alternating with "low-keyed" periods when they become aware that mother is absent from the room (Mahler 1972). At these times gestural and performance motility are reduced, interest in their surroundings diminishes, and they seem inwardly preoccupied. This low-keyed state may be inferred when comfort from another person may cause the child to burst into tears, and the state disappears with mother's return. Mahler compares this "dampened down" state to a miniature anaclitic depression and believes that during this period of quiescence the child is attempting to hold onto the memory of the mother by "imaging" (Rubenfine 1961). This is an early phase of the subsequently developed stage of object constancy during which the introjected memory of the mother can easily be maintained.

Patients who eventually manifest manic-depressive illness may have a desynchronization in the area of affective development. The early histories of many manic-depressive patients clearly indicate an interference with the capacity to dampen down, a developmental milestone which should be accomplished by two years of age. This is the possible result of some genetic-physiological impairment in the switching mechanisms as described by Bunney, Goodwin, Davis, and Fawcett (1968) and Bunney, Goodwin, and Murphy (1972) in which rapid and reversible changes from mania to depression and vice versa involve neurotransmitter (i.e., biogenic amine) function at the adrenergic nerve

257

endings or some instability of the neuronal membrane. More recently, genetic studies have not confirmed linkage (Gershon 1978) but did find a history of subclinical affective disturbance in childhood (McKnew, Cytryn, Efron, Gershon, and Bunney 1979).

Childhood and Manic-Depressive Illness

Arieti (1959) and Cohen, Baker, Cohen, Fromm-Reichman, and Weigert (1954) described early childhood patterns of manic-depressive adults and saw them as repressed children dominated by strong but changeable parents. Anthony and Scott (1960) questioned whether manic-depressive illness ever occurred in a clinically recognizable form in the younger child but were "prepared to admit . . . that certain 'embryonic' features may make a transient appearance in the very early years." They believed that there was a "manic-depressive tendency" that was latent in the susceptible individual and existed in an internalized form.

BEHAVIORAL PROFILE

My review of early developmental histories of diagnosed manic-depressive children and adolescents has revealed a behavioral profile usually consisting of all or most of the following characteristics:

1. Early evidence of affective instability. As early as one year of age parents recognize a pattern of affective extremes.

2. Dysphoric reactions to early stages of separation-individuation. The child has little ability to dampen down or achieve a low-keyed state. Separations usually lead to exaggerated reactions to loss frequently manifested as temper tantrums or periodic hyperactivity.

3. Dilation of the ego with persistence of grandiose and idealizing self-structures owing to failure of normal transformations of narcissism. This may manifest itself as an outgoing, dramatic quality with a theatrical flair. Many histories reveal early interest in acting and an easy willingness to perform.

4. Infantile circadian patterns tend to persist with reactions governed by inner, affective impulses rather than shifting to the environmental patterns of the family. Bizarre eating and sleep patterns and impulsivity may continue in spite of all efforts to enforce normal daily rhythms.

5. There is very frequently a family history of affective disorder. In

addition to the presence of bipolar and unipolar patterns, equivalent states such as alcoholism or compulsive gambling may be elicited.

MANIC-DEPRESSIVE DISORDER IN A PRESCHOOL-AGED CHILD

Jody was first seen at age three because of hyperactivity, low frustration tolerance, impulsive and destructive behavior, and inability to concentrate. The second of three children, she was active at birth and her care was considered difficult. She slept in short spurts and ate poorly. Coordination was good, walking developed at fourteen months, but she was seen as hyperactive, impulsive, and uncontainable.

Mother sought psychiatric evaluation at age two because Jody changed moods very rapidly. While playing and without apparent reason she would hit, bite, scratch, and become destructive. On one occasion mother was reading her a story and Jody suddenly turned and bit her. During these occasional periods of irrational behavior she responded to no one and was very destructive. When frustrated she would roll around on the floor flailing her arms and legs, and was difficult to reach verbally. Mother described several incidents when Jody would start crying and tell her she felt "bad inside" and wished she could die.

At other times, for long periods, she was likable, warm, friendly, and outgoing. She had a difficult time in nursery school and kindergarten with separation and relating to other children. However, her relationships with teachers were positive and her work was capable and creative.

The parents were cooperative and well motivated. Mother insisted that there was something wrong with Jody even though assured by her pediatrician and a psychiatric evaluation that Jody was developing normally. Mother described herself as a rather cyclothymic individual with mood swings, accentuated when fatigued. A maternal aunt (mother's sister) manifests wide mood swings and has had some manic psychotic episodes. Both maternal grandparents suffer from severe emotional difficulties; grandfather is a depressive with years of treatment and grandmother is described as a classic manic-depressive.

Jody was receiving weekly psychotherapy from age three with some overall improvement. At the age of five years, after an upsetting incident, she became agitated, hyperactive, and demanding and remained in this agitated state for several months. She regressed to provocative, destructive behavior and appeared dilated and hypomanic. In school she was destructive, fought with her peers, and insulted and attacked close friends. After several months of close consultation with the family and the use of tranquilizers, Jody calmed down and resumed her better-integrated state. Several months later a similar episode was precipitated.

It was at this point that it occurred to me that we might be dealing with a bipolar, alternating mood state which was rooted in biological vulnerabilities and triggered by depressive reactions. The affective crisis resembled the dilated, hypomanic state of the adult and had many characteristics of a periodic reaction unrelated to reality stress.

Therefore, at age five and one-half, a decision was made to attempt to treat these alternating affective states with lithium carbonate. An evaluation of her cardiac, renal, and thyroid systems was undertaken and proved normal except for the discovery that the patient had manifested a periodic "salt hunger" for many years and would eat large quantities of table salt. At the point Jody cycled into a state of manic behavior, lithium carbonate, 900 mg daily, was started on an outpatient basis. Within two weeks with monitoring of the blood lithium level every three days and adjusting the lithium intake to assure a blood level of 0.8–1.2 meq/liter, a noticeable leveling off of the manic affective state occurred and the patient was able to resume her usual activities without the destructive, agitated symptoms. In addition the salt craving seemed to disappear.

Jody has remained on lithium carbonate, 900 mg daily, for the past twelve years and has periodically received psychotherapy. There have been brief recurrences of the periodic cyclic manic episodes when she stopped her lithium impulsively. In general we see a child who continues to function in school and at home. While there was a remarkable amount of immaturity present, there has been a gradual improvement in function, but patient is considered a borderline personality with difficulties in object relationships and self-esteem.

We believe that Jody is an example of juvenile manic-depressive disorder. The onset of the illness was recognized by age two by the mother, but distinct phasic disturbance was not seen until age five.

Prior to this, distinct, episodic moods with erratic, disintegrative behavior were seen to alternate with periods of highly integrated behavior. Intellectual functioning has always remained intact. The affective episodes seem to have been precipitated by loss reactions which overwhelmed the ego and resulted in a shift to affective solutions (Feinstein 1967).

MANIC-DEPRESSIVE DISORDER IN A LATENCY AGED CHILD

Jan, the second of three children, was first seen at age ten after she had an emotional outburst which upset the school and her parents. She was described as being restless, provocative, constantly bickering, excessively curious, and functioning poorly in school. Described as always being bright and precocious, she was born eleven months after her older sister. She seemed happy and alert for the first few years and related to her sister as though she were a twin, and parents treated them as such.

She began manifesting symptoms of excessive reactivity, hyperactivity, and irritability at age three, following the birth of her younger brother. This was a difficult time for the family. Father failed in his business in California. Mother was struggling with severe separation anxiety and insisted on a move back to Chicago, where they moved in with the maternal grandparents. Jan had a poor relationship with her grandmother, was irritable and negativistic, apparently suffering from the birth of the brother, the move, and her mother's depression.

Jan's symptomatic behaviors continued for several years and interfered with her early school adjustment. She was described as hyperactive and isolated. A diagnostic evaluation at age five revealed an IQ of 144 with projective test results which described her as "unusual." She perceived her parents as "mad" and was preoccupied with death. Psychiatric evaluation found her constricted, anxious, and angry, but affectless on the surface. Psychotherapy was advised but not carried out.

Jan's school adjustment has continued to be difficult. Under stress she becomes "paranoid" and "glazed over" as she withdraws. She has a short attention span and does not concentrate.

Mother described her behavior as having a definite cyclic pattern. These phases last several months and the "bad cycle" is characterized by frenetic activity, an inability to stop talking, and increased difficulty with relationships.

In the family, the paternal grandmother died early, and paternal grandfather had a stroke and a severe depression before death. Maternal great-grandfather is reported to have had a senile depression. Maternal grandmother is described as unstable and has had depressive episodes.

In psychiatric examination, Jan, a petite, attractive ten-year-old, was precocious and dramatic. She was very feminine and seductive and made herself comfortable. She inspected the office in a dilated fashion, commenting on the furniture, the "original" paintings, and tiny details of my clothing. She quoted television commercials, wisecracked about her teachers and school, and offered to share her chewing gum with me. She talked about feeling "high" and said she liked the sensation of feeling "drunk."

Her general speech was a flight of ideas, with rapid, loose associations. Thought content was not distorted and sensorium was clear. She discussed her difficulty in controlling affects and reported she frequently cannot stop laughing but handles it by acting "gruffy." She described herself as an anxious person who did not bother others with her fears. "I'm just a chicken. I just sit in bed and worry half the night."

A tentative diagnosis of manic-depressive disorder was made and, after a medical workup, lithium carbonate, 900 mg daily, was prescribed. Patient was seen in once weekly psychotherapy with a gradual leveling off of dilated affect. Jan was able to go to camp for two weeks and had no separation anxiety. She remained outgoing and vivacious, but there were no violent affective swings. Long-term follow-up has included a manic episode at age sixteen after stopping medication. Independent evaluation confirmed the presence of manic-depressive illness. Patient resumed lithium therapy and is continuing with her education, but her personality development is immature and unstable.

Adolescence and Manic-Depressive Disorder

The longitudinal, observational approach has confirmed the etiological importance of early infantile development, the oedipal period, and latency to psychic growth. Adolescence as a developmental stage is now considered to have the same degree of significance as an etiological precursor of later development. This developmental work, which has been described by Blos (1967) as a recapitulation of the separation-individuation tasks, makes the adolescent vulnerable not only to normal everyday stress but also to unresolved conflicts from infancy and childhood. Other descriptions of the developmental work during adolescence include a liquefaction of the ego (Eissler 1958) and partial regression of the ego to the stage of undifferentiated object relationships in the service of ego mastery (Freud 1958; Geleerd 1961). This major reworking of the ego defenses at the service of character synthesis renders the pubertal adolescent susceptible to a breakdown of defenses and an emergence of symptoms.

The emergence of symptomatic manic-depressive illness during adolescence is more common than during childhood. Again, the early manifestations of the affect-based illness do not conform to the traditional descriptions but rather reflect the developmental level and the particular vicissitudes with which an adolescent is dealing. In addition, the amount of bipolar affective instability may be dependent on the genetic configuration and the quality of early character development.

CLINICAL FEATURES

Manic-depressive illness may emerge during puberty and adolescence manifesting some of the following symptoms:

1. Severe adolescent rebellion manifested by negativism, overconfidence, and an insistence on a feeling of well-being.

2. Exaggerated self-esteem with grandiose conceptions of physical, mental, and moral powers and overcommitment to adolescent tasks.

3. Heightened motor activity manifested by restlessness, hyperactivity, and in some examples by the compulsive overactivity of anorexia nervosa. Several patients with anorexia nervosa were later discovered to have manic-depressive illness, and this should be thought of and ruled out in every case of anorexia.

4. Exaggeration of libidinal impulses may surface as a sudden change from an inhibited child to an aggressive, sexually acting-out adolescent. Puberty, particularly in girls, may be seen as a great threat to the body image. In one case a period of amenorrhea after menarche eventuated into a manic-depressive breakdown with delusions of being pregnant.

5. Gradual emergence of a cyclic, bipolar pattern of affect disorder but often manifesting itself as marked instability with short periods of

depression and mania rather than the longer periods typical of adult manic-depression. Suicidal ideation is frequently noted.

MANIC-DEPRESSIVE DISORDER IN AN ADOLESCENT

Art is a twenty-one-year-old white male admitted with a manic-affective state. While preparing to transfer to a college away from home, his behavior became expansive and dilated, increasing in mood until he was in a classical manic frenzy with agitation, flight of ideas, pressure of speech, and an inability to control affects.

Patient, who has been known to our institution from age fourteen, has been under continuous psychiatric treatment in various hospitals, residential treatment centers, and outpatient facilities. In the two years prior to the current episode, he attended a junior college and remained in treatment with a social worker at a child-care agency. Various diagnoses were made from schizophrenia to character and neurotic disorders. Some descriptions of hypomanic behavior were scattered through the descriptive material, and one psychiatrist mentioned manic-depressive psychosis as part of the differential diagnosis. The psychological studies all struggled diagnostically because the schizophrenic behavior was contrasted with an absence of a thought disorder.

His parents report that Art had marked difficulty with affective controls from infancy. The second of five children, he had a difficult birth and had trouble sucking at first. While a good eater eventually, he required three to four bottles of milk during the night through his second year. Teething was an ordeal with continuous irritability. He reacted poorly to aspirin and barbiturates. He was a very active child, constantly in motion. He weaned with difficulty at age two, crying continuously for nights. He used a pacifier until four and sucked his thumb voraciously until adolescence.

Art had severe separation anxiety which became agitated if parents went on a vacation. After their return he would take weeks to settle down, requiring mother to sit with him for hours while he fell asleep.

A nursery school teacher described him at age four as having "peculiar mood changes." He would alternate between being "the life and soul and leader of an activity and suddenly without apparent cause would withdraw, put on his jacket, and suck his thumb in a corner." This pattern persisted throughout early life until overt symptoms of severe anxiety, temper tantrums, and, retrospectively, manic states began at age eleven following the death of a close relative and prior to a move to the United States from another country.

Paternal grandfather was described as a depressive character. Maternal grandfather at the age of forty-five suddenly left his business and became a compulsive gambler and alcoholic. He became alienated from his family and deteriorated.

Patient was placed on lithium carbonate, requiring doses as high as 2,400 mg daily until the manic state was controlled. This case represents an example of manic-depressive illness which was not recognized early and seems retrospectively to fulfill the criteria of juvenile manic-depressive illness. Long-term follow-up has confirmed the diagnosis of manic-depression and, after a stormy course, patient has accepted his illness and continued therapy. He is making a good adjustment although he remains vulnerable to cyclic affective states.

Diagnostic Aspects of Manic-Depressive Disorder

The identification of manic-depressive disorder in childhood has been a matter of some controversy, subject to changes in diagnostic fashion (Anthony and Scott 1960). This ambiguity stems from a multiplicity of sources, both theoretical and practical. Traditional analytic thinkers have been particularly reluctant to acknowledge the existence of childhood affective disorders because, by psychoanalytic definition, clinical depression presupposes the development of superego structures. Psychodynamic theorists such as Klein, meanwhile, have postulated mania as an inherent infantile coping mechanism—not necessarily an aberrant state.

Resolution of this conflict has not been forthcoming, in part because of inconsistent diagnostic criteria for assessing affective illness and a concomitant lack of observational agreement. Failure to identify depressive equivalents in the behavior-disordered child is one such limitation. Flight of ideas and pressured speech, commonly associated with manic-depression, have been considered by others to be a pathognomic of schizophrenia (Carlson 1979). Similarly, such behavioral characteristics as distractibility, lability of affect, and irritability—which would seem to be definitional of manic-depressive disorder—are often interpreted as hyperactivity, clearly not a psychotic state.

The criteria usually employed for the diagnosis of manic-depressive illness reflect Kraepelin's (1921) early descriptive studies. By utilizing end states, such as a full-blown manic episode, as criteria, this system overlooks important developmental changes in affect and thus would seem to preclude the diagnosis of manic-depressive illness in children. The diagnostic requirement that there should be both a distinct and marked phasic disturbance of affect (Redlich and Freedman 1966) and evidence of a state approximating the classical description (Anthony and Scott 1960) frequently delays the diagnosis for many years.

Klein (1934) contends that in early development the child passes through a transient manic state which she considers a defense against early infantile depression. The basis for this inference was her observation of the infant's feeling of omnipotence and control over objects. In normal children, however, this natural overreaction typically disappears by the age of two as they develop a sense of separateness from mother and a self-concept. The persistence of mood extremes, coupled with a family history of affective disorder, could be considered consistent with early indications of affective illness.

Davis (1979) describes what he calls a specific manic-depressive variant syndrome of childhood which requires the presence of affective storms; a family history of affective disorder; mental, physical, or verbal overactivity; troubled interpersonal relationships; and no formal thought disorder in children who respond to lithium carbonate.

The frequency of breakdown in manic-depressive illness increases with the development of puberty and the onset of adolescence. Again, the affective reactions are age appropriate and emphasize those defenses which are critical at a particular stage of life.

The question of the timing of the breakdown is of great interest. The loss of a parent and the transition from childhood to adolescence are both considered major demands on the gradually emerging adolescent ego. Mourning and progression through transitional developmental states require the capacity to utilize ego defenses in the mastery of the loss of loved objects (mother, childhood). A fundamental defect in the affect system, probably genetically determined, overwhelms the ego defenses, and the resultant affective reactions may be characterized as manic-depressive, essentially indicating exaggerated or blocked capacities to deal with the normal affective response to the perception of a loss. If the intensity of the stimulation is too great or the environmental supports are sadomasochistic rather than accepting and supportive, an alteration of consciousness may result, manifested by psychotic thinking or behavior.

Schizophrenia in adolescents is frequently a difficult diagnosis to make and, as Masterson (1967) points out, only in 25 percent of seriously disturbed adolescents can the diagnosis be made at the onset; the long-term picture of the disease process emerges slowly during the diagnostic and therapeutic process. Stone (1971) discusses the dilemmas of making a definite diagnosis of manic-depressive illness and the present tendency to call a patient "schizophrenic till proven otherwise." The diagnosis of manic-depressive illness in adolescents is made keeping in mind adolescent behavioral equivalents of the classical end results of a bipolar affective disorder.

Anthony and Scott (1960) believe that a genetic clock is operative in an individual who is genetically predisposed or environmentally handicapped. Gershon (1978) reviewed genetic markers used in studies of psychiatric illness and studied red-green color blindness, Xg blood group antigen, and histocompatibility lymphocyte antigen (HLA). The evidence has been against close linkage for each of these markers. The most promising prediction of vulnerability in adult life is the presence of subclinical disturbance in childhood (McKnew et al. 1979).

Treatment of Juvenile Manic-Depressive Illness

A major advance in the treatment of the manic-depressive disorders is the present extensive use of lithium carbonate. First described by Cade (1949), who noted that lithium salts seemed efficacious in treating acute affective disorders of the manic-depressive type, lithium now appears equally effective as a prophylactic agent in preventing or minimizing recurrences (Baastrup and Schou 1967). Lithium carbonate is considered a safe drug and functions without blunting of perception or intellect (Kline 1969; Schlagenhauf, Tipin, and White 1966; Schou 1959, 1968). The common toxic symptoms of the fine hand tremor, anorexia, nausea, and diarrhea rapidly disappear if the dosage is reduced (Wolpert and Mueller 1969).

Annell (1969) described the use of lithium in twelve children from the age of seven upward. Only two adolescent patients (ages fourteen and sixteen) manifested typical signs of a manic state. All others demonstrated various symptom complexes (sleep disorders, night terrors, and vegetative disorders, for example, stomachaches and headaches) but many had histories of manic-depressive illness in their families which led to the idea of trying the medication on an empirical basis. The cases selected for that study were characterized by the sudden change between normalcy and depression, or between depression and hyperactivity, that has been described as typical of the bipolar type of depression found in the manic-depressive psychosis (Perris 1969).

The use of lithium carbonate has been reported in young children and adolescents with promising results (Carlson 1979; Feinstein and Wolpert 1973; Youngerman and Canino 1978). Careful medical cooperation is necessary, and the dosage and lithium blood-level studies must be carefully monitored. Even though the use of lithium in cases of affective illness frequently leads to a rapid resolution of the manic attack, the importance of concomitant psychotherapy should not be overlooked.

CLINICAL MANAGEMENT

A thorough medical survey should be conducted in children and adolescents with careful attention to cardiac, renal, liver, and thyroid function. An electroencephalogram should be secured if there is any history of convulsive disorder since lithium may lower the convulsive threshold. Continuous monitoring of thyroid function is necessary because of the thyroid-suppressing effects of lithium. None of our series has been affected, but several adults being followed have developed hypothyroidism.

The average dosage of lithium ranges from 900 mg to 1,800 mg (or higher) depending on the blood level. The general therapeutic range is 0.8–1.4 meq/liter with the most comfortable range between 1.0 and 1.2 meq/liter. Patients in a manic phase usually require a higher dosage to maintain therapeutic levels, but that level can be reduced with symptom remission (Carlson 1979).

Lithium carbonate is now available as tablets, capsules, and in the liquid as lithium citrate. Well absorbed by the gastrointestinal tract, the blood level peaks in two hours after ingestion, and half-life in adolescents is eighteen to twenty-four hours. Many children complain of gastric irritation, and it is recommended that lithium be taken with food; smaller, more frequent doses may minimize the distress, or slow-release preparations may be effective. Weekly lithium levels should be obtained for the first month or until a stable therapeutic dose is achieved; then monthly or bimonthly.

Side effects are minor (nausea, fine tremor, polyuria, polydipsia, weight gain, and toxicity) and are usually controlled by slight dosage reduction (Carlson 1979). Uncontrolled symptoms of affective disorder or psychotic reaction may require additional use of tranquilizers and antidepressants with appropriate attention to the toxic effects of these drugs, especially haloperidol.

PSYCHOTHERAPY

Our long-term experience with a group of childhood and adolescent manic-depressives has led us to recommend ongoing supportive psychotherapy as well as more intensive psychoanalytic psychotherapy in the presence of developmental defect. The affective lability of childhood may be considered a traumatic factor in early development and often results in developmental interferences resulting in borderline personality organization. Many of our study group demonstrated personality organization, as described by Kernberg (1978), Masterson (1978), and Schwartzberg (1978), manifesting broad interference with self-development and distortions in object relationships.

Conclusions

The examples presented describe children and adolescents with periodic alternating affective disorders who can be considered cases of juvenile manic-depressive illness. Manic-depressive disorder may appear in early childhood, manifesting itself as erratic, rapidly shifting mood behavior with a basic intactness of intellect. The apparent lack of precipitating trauma may be explained by the enormous sensitivity of these patients to loss or the fear of loss which triggers a distinct, affective episode.

The effectiveness of lithium carbonate makes the early diagnosis of manic-depressive disorder necessary. Lithium carbonate is a useful drug in the treatment of juvenile manic-depressive illness, and its use is described along with the definite need for psychotherapy to facilitate acceptance of the disorder and to avoid characterological defect.

REFERENCES

Annel, A. L. 1969. Lithium in the treatment of children and adolescents. *Acta Psychiatrica Scandinavica* (suppl.) 207:19–33.

Anthony, E. J., and Scott, P. 1960. Manic-depressive psychosis in childhood. *Journal of Child Psychology and Psychiatry* 1:53–72.

Arieti, S. 1959. Manic-depressive psychosis. In S. Arieti, ed. *American Handbook of Psychiatry*. New York: Basic.

Baastrup, P. D., and Schou, M. 1967. Lithium as a prophylactic agent: its effect against recurrent depressions and manic-depressive psychosis. *Archives of General Psychiatry* 17:162–172.

Blos, P. 1967. The second individuation process of adolescence. *Psychoanalytic Study of the Child* 22:162–186.

Bunney, W. E., Jr.; Goodwin, F. K.; Davis, J. M.; and Fawcett, J. A. 1968. A behavioral-biochemical study of lithium treatment. *American Journal of Psychiatry* 125:499–512.

Bunney, W. E., Jr.; Goodwin, F. K.; and Murphy, D. L. 1972. The "switch process" in manic-depressive illness. III. Theoretical implications. *Archives of General Psychiatry* 27:312–317.

Cade, J. F. 1949. Lithium salts in the treatment of psychotic excitement. *Medical Journal of Australia* 36: 349–352.

Carlson, G. A. 1979. Lithium use in adolescents: clinical indications and management. *Adolescent Psychiatry* 7:410–418.

Cohen, M. D.; Baker, G.; Cohen, R. A.; Fromm-Reichmann, F.; and Weigert, E. V. 1954. An intensive study of twelve cases of manic-depressive psychosis. *Psychiatry* 17:103–137.

Davis, R. E. 1979. Manic-depressive variant syndrome of childhood. *American Journal of Psychiatry* 136:702–705.

DSM III. 1980. *Diagnostic and Statistical Manual of Mental Disorders*. 3d ed. Washington, D.C.: American Psychiatric Association.

Eissler, K. R. 1958. Notes on problems of technique in the psychoanalytic treatment of adolescents. *Psychoanalytic Study of the Child* 13:223–254.

Feinstein, S. C. 1967. Aggression and adolescence. *Bulletin of the Chicago Society for Adolescent Psychiatry* 1:1–8.

Feinstein, S. C. 1973. Diagnostic and therapeutic aspects of manic-depressive illness in early childhood. *Early Child Development and Care* 3:1–12.

Feinstein, S. C. 1980. Why they were afraid of Virginia Woolf: perspectives on juvenile manic-depressive illness. *Adolescent Psychiatry* 8:332–343.

Feinstein, S., and Wolpert, E. 1973. Juvenile manic-depressive illness: clinical and therapeutic considerations. *Journal of the American Academy of Child Psychiatry* 12:123–136.

Freud, A. 1958. Adolescence. *Psychoanalytic Study of the Child* 13:255–278.

Freud, S. 1923. The ego and the id. *Standard Edition* 19:13–66. London: Hogarth, 1961.

Geleerd, E. R. 1961. Some aspects of ego vicissitudes in adolescence. *Journal of the American Psychoanalytic Association* 9:394–405.

Gershon, E. S. 1978. Genetic markers in affective illness. *Continuing Medical Education Syllabus and Scientific Proceedings.* Annual Meeting American Psychiatric Association. Abstract 223:109. Washington, D.C.: American Psychiatric Association.

Kernberg, O. F. 1978. The diagnosis of borderline conditions in adolescence. *Adolescent Psychiatry* 6:298–319.

Kestenbaum, C. J. 1980. Adolescents at risk for manic-depressive illness. *Adolescent Psychiatry* 8:344–366.

Klein, M. 1934. The psychogenesis of manic-depressive states. *Contributions to Psycho-Analysis.* London: Hogarth.

Kline, N. S. 1969. Lithium: the history of its use in psychiatry. In *Modern Problems in Pharmacology.* Vol. 3. White Plains, N.Y.: Phiebig.

Kraepelin, E. 1904. *Lectures on Clinical Psychiatry.* London: Balliere, Tindall & Cox. In E. Wolpert, ed. *Manic-Depressive Illness.* New York: International Universities Press, 1977.

Kraepelin, E. 1921. *Manic-Depressive Insanity and Paranoia.* London: Livingstone. In E. Wolpert, ed. *Manic-Depressive Illness.* New York: International Universities Press, 1977.

McKnew, D. H.; Cytryn, L.; Efron, A. M.; Gershon, E. S.; and Bunney, W. E., Jr. 1979. Offspring of patients with affective disorders. *British Journal of Psychiatry* 134:148–152.

Mahler, M. 1972. On the first three subphases of the separation-individuation process. *International Journal of Psycho-Analysis* 53:333–338.

Masterson, J. F. 1967. *The Psychiatric Dilemma of Adolescence.* Boston: Little, Brown.

Masterson, J. F. 1978. The borderline adolescent: an object relations view. *Adolescent Psychiatry* 6:344–359.

Perris, C. 1969. The separation of bipolar (manic-depressive) from unipolar recurrent depressive psychosis. *Behavioral Neuropsychiatry* 1(8): 17–24.

Redlich, F., and Freedman, D. 1966. *The Theory and Practice of Psychiatry.* New York: Basic.

Rubenfine, D. L. 1961. Perception, reality testing, and symbolism. *Psychoanalytic Study of the Child* 16:73–89.

Schlangenhauf, J.; Tipin, J.; and White, R. B. 1966. The use of lithium carbonate in the treatment of manic psychoses. *American Journal of Psychiatry* 123:201–205.

Schou, M. 1959. Lithium in psychiatric therapy: stock-taking after ten years. *Psychopharmacology* 1:65–78.

Schou, M. 1968. Special review: lithium in psychiatric therapy and prophylaxis. *Journal Psychiatric Research* 6:67–95.

Schwartzberg, A. Z. 1978. Overview of the borderline syndrome of adolescence. *Adolescent Psychiatry* 6:286–297.

Stone, M. H. 1971. Mania: a guide for the perplexed. *Psychotherapy and Social Science Revue* 5(10): 14–18.

Wolpert, E. 1975. Manic-depressive illness as an actual neurosis. In E. J. Anthony and T. Benedek, eds. *Depression and Human Existence*. Boston: Little, Brown.

Wolpert, E. A., and Mueller, P. 1969. Lithium carbonate in the treatment of manic-depressive disorders. *Archives of General Psychiatry* 21:155–159.

Youngerman, J., and Canino, I. 1978. Lithium carbonate use in children and adolescents: a survey of the literature. *Archives of General Psychiatry* 35:216–224.

20 THE OFFSPRING OF BIPOLAR
MANIC-DEPRESSIVES: CLINICAL FEATURES

LEO KRON, PAOLO DECINA, CLARICE J. KESTENBAUM, SUSAN FARBER,
MARGARET GARGAN, AND RONALD FIEVE

There is a higher incidence of psychopathology among the children of psychiatrically disturbed parents than in the general population (Rutter 1977). This is particularly so with regard to affective disorders where, according to Winokur, Clayton, and Reich (1969), offspring are at an increased risk for developing minor depression, cyclothymia, sociopathy, and alcoholism and where genetic factors are strongly implicated (Kallman 1954; Slater 1936; Stenstedt 1952). Familial studies have found that morbidity risk rates for affective illness in the first-degree relatives of bipolar probands are between 10 percent and 40 percent, with more than one-third of these at risk for bipolar illness (Angst 1966; Gershon, Dunner, and Goodwin 1971; James and Chapman 1975; Perris 1966; Smeraldi, Negri, and Melicaam 1977; Winokur and Clayton 1967; Zerbin-Rudin 1971). Substantially higher rates of affective pathology are found when direct rather than indirect methods are used to evaluate relatives (Waters and Marchenko-Bouer 1980).

The average age of onset of manic-depressive illness is over thirty years, although more than one-third of bipolar cases have an early onset between the ages of ten and nineteen (Mendlewicz, Fieve, Rainer, and Fleiss 1973; Winokur et al. 1969). Carlson and Strober (1978) have further suggested that affective disorder is underdiagnosed in adolescence, and its initial expression is often mistaken for an adjustment reaction or schizophrenia. True bipolar illness, however, as classically described (Kraepelin 1921) with its biphasic periodicity and its elation, is extremely rare below the age of twelve. No cases of mania or hypomania have been found in the studies of juvenile offspring (Greenhill and Shopsin 1979; Kuyler, Rosenthal, Igel, Dunner, and Fieve 1980; McKnew, Cytryn, Efron, Gershon, and Bunney 1979; O'Connell, Mayo, O'Brien, and Misrsheidaie 1979), including the study reported here. Reviewing the twenty-eight cases of childhood bipolar illness which have been reported up to that time, Anthony and Scott (1960) found only three, all eleven years old, that met their criteria for a bipolar diagnosis.[1] Feinstein and Wolpert (1973) reported the case of a girl seeming to fit these criteria, whose intermittent impulsivity, distractibility, hyperactivity, and destructive behavior first brought her to treatment at the age of three. Affective swings continued with increasing severity until she was placed on lithium at age six and a half. Davis (1979) has described a bipolar syndrome in childhood characterized by hyperactivity and affective storms. Nevertheless, the period around puberty seems to be a necessary prelude to the development of the classic bipolar picture as we are familiar with it in adults.

Are there, however, clinical features which predate the onset of the full clinical syndrome and which can be thought of as premorbid or as an early expression of a bipolar diathesis?

Anthony and Scott (1960) suggested that a latent tendency to manic-depressive illness could be seen in an internalized, psychodynamic form in early life prior to the external expression of the tendency in the overt psychotic state later in life. Feinstein (1980; Feinstein and Wolpert 1973) hypothesized that the bipolar diathesis resulted in "a fundamental defect in the affect system which when overstimulated begins a discharge pattern that does not easily lend itself to autonomous emotional control." The expression of this vulnerability is affected by development and in children is associated with clear affective instability, hypersensitivity to loss, and the development of expansive, grandiose, and exhibitionistic personality traits. Kallman (1954), Kraepelin (1913), Leonhard (1968), and others have formulated relationships between personality and later-developing affective subtypes, such that diluted forms characterized as hypomanic, hypomelancholic, and cyclothymic are found premorbidly in those (including relatives) who later become manic, depressed, and bipolar, respectively. A consensus seems particularly to exist regarding the presence of premorbid features in adults later developing depression.

Psychiatric clinicians from different countries and apparently uninfluenced by each other's writings (Japan, United States, Switzerland, and Germany) have promulgated remarkably similar personality constellations to be part of the premorbid state in depression (Von Zerssen

274

1977). Patients are described as rigid, orderly, conscientious, conventional, dependent, inhibited, obsessive, pessimistic, insecure, and sensitive. These and similar characteristics (introversion, neuroticism) have also been found using self-rating questionnaires and personality inventories in which depressed and control groups have been compared (Kendell and Discipio 1970; Von Zerssen 1977).

Data regarding the premorbid characteristics of bipolar manic-depressives are less consistent. Retrospective clinical descriptions of these patients reveal variable premorbid pictures. They have been described as having depressive features, hypomanic-expansive features, impulsivity, obsessionality, and other nonspecific behavioral and affective symptomatology. Often, however, there is no evidence of disturbed functioning or psychopathology severe enough to attract psychiatric attention. In fact, many patients who go on to develop bipolar illness seem to function normally if not at a superior level (Berg, Hullin, Allsopp, O'Brien, and MacDonald 1974; Cohen, Baker, Cohen, Fromm-Reichmann, and Weigert 1954; Davenport, Adland, Gold, and Goodwin 1979; Kestenbaum 1980).

Observations on families in which there is a multigenerational expression of bipolar illness (Davenport et al. 1979) revealed several instances in which the premorbid functions were at least above average and in some cases superior, and others in which they were pathological with nonspecific affective and behavioral disturbances. Findings from the intensive psychotherapy of manic-depressives portray them in childhood as highly functioning, extroverted, ambitious, and sociable, although having superficial relationships with unmet dependency needs and a rigid adherence to conventional values and achievement (Cohen et al. 1954; Fromm-Reichmann 1949; Gibson, Cohen, and Cohen 1959).

Using personality inventories, bipolar patients have been differentiated premorbidly from unipolars on scales of extroversion, sociability, and activity but not significantly different from the general population on any scale except obsessionality (Hirschfeld and Klerman 1979; Perris 1966; Von Zerssen 1977).

Several studies of bipolar offspring have been undertaken, employing variable methodologies and revealing rates of psychopathology ranging from 33 to 45 percent (Greenhill and Shopsin 1979; Kuyler et al. 1979; McKnew et al. 1979; O'Connell et al. 1979). In those studies where children were assessed by parental questionnaire only, pathology was not easily categorized and included diverse personality, behavior, and learning disorders, as well as depression, although affec-

275

tive symptoms seemed to be minimized (Greenhill and Shopsin 1979; Kuyler et al. (1980). Where bipolar offspring were directly examined, depression was diagnosed in as many as 25–45 percent of the children (McKnew et al. 1979; O'Connell et al. 1979). Evidence of biphasic mood fluctuation over time was noted by McKnew et al. (1979).

There is an enlarging literature associating affective (bipolar) illness with disorders of cerebral laterality (Flor-Henry 1979; Lishman and McKeekan 1976). Kestenbaum (1979) suggested that such a disorder may be seen in children at risk for affective illness, as manifested in a psychological test pattern in the WISC-R with verbal scores significantly higher than performance scores. The aims of this study were to test this hypothesis as well as to clinically assess the offspring of bipolar parents blindly compared to matched normal controls.

Subjects and Methods

Eighteen bipolar patients (BP), diagnosed according to research diagnostic criteria (RDC) (Spitzer, Endicott, and Robins 1978) and who had children between the ages of seven and fourteen years, were randomly selected from an outpatient clinic.[2] Of the adult probands, eleven were classified as Bipolar I (BP I) (that is, having a cyclical affective disorder including hospitalizations for mania), and seven were classified as Bipolar II (BP II) (that is, having a cyclical affective disorder including hospitalizations for depression only) (Fieve 1975). The experimental group was composed of their thirty-one children, seventeen girls (mean age=11.4 years) and fourteen boys (mean age=10.5 years). The control sample consisted of eighteen children, nine boys (mean age=11.4; range=9.7–13.8) and nine girls (mean age=11.3 years; range=7–14.6), who had a negative history for any affective illness in first-degree relatives and bipolar illness in second-degree relatives. The two samples were similar with regard to age, sex, and socioeconomic status.

The assessment of each child included a semistructured interview with the child and his primary caretaker, psychological testing, and a determination of handedness. The child's interviewer and tester were blind to parental reports and parental diagnosis. The parental interview elicited information regarding pregnancy, development, current symptomatology, and functioning. A motoric lateralization questionnaire (Raczkowski, Kalat, and Nebes 1974) was completed by the parent, assessing preference for unimanual tasks. Each child's semistructured interview was scored according to the Mental Health Assessment Form (Kestenbaum and Bird 1978) and involved an inquiry into all areas of the child's life and functioning, including assets as well as pathology. Items from the "Kiddie-SADS" (Chambers, Puig-Antich, and Tabrizi 1978) were incorporated to assess in greater detail disturbances in mood and other areas of evident psychopathology. The overall functioning of each child was assessed with the Global Assessment Score (GAS) (Spitzer, Endicott, and Gibbon 1973). Psychological testing, including projectives and the WISC-R, was administered to each child.

After each interview, clinical observations were recorded in a form congruent with RDC/DSM III diagnostic criteria.

Results

Significant differences between the experimental and control groups were found with regard to the nature and extent of psychopathology, IQ findings on the WISC-R, and laterality as manifested in handedness.

HANDEDNESS

A statistically significant difference ($P<.05$) between experimental and control groups was found with regard to handedness. In the experimental group, nine children (six boys and three girls) were classified as left-handers. In the control group, only one of eighteen children was classified as left-handed.

WISC-R

A repeated measure analysis of variance was conducted on verbal and performance IQ scores with group and sex as between-subject variables. An interaction was obtained between subject group and verbal performance IQ scores. As indicated in table 1 and confirmed by post hoc comparison, experimental and control children did not differ with regard to their verbal IQ scores. The mean performance IQ scores of the experimental children, however, were significantly less than those of controls ($P<.05$). Within the experimental group—that is, children of bipolar parents—a mean discrepancy of 8.2 was found as compared to a mean discrepancy of only 1.9 in the experimental group ($P<.05$).

TABLE 1

	Experimental Children*		Control Children†	
	Mean	SD	Mean	SD
Full IQ	116.2 ±	13.8	121.9 ±	7.8
Verbal IQ............	118.4 ±	14.3	120.5 ±	9.8
Performance IQ	110.2 ±	13.9	118.6 ±	9.2

*Mean verbal/performance discrepancy = 8.2; 39 percent had a verbal/performance discrepancy of more than 15 points.
†Mean verbal/performance discrepancy = 1.9; 11 percent had a verbal/performance discrepancy of more than 15 points ($P<.05$).

The finding of this verbal/performance discrepancy in the experimental children was a rather strong effect. By population norms (Kaufman 1979), a discrepancy in this direction equal to or greater than fifteen points is expected in less than 13 percent of children. In our control group, 11 percent, or two children out of eighteen, manifested a discrepancy of this magnitude. In the experimental group, 39 percent, or twelve children out of thirty-one, showed this large discrepancy. The discrepancy was examined as a function of the status of parents as BP I or BP II. Children of BP I parents showed a greater mean discrepancy (10.6) than children of BP II probands (4.4). This effect, possibly because of small sample size, was marginally significant. There was a trend for the left-handed group to evidence the verbal/performance discrepancy to a greater extent than the right-handers. However, this effect did not reach statistical significance.

Clinical Characteristics and Psychiatric Diagnoses

Preliminary analysis of scales derived from the Mental Health Assessment Form found that the experimental group was significantly differentiated from the control group ($P=.05$) with regard to scales of depression, overactivity, overproduction of florid fantasy, and attractiveness. There was also a nonsignificant trend to be more distractible, irritable, impulsive, anxious, and histrionic, and a greater tendency to demonstrate depressive equivalents (for example, delinquency). Relationships with other family members and peers tended to be disturbed and overly aggressive. There were, moreover, positive attributes which discriminated the two groups: the experimental group was rated

278

as more attractive and intelligent, most likely on the basis of high verbal ability. Some of the experimental children seemed to have more hobbies and interests than the comparison group.

Only one child of the control group warranted a diagnosis, that of depression. As indicated in table 2, of the sixteen children in the experimental group who received DSM III/RDC diagnoses, eight children (five girls and three boys) had depressive disorders (two major and six minor). Of these eight children, four received additional diagnoses: two were attention-deficit disorder without hyperactivity and two were overanxious disorder. Of the eight children who received diagnoses other than depression, one was an overanxious disorder, two were conduct disorders, and the remaining five children (four boys and one girl) exhibited psychiatric symptomatology which, although severe, could not be satisfactorily diagnosed by DSM III/RDC criteria. They were labeled RDC undiagnosable, even though in some instances at least two DSM III/RDC diagnoses could be applied but without reflecting accurately the extent and nature of the pathology involved. Likewise, several of the undiagnosed and functional children demonstrated characteristics at a state and trait level, suggestive of a diagnosis but without satisfying the required DSM III/RDC criteria.

All the cases were then reviewed by the three project psychiatrists to explore the presence of any clinical patterns of developing traits. Three

TABLE 2
DSM III/RDC DIAGNOSES OF EXPERIMENTAL
CHILDREN
$(N=31)$*

Primary Diagnosis	Number of Children
Depression†	8
Attention deficit disorder	2
Overanxious disorder	2
Conduct disorders	2
Overanxious disorder	1
RDC undiagnosable	5

*Fifteen children without DSM III/RDC diagnosis (10 girls, 5 boys); sixteen children with DSM III/RDC diagnosis (7 girls, 9 boys).
†Four of these children received two diagnoses.

broad clinical groups were recognized into which twenty-five of the thirty-one children could be placed by unanimous consensus. These groups were identified as extroverted, inhibited, and impulsive. A fourth miscellaneous category was added (see table 3). Each group contained children at various levels of functioning, the most dysfunctional group being the impulsive. Characteristics of children in the extroverted and inhibited groups resembled those frequently described in association with affective illness. In fact, five of the nine children assigned to the inhibited group also warranted a diagnosis of depression.

Although a verbal/performance discrepancy on the WISC-R discriminated the experimental group from the control group, there was no relationship between this discrepancy and psychiatric diagnosis. There was, however, a significant association ($P > .05$) between this verbal/performance discrepancy and the extroverted group of children. Furthermore, children within this extroverted group manifested verbal/performance discrepancies that were approximately three times as large as experimental children placed in the other three groups. Some anecdotal material will illustrate the above clinical findings.

TABLE 3

Group and Characteristics*	Examples
Extroverted ($N = 10$):†	
Extroverted	Outgoing
	Energies are directed outside, active
	in school, hobbies, etc.
	Sociable
	Alloplastic
Expressive	Verbal (at extreme, pressured and verbose)
	Creative, artistic
	Easy access to fantasy, dreams, magical thinking
	Imaginative
Exhibitionistic	Attention seeking (audience oriented)
	Histrionic (dramatic, seductive), particularly in girls
	Joking, clowning behavior
	Bravado, counterphobic behavior (particularly in boys)
Immature (with respect to behavior)	Overly dependent
	Increased separation anxiety
	Requiring much reassurance
	Regressive play and behavior

TABLE 3 (*Continued*)

Group and Characteristics*	Examples
Egocentric	Self-involved
	Self-overvaluation and expansiveness
	Unempathic
	Manipulative
Inhibited (*N*=9):	
Inhibited	Constricted, low keyed
	Unsociable
	Lack of spontaneity
	Autoplastic
Obsessive	Orderly, controlled
	Intellectualized (affects avoided and isolated)
	Perfectionistic
	Unimaginative (with poor access to fantasy, dream life)
Cautious	Shy
	Guarded
	Wary of rejection
	Vulnerable self-esteem
	Pessimistic
Pseudomature	Parentified
	Reliable
	Conscientious
	Conventional
Anxious	Tense
	High strung
	Irritable
	Fearful (with phobic trends)
Impulsive (*N*=6):	
Impulsive	Poor impulse control
	Low frustration tolerance
	Acts without thinking
Hyperactive	Fidgety and restless
	Always on the go
Distractible	Easily distracted
	Unable to concentrate in school
Aggressive	Fights with peers and siblings
	Struggles with parents frequently
	Prominent aggressive themes in fantasies and dreams
Conduct disorders	As defined by DSM III
Other (*N*=6):	
Other clinical presentations not classifiable in above groups	One case; overanxious disorder

*To be placed within one of the groups each child demonstrated at least four of its characteristics.

†The extroverted group is significantly associated with a verbal/performance discrepancy greater than fifteen points ($P<.05$).

Clinical Anecdotes

CASE EXAMPLE 1

Fred demonstrates characteristics of the extroverted group of children and has a large verbal/performance discrepancy of twenty-five points. He received no psychiatric diagnosis and is reported to be functioning well.

Fred is a pleasant, warmly related twelve-year-old whose father is diagnosed as Bipolar I. He is bright, articulate, and dramatic. He is moderately overactive and somewhat pressured in speech.

Developmental history reveals him to have been a premature infant with nonspecific feeding problems. He suffered from childhood asthma. Noteworthy in his development was an unusual precocity in the acquisition of language. Currently Fred functions well in school, excels in reading, and is active outside of school, filling his time with numerous interests. He likes to draw and paint, plays the trombone, avidly collects comic books, lifts weights, and earns extra money with a paper route. He likes nothing more, however, than to ride down the street on his unicycle, attracting everyone's attention. He performs for audiences and sees himself as a clown, which at school sometimes results in reprimands. Yet he also reproaches himself for being what he calls too "egocentric" (by which he means that he thinks too much of himself). He thinks that his parents would describe him as good-natured, smart, funny, alive, and always on the go. In fact, this is the way they describe him, although they add to the observation of his exceptionally confident manner and "big ego" that he is unempathically manipulative.

Coexisting with his exhibitionism and grandiosity, there is evidence of pronounced damage to his self-esteem. He often feels "awkward, like a schlepp" and is concerned that he "sounds stupid." He often thinks that people do not like him, think him foolish, and laugh at him rather than with him. Psychological projectives reveal a "pervasive sense of vulnerability" with a "poor self-esteem . . . defended by exhibitionism."

Fred does not like to have sad feelings and tries to avoid them through activity, by "doing something." He also noted, curiously, that although he felt "scared" initially on hearing of his mother's recent hysterectomy, he soon thereafter reacted by feeling in "high spirits." He expressed some awareness of the inappropriateness of this reaction.

Overtly Fred is mildly symptomatic. He is occasionally enuretic, overeats, and suffers from frequent "stomachaches." When his parents are away he becomes preoccupied with their safety. Less now than when he was younger, Fred feels afraid of becoming lost when he is in a large crowd. He has many dreams of being chased, once by an ambulance and once by a man in a hearse.

Fred, therefore, demonstrates several characteristics of the extroverted group of children. He is extroverted, exhibitionistic, expressive, egocentric, and expansive. In fact, were he an adult he would actually satisfy the DSM III criteria for a narcissistic personality. He also demonstrates hypomanic reactions to feared loss and threats to his self-esteem typical of the adult bipolar patient. These seem to place Fred at risk for the development of overt affective pathology as further development takes place, even though at this time there is no grossly perceptible disturbance of functioning.

CASE EXAMPLE 2

As opposed to Fred, whose GAS is 70, his thirteen-year-old brother Tim functions poorly with a GAS of 41. He is one of those children who, although quite symptomatic, was categorized as RDC undiagnosable. He warrants the DSM III diagnosis of a moderately severe socialized conduct disorder and probably attention deficit disorder, but it was felt that these did not reflect accurately the nature and extent of his pathology, particularly with regard to his faulty ego functioning (that is, reality sense).

Tim demonstrated characteristics of the impulsive group of children. Although maintaining an air of bravado, he is quite anxious, with pressured speech. He has a low tolerance for frustration. He was described by his parents as extremely active since birth and was diagnosed as hyperactive by his pediatrician prior to entering school. He has always been slow to learn and is currently in danger of failing despite an IQ in the average range (full scale 107).

Tim fights frequently, has been caught stealing a bike, but continues to steal and shoplift. He relates this boastfully and without guilt. Likewise, he takes pride in his athletic skills and in his reputation as an aggressive player. He states that he is unafraid. He is often angry, argues constantly with his parents, and has recently been planning to run away from home.

He feels sad often when he is alone but prefers to "celebrate" when these feelings come on. He likes to "be on the move." For release he will jump on his motorbike—which is, incidentally, unlicensed—and will take a long "joy ride." Sometimes when he is alone or in a small room he becomes quite frightened and has the feeling that he is "floating in space." During the interview he complained that the walls were too white and seemed to be "coming in" on him. At these times he becomes anxious and there is a loss in his sense of reality.

In addition to a learning disability, psychological tests reveal that Tim experiences "high levels of anxiety associated with pre-occupations of violence and bodily damage which intrude into his secondary process thinking." Tim is placed in the impulsive group and seems well on the way, at least, to sociopathy.

CASE EXAMPLE 3

Gloria, age eleven, and Alice, age nine, live with their mother, who bears a diagnosis of Bipolar I. The parents are separated. Both girls are good students, but Alice is socially more successful. She is outgoing and spontaneous, and has many friends. Although she seems somewhat immature, insofar as she is overly dependent on her mother, she is quite precociously interested in boys and heterosexuality. She is histrionic, likes to "joke around," and when sad takes solace in an active and romantic fantasy life which includes imaginary playmates, boyfriends, and babies.

Alice received a GAS of 72, was categorized as extroverted, and did not warrant a psychiatric diagnosis. Gloria, on the other hand, demonstrated characteristics of the inhibited group. She received a GAS of 55 and, although an excellent student, was very symptomatic in several areas of functioning. She satisfied RDC for the diagnosis of a depressive disorder and experienced anxiety generalized and severe enough to meet the DSM III diagnosis of an overanxious disorder. This anxiety, however, was considered to be related to the syndrome of depression.

As opposed to Alice, who was seductively clad in a rather skimpy tube top, Gloria was covered, chin to ankle, by a floor-length, long-sleeved dress. She sat rigidly. Her hands fidgeted constantly and she smiled stiffly and inappropriately, not succeeding in concealing her considerably depressed affect. At times she seemed near to tears but the smile remained.

The attainment of developmental milestones was unremarkable, and Gloria is described as always being somewhat tense and irritable. There was one episode of febrile seizures at approximately twelve months. Both mother and Gloria agree that she experiences mood swings, synchronous with those of mother, especially with regard to depression. Mother sees Gloria as being much like her, yet there is some role reversal during the mother's depressions. Gloria is "eleven going on forty," as her mother states, perfectionistic, pseudomature, conscientious, orderly, and quite obsessional. Frequently at home she must check and recheck the doors at night to be sure that they are closed. She has difficulty getting to sleep, experiences visual and auditory illusions, and is troubled by frequent nightmares. She is phobic, frightened of the dark and insects.

As opposed to Alice, Gloria has only one friend and sometimes will resort to playing with her younger sister's friends. She is ashamed of this. Occasionally she loses interest in her usual activities and spends much time all by herself. She observes that at times she is uncomfortable and sad feelings come upon her for no apparent reason. At these times, she will lie in bed waiting for them to disappear. She would prefer to remain young and is pessimistic about the future; at times she wishes she were dead.

Projective tests reveal depression associated with preoccupation with abandonment, persecutory, and sadistic fantasies.

Discussion

A most striking finding of our study was the substantiation of Kestenbaum's (1979) clinical impressions, associating a verbal/performance discrepancy on the WISC-R with bipolar offspring. Atypical patterns in the WISC-R, with verbal IQ significantly higher than performance IQ (found in our study to be associated with bipolar offspring), have been reported in adult bipolars as well. The reverse pattern, where performance IQ is higher than verbal IQ, has been reported in the offspring of schizophrenics and the offspring of patients with mixed psychiatric disorders (Gruzelier, Mednick, and Schulsinger 1979; Kestenbaum 1980).

285

The findings of left-handedness as significantly related to bipolar offspring have never before been reported. However, left-handedness has been found to be associated with endogenous psychoses in adults, especially schizoaffective and bipolar (Flor-Henry 1979; Lishman and McKeekan 1976).

The findings of the verbal/performance discrepancy and the left-handedness are consistent with the hypothesis that a disturbance and/or imbalance in lateralized brain function may be present in some bipolar patients.

The difference in diagnosable psychopathology between the experimental and control groups is substantial. While only one of the children in the control group received a diagnosis, 52 percent of the experimental group received RDC/DSM III diagnoses. There were no cases of mania or hypomania, but 25 percent of the experimental children were found to be depressed. These findings are consistent with previous studies (Greenhill and Shopsin 1979; Kuyler et al. 1980; McKnew et al. 1979; O'Connell et al. 1979; Waters and Marchenko-Bouer 1980), underscore the affective vulnerability of bipolar offspring, and are supportive of the contention that direct examination of the offspring yields more specific psychiatric diagnoses than parental reports (McKnew et al. 1979). In several instances parental reports reflected denial of significant depression in their children.

Preliminary attempts to classify the experimental children according to developing traits found them to fall into four broad groups—extroverted, inhibited, impulsive, and miscellaneous (table 3). Features of the inhibited group are similar to those described in the literature to be associated with states premorbid to depression in adults (that is, obsessiveness, conventionality, conscientiousness, inhibition, pessimism, and insecurity) (Hirschfeld and Klerman 1979; Kendell and Discipio 1970; Von Zerssen 1977). The fact that five out of nine children assigned to that group also warranted a diagnosis of depression is consistent with the contention that a relationship exists between these character traits and depression in childhood as well.

Likewise, the features associated with the extroverted group of children have been described in individuals who later develop bipolar illness (Cohen et al. 1954; Davenport et al. 1979; Fromm-Reichmann 1949; Gibson et al. 1959; Kallman 1954; Kraepelin 1913; Leonhard 1968; Stone 1980; Von Zerssen 1977) and are seen in extremely exaggerated forms as part of the adult hypomanic/manic syndrome. It is with this group that the verbal/performance discrepancy is significantly associated. The discrepancies in this group are approximately three times as large as in the other experimental groups. Since a greater verbal/performance discrepancy in the children was associated with having a Bipolar I parent (that is, one with a more pronounced manic component), an important relationship could exist between the verbal/performance discrepancy and the degree of a tendency toward mania in the children as well.

The impulsive group of children was the most dysfunctional, having behavioral and learning disabilities which have been associated with sociopathy in later life.

Conclusions

Twenty-five of the thirty-two experimental children could be placed in one of three groups (extroverted, inhibited, impulsive) which might reflect a variable tendency toward the later development of one of those entities considered as part of the affective spectrum of disorders and found in the relatives of affectively ill probands (that is, cyclothymia, depression, sociopathy, and alcoholism) (Winokur 1973). Further studies are needed to delineate more clearly the nature of these too-broad groupings and to follow these children into adulthood. Studies should not, however, limit themselves to looking only at offspring with overt affective pathology to locate traits reflecting future affective vulnerability. In accord with reports of normal nondysfunctional adjustments prior to the onset of bipolar illness (Berg et al. 1974; Kestenbaum 1980; Perris 1966; Von Zerssen 1977), most of the experimental children were not considered by their parents to be dysfunctional or to have emotional difficulties. This was particularly true of the extroverted group of children in whom traits possibly related to future bipolar pathology are consistent with parental expectations and parental denial.

Whether and when a child actually goes on to an affective decompensation is probably dependent on the extent of an affective vulnerability determined by gene-environment interaction. However, one hypothesis generated by this study and requiring prospective studies for confirmation is that a child grouped in one of the three groups is more likely under stress to develop the homologous affective spectrum disorder in later life. Thus, a child from the extroverted group might be more likely to develop an affective disorder where hypomanic or manic episodes are relatively pronounced. Or a child from the inhibited group

287

might be more likely to be depressed and a child from the impulsive group more prone to sociopathy later in life. Further studies are likewise required to investigate the possibly important role of the verbal/performance discrepancy as a reliable marker in some children at risk for bipolar illness.

1. Anthony and Scott's (1960) criteria for diagnosis of manic-depressive illness in childhood are: (1) classical clinical description (as given by Kraepelin, Bleuler, Meyer, and others); (2) positive family history of a manic-depressive "diathesis"; (3) an early tendency to manic-depressive reactions as manifested in: (*a*) cyclothymic tendencies, and (*b*) manic or depressive pyrexial reactions; (4) evidence of clinical periodicity or recurrence; (5) diphasic swings of mood; (6) endogenous character (clinical course minimally related to environmental events); (7) severity of illness substantial as indicated by a need for inpatient treatment, heavy sedation, or ECT; (8) an abnormal underlying personality of an extroverted type; (9) absence of evidence of other abnormal conditions (that is, schizophrenia, organic states, etc.); and (10) the diagnostic evidence based on current, not retrospective, assessments. Five or more criteria are required to make the diagnosis.

2. Foundation for Depression and Manic-Depression, New York.

REFERENCES

Angst, J. 1966. *Zur Atiologie und Nosology Endogener Depressiver Psychosen*. In Monographien aus dem Gesamtgebiete der Neurologie und Psychiatrie, no. 112. Berlin: Springer.

Anthony, J., and Scott, P. 1960. Manic-depressive psychosis in childhood. *Journal of Child Psychology and Psychiatry* 1:53–72.

Berg, I.; Hullin, R.; Allsopp, M.; O'Brien, P.; and MacDonald, R. 1974. Bipolar manic depressive psychosis in early adolescence: a case report. *British Journal of Psychiatry* 125:416–417.

Carlson, G. A., and Strober, M. 1978. Manic depressive illness in early adolescence: a study of clinical and diagnostic characteristics in six cases. *Journal of the American Academy of Child Psychiatry* 17:138–153.

Chambers, W.; Puig-Antich, J.; and Tabrizi, M. A. 1978. The ongoing development of the Kiddie-SADS (Schedule for Affective Disorders and Schizophrenia for School-Age Children). Read at the American Academy of Child Psychiatry Annual Meeting, San Diego.

Cohen, M. B.; Baker, G.; Cohen, R. A.; Fromm-Reichmann, F.; and Weigert, E. V. 1954. An intensive study of twelve cases of manic-depressive psychosis. *Psychiatry* 17:103–137.

Davenport, Y.; Adland, M.; Gold, P.; and Goodwin, F. K. 1979. Multi-generational families. *American Journal of Orthopsychiatry* 49:24–35.

Davis, R. 1979. Manic-depressive variant syndrome of childhood: a preliminary report. *American Journal of Psychiatry* 136:702–705.

Feinstein, S. C. 1980. Why they were afraid of Virginia Woolf: perspectives on juvenile manic-depressive illness. *Adolescent Psychiatry* 8:332–343.

Feinstein, S. C., and Wolpert, E. A. 1973. Juvenile manic-depressive illness: clinical and therapeutic considerations. *Journal of the American Academy of Child Psychiatry* 12:123–136.

Fieve, R. 1975. Primary affective disorder. In F. Flach and S. Draghi, eds. *The Nature and Treatment of Depression*. New York: Wiley.

Flor-Henry, P. 1979. Laterality, shifts of cerebral dominance, sinistrality, and psychosis. In J. Gruzelier and P. Flor-Henry, eds. *Hemisphere Asymmetries of Function in Psychopathology*. Amsterdam: Elsevier–North-Holland.

Fromm-Reichmann, F. 1949. Intensive psychotherapy of manic-depressives, part II. *Confinia Neurologica* 9:158–165.

Gershon, B.; Dunner, D.; and Goodwin, R. 1971. Toward a biology of affective disorders. *Archives of General Psychiatry* 25:1–15.

Gibson, R. W.; Cohen, M. B.; and Cohen, R. A. 1959. On the dynamics of the manic-depressive personality. *American Journal of Psychiatry* 115:1101–1107.

Greenhill, L., and Shopsin, B. 1979. Survey of mental disorders in the children of patients with affective disorders. In J. Mendelwicz and B. Shopsin, eds. *Genetic Aspects of Affective Illness*. New York: Spectrum.

Gruzelier, J.; Mednick, S.; and Schulsinger, F. 1979. Lateralized impairments in the WISC profiles of children at genetic risk for psychopathology. In J. Gruzelier and P. Flor-Henry, eds. *Hemisphere Asymmetries of Function in Psychopathology*. Amsterdam: Elsevier–North-Holland.

Hirschfeld, R., and Klerman, G. 1979. Personality attributes and affective disorders. *American Journal of Psychiatry* 136:67–70.

James, N. M., and Chapman, C. J. 1975. A genetic study of bipolar affective disorder. *British Journal of Psychiatry* 126:449–456.

Kallman, F. S. 1954. Genetic principles in manic-depressive psychosis. In J. Zubin and P. Hoch, eds. *Depression*. New York: Grune & Stratton.

Kaufman, A. S. 1979. *Intelligence Testing with the W.I.S.C.-R.* New York: Wiley.

Kendell, R. E., and Discipio, W. J. 1970. Obsessional symptoms and obsessional personality traits in patients with depressive illness. *Psychological Medicine* 1:65–72.

Kestenbaum, C. J. 1979. Children at risk for manic-depressive illness: possible predictors. *American Journal of Psychiatry* 136:1206–1208.

Kestenbaum, C. J. 1980. Adolescents at risk for manic-depressive illness. *Adolescent Psychiatry* 8:344–366.

Kestenbaum, C. J., and Bird, H. R. 1978. A reliability study of the mental health assessment form for school age children. *Journal of the American Academy of Child Psychiatry* 17(2): 338–347.

Kraepelin, E. 1909–1913. *Psychiatrie*. Vols. 1 and 3. Leipzig: Barth.

Kraepelin, E. 1921. In G. M. Robertson, ed. *Manic Depressive Insanity and Paranoia*. Edinburgh: Livingstone.

Kuyler, P.; Rosenthal, L.; Igel, G.; Dunner, D.; and Fieve, R. 1980. Psychopathology among children of manic depressive patients. *Biological Psychiatry* 15(4): 589–596.

Leonhard, K. 1968. *Aufteilung der Endogenen Psychosen*. 4th ed. Berlin: Akademie-Verlag.

Lishman, W. A., and McKeekan, E. R. L. 1976. Hand preference patterns in psychiatric patients. *British Journal of Psychiatry* 129:158–166.

McKnew, D.; Cytryn, L.; Efron, A.; Gershon, D.; and Bunney, W. 1979. Offspring of patients with affective disorders. *British Journal of Psychiatry* 134:148–152.

Mendlewicz, J.; Fieve, R.; Rainer, J. D.; and Fleiss, J. L. 1973. Manic-depressive illness: a comparative study of patients with and without a family history. *British Journal of Psychiatry* 120:523–530.

O'Connell, R. A.; Mayo, J. A.; O'Brien, J. D.; and Misrsheidaie, F. 1979. Children of bipolar manic-depressives. In J. Mendlewicz and B. Shopsin, eds. *The Genetics of Affective Disorder*. New York: Spectrum.

Perris, C. 1966. A study of bipolar and unipolar recurrent depressive psychoses. *Acta Psychiatricia Scandinavica* (suppl.) 42:68–82.

Raczkowski, D.; Kalat, J. W.; and Nebes, R. 1974. Reliability and validity of some handedness questionnaire items. *Neuropsychologica* 12:43–47.

Rutter, M. 1977. Other family influences on development. In M. Rutter and L. Hersov, eds. *Child Psychiatry: Modern Approaches*. London: Blackwell.

Slater, E. 1936. The inheritance of manic depressive insanity. *Proceedings of the Royal Society of Medicine* 29:981–990.

Smeraldi, E.; Negri, F.; and Melicaam, A. 1977. A genetic study of affective disorder. *Acta Psychiatrica Scandinavica* 56:382–398.

Spitzer, R. L.; Endicott, J.; and Robins, E. 1978. Research diagnostic criteria. *Archives of General Psychiatry* 35:773–782.

Spitzer, R. L.; Endicott, J.; and Gibbon, M. 1973. *Global Assessment Scale*. New York: Biometrics Research, New York State Department of Mental Hygiene.

Stenstedt, A. 1952. *A Study in Manic-Depressive Psychosis*. Copenhagen: Munksgaart.

Stone, M. H. 1980. *The Borderline Syndrome*. New York: McGraw-Hill.

Von Zerssen, D. 1977. Premorbid personality and affective psychoses. In G. D. Burrows, ed. *Handbook of Studies on Depression*. New York: Excerpta Medica.

Waters, B. G. H., and Marchenko-Bouer, I. 1980. Psychiatric illness in the adult offspring of bipolar manic-depressives. *Journal of Affective Disorders* 2:119–126.

Winokur, G. 1973. Diagnostic and genetic aspects of affective illness. *Psychiatric Annals* 3:6–20.

Winokur, G., and Clayton, P. 1967. Family history studies: two types of affective disorders separated according to genetic and clinical factors. In J. Wortis, ed. *Recent Advances in Biological Psychiatry, Volume 9*. New York: Plenum.

Winokur, G.; Clayton, P.; and Reich, T. 1969. *Manic Depressive Illness*. St. Louis: Mosby.

Zerbin-Rudin, A. 1971. Genetische Aspeckte der Endogenen Psychosen. *Fortschritte der Neurologie, Psychiatrie und ihrer Grenzgebiete* 39:459–494.

21 FANTASY IN CHILDHOOD DEPRESSION AND OTHER FORMS OF CHILD PSYCHOPATHOLOGY

DONALD H. MC KNEW, JR., LEON CYTRYN, MARTINE LAMOUR,
AND ALAN APTER

Several years ago the senior authors proposed a tripartite classification of childhood depression, that is, chronic, acute, and masked depressive reactions (Cytryn and McKnew 1972). The children in the first two categories exhibited frank symptoms of depression such as sad mood, anhedonia, despair, agitation or retardation, sleep and feeding disturbances, and suicidal ideation. In addition, their fantasy material was dominated by themes of thwarting, frustration, being trapped, physical injury, death, and suicide. The fantasy was elicited during the psychiatric interviews by commonly used means of child examination such as content of dreams, television, stories, movies, books, three wishes, Despert fables, drawings accompanied by storytelling, and sometimes TAT cards.

We were struck by the fact that many children who presented with symptoms of nondepressive psychopathology such as hyperactivity, antisocial behavior, phobias, obsessive compulsive disorder, and psychosomatic illness had a thematic fantasy pattern similar to that of children with overt depressive syndromes. In addition, many of these children exhibited occasional overt depressive mood and behavior as well as depressive verbalization. Such occurrences were usually brief, lasting a few hours, following which the child usually returned to his or her habitual behavior and symptom patterns.

We labeled these children as having masked depressive reaction. Such diagnosis was based on inference, that is, depressive fantasy and occasional overt depressive symptoms of short duration.

Since our original publication, the existence of overt depressive illness in childhood has become widely recognized by psychiatric researchers and practitioners (Cytryn and McKnew 1979, 1980). However, the concept of masked depression as a diagnostic syndrome *sui generis* has been questioned and criticized as vague, subject to interviewer bias, and above all as lacking clear-cut operational criteria which are being increasingly emphasized as the best way of obtaining reliability and validity of a diagnostic category (Carlson and Cantwell 1980). We ourselves became concerned, lest masked depressive reaction be used as a wastebasket diagnosis, following such examples as "atypical" child (Cytryn, McKnew, and Bunney 1980). In addition, in following the children diagnosed as having a masked depressive reaction, for periods ranging from four weeks to ten years, it became obvious that most of them did not develop a clear-cut affective disorder of significant duration but, rather, continued with the same overt psychopathological pattern which predominated at the time of the original diagnosis.

Recently, we reevaluated (Cytryn and McKnew 1980) our original nosology of childhood depression in an attempt to bring it into line with diagnostic systems developed by other investigators, as well as with adult criteria of affective disorders. In this reassessment we concluded that, on clinical grounds, maintaining the diagnostic category of masked depression of childhood is no longer tenable.

In order to obtain further proof of this largely clinical decision, this study was undertaken to explore the relationship of depressive fantasy in children to (1) the diagnosis of clinical depression as obtained by recognized operational criteria and (2) general psychopathology as evaluated by the same operational criteria.

Methods

As a part of a follow-up study of eighteen children of manic-depressive parents and six children of normal control parents, we used a variety of diagnostic measures as recommended by Raskin (1973): (1) Weinberg criteria (Weinberg, Rutman, and Sullivan 1973); (2) DSM III (1980); (3) the Achenbach child behavior checklist (Achenbach and Edelbrock 1973); and (4) the Children's Affective Rating Scale (CARS) (McKnew, Cytryn, Efron, Gershon, and Bunney 1979), shown in table 1. The scores obtained in all these instruments in the above study were subjected to a statistical analysis in order to ascertain the correlation of

293

TABLE 1
CHILDREN'S AFFECTIVE RATING SCALE (CARS)

Item	Description
Mood and behavior	*Low*—Looks sad, mildly dejected, some hesitancy in social contact.
	Moderate—Dejected, occasionally tearful, voice monotonous.
	High—Extremely sad posture and facial expression, occasional crying, slow speech, monotonous voice. Difficult to contact or relate to, stays to himself; lacks responsiveness to environment. Serious disturbances of appetite and sleep.
Verbal expression	*Low*—Talks of being disappointed, thwarted, excluded, blamed, criticized.
	Moderate—Talks of being unloved, worthless, unattractive, lost, ridiculed, rejected, sad, crying.
	High—Talks of suicide, being killed, abandoned, hopeless.
Fantasy	*Low*—Disappointed, thwarted, mistreated, excluded, blamed, criticized.
	Moderate—Mild physical injury, loss of material possession, being lost, ridiculed, rejected.
	High—Suicide, being killed, mutilation, loss of significant person.

NOTE.—Scored on a ten-point scale.

the fantasy segment of the CARS (CARS III) with the diagnostic instruments listed and the ability of the same fantasy segment (CARS III) to differentiate between subgroups of patients diagnosed by the DSM III. The Pearson R correlation coefficient was used.

Results

There was no significant correlation between the fantasy segment of the CARS (CARS III) and the depression factor of the Achenbach scale, DMS III–depressive disorders, and the Weinberg criteria (see tables 2 and 3). However, there was a significant correlation of this segment with the DSM III–total psychopathology.

Further analysis showed that the fantasy segment of the CARS could not distinguish between normal versus depressed children as diagnosed by the DSM III, nor could it distinguish depressed children from those with general psychopathology. However, the same segment could distinguish normal children from those with general psychopathology. (All were diagnosed by DSM III criteria.)

294

TABLE 2
CORRELATIONS BETWEEN DEPRESSIVE FANTASY (CARS III) AND
VARIOUS DIAGNOSTIC INSTRUMENTS
($N = 24$; Pearson R)

	R	P
Weinberg	.1953	.23
DSM III (depressive disorder)	.2085	.20
DSM III (all psychopathology)	.3554	.03*
Achenbach (depressive factor)	.2510	.12

*Statistically significant.

TABLE 3
ABILITY OF DEPRESSIVE FANTASY (CARS III) TO DISTINGUISH
SUBGROUPS OF PATIENTS ON DSM III
($N = 24$; Pearson R)

	R	P
Normal vs. depressed children	.2713	.18
Depressed vs. children with other psychopathology	.2267	.28
Normal vs. children with any psychopathology	.3513	.03*

*Statistically significant.

Discussion

The results indicate that depressive fantasy as measured by the fantasy segment of the CARS is not significantly related to the various operational diagnoses of depression in children as measured by the instruments previously mentioned. It also appears unable to distinguish between depressed and nondepressed children. However, it does correlate significantly with general psychopathology, and it also distinguishes between normal children and those with psychopathology.

In scanning the literature on fantasy, one is struck by the relative paucity of information relating fantasy to psychopathology in children. To cite just two examples, the *Psychoanalytic Study of the Child* had only eight papers dealing with fantasy in its first twenty-five volumes, while Anna Freud's *Psycho-Analytical Treatment of Children* (1946) contains only two dreams. Sigmund Freud and other psychoanalytic writers saw fantasy as serving the function of fulfillment of secret and repressed wishes derived from undischarged, instinctual tensions. Freud (1900) maintained that daydreams or fantasies share with night dreams the function of wish fulfillment. However, unlike the latter, only some fantasies operate on an unconscious level governed by the primary process while many operate on a preconscious level, subject to secondary-process thinking mechanisms.

In discussing dreams of depressed adults, Beck (1967) describes the frequency of such themes as being thwarted, trapped, ridiculed, disappointed, hurt, or killed. He considers such dreams as specific to depressed patients, though to the best of our knowledge there was no systematic study attempting to investigate the frequency of such themes in dreams of normal controls as well as in adults with nondepressive psychopathology. Even if Beck's assumption is correct, it is unknown whether, in the daydreams or fantasies of these patients, such depressive themes also predominate.

Freud (1900) further related dream content to specific psychiatric diagnoses such as hysteria, obsessions, schizophrenia, depression, and organic brain disease, as well as absence of psychopathology and even sex of the dreamer. These studies, however, were largely based on clinical impressions rather than a systematic, controlled research design.

In an excellent review, Silberfeld (1978) examined the concept of fantasy as elaborated by various investigators in the late nineteenth and twentieth centuries with frequently widely differing viewpoints. Klinger (1975) challenges the dichotomy between dreams and fantasy as maintained by many classical psychoanalysts. He considers dreams and fantasies as parts of continuous streams of mental activities, each blending imperceptibly into the other. Unlike Freud and his early followers, he views fantasies as reflecting the thoughts and themes typical of a given age group, rather than related to instinctual drives. Klinger goes on to say that fantasy is closely related to the child's self-image but only loosely related to the child's overt behavior. Furthermore, he believes that neither dreaming nor fantasy is helping the child to find solutions to his problem. Winnicott (1971), though representing the more classical view of the split between dreams and fantasy, shares Klinger's notion that fantasies merely reflect the here and now and are devoid of future orientation or personal invested meaning.

On the other hand, many investigators emphasize the usefulness of fantasy in helping the child in anticipating goals and action, solutions to external conflicts, rehearsal for adult roles, and achievement of mastery by creativity (Greenacre 1959). Gould (1973) stressed the fantasy as a necessary stage of intellectual development and warned that interference with the spontaneous development of fantasy may make it very difficult to integrate affects and ego functions.

Gould and several other authors recognized the existence in the child's fantasy of frightening themes, such as destruction, death, disintegration, helplessness, injury, and loss or pain. However, she links these negative themes, not to psychopathology, but to a child's relative inability to distinguish between real and pretend danger. She sees such fantasies as helping the child in the maturation process by eventually leading to reality testing and a distinction between the real and imaginary world.

Conclusion

Some investigators stress the interrelationship between the content of fantasy and dreams and the child's level of psychic development. Our study suggests that we must take into account, not only the content of the fantasy, but also how much of a child's thinking is dominated by it as measured by appropriate rating instruments. Thus, there may be a threshold in the child's fantasy life. When this threshold is exceeded and the child's thinking is flooded by excessive affects, unsolved problems, and conflicts, it will reflect the child's general inability to cope and manifest itself in a variety of psychopathological symptoms.

Most clinicians working with children are aware that fantasy plays a sizable role in any child's psychic life. Our study reinforces this concept by indicating a meaningful relationship between childhood fantasy and psychopathology. It would seem advisable not to ignore childhood fantasy but, rather, to explore further its relationship to the normal and disturbed psychic life of the child and to assess its potential usefulness in the diagnostic assessment of children.

REFERENCES

Achenbach, T. M., and Edelbrock, C. S. 1973. The classification of child psychopathology; a review and analysis of empirical efforts. *Psychological Bulletin* 85:1275–1301.
Beck, A. T. 1967. Patterns in dreams of depressed patients. In *Depression*. New York: Harper & Row.

Carlson, G. A., and Cantwell, D. A. 1980. Unmasking masked depression. *American Journal of Psychiatry* 137:445–449.

Cytryn, L., and McKnew, D. H. 1972. Proposed classification of childhood depression. *American Journal of Psychiatry* 129:149–155.

Cytryn, L., and McKnew, D. H. 1979. Affective disorders in childhood. In J. L. Noshpitz, ed. *Basic Handbook of Child Psychiatry.* New York: Basic.

Cytryn, L., and McKnew, D. H. 1980. Affective disorders in childhood. In H. I. Kaplan, A. M. Freedman, and B. J. Sadock, eds. *Comprehensive Textbook of Psychiatry III.* 3d ed. Baltimore: Williams & Wilkins.

Cytryn, L.; McKnew, D. H.; and Bunney, W. E., Jr. 1980. Diagnosis of childhood depression: a reassessment. *American Journal of Psychiatry* 137:22–25.

Diagnostic and Statistical Manual of Mental Disorders (DSM-III). 1980. Washington, D.C.: American Psychiatric Association.

Freud, A. 1946. *The Psycho-Analytical Treatment of Children.* London: Imago.

Freud, S. 1900. The interpretation of dreams. *Standard Edition,* vols. 4–5. London: Hogarth, 1953.

Gould, R. 1973. *Child Studies through Fantasy.* New York: Quadrangle.

Greenacre, P. 1969. Play and creative imagination. *Psychoanalytic Study of the Child* 14:61–80.

Klinger, E. 1975. *The Structure and Function of Fantasy.* New York: Delta.

McKnew, D. H.; Cytryn, L.; Efron, A. M.; Gershon, E. S.; and Bunney, W. E., Jr. 1979. Offspring of patients with affective disorders. *British Journal of Psychiatry* 134:148–152.

Raskin, A. 1973. Depression in children: fact or fallacy. In R. G. Schulterbrandt and A. Raskin, eds. *Depression in Childhood.* New York: Raven.

Silberfeld, M. 1978. The idea of fantasy. *Psychiatric Journal of the University of Ottawa* 3:81–86.

Weinberg, W. A.; Rutman, J.; and Sullivan, L. 1973. Depression in children referred to an educational diagnostic center: diagnosis and treatment. *Journal of Pediatrics* 83:1065–1072.

Winnicott, D. W. 1971. *Playing and Reality.* London: Tavistock.

22 PREDICTORS OF BIPOLAR ILLNESS IN ADOLESCENTS WITH MAJOR DEPRESSION: A FOLLOW-UP INVESTIGATION[1]

MICHAEL STROBER AND GABRIELLE CARLSON

A major trend in child psychiatry is the increased prominence devoted to the study of affective disorders and their relation to adult psychopathology (Gittleman-Klein 1977; Puig-Antich 1980). This departure from theoretical tradition has been encouraged by advances in the therapeutic pharmacology and prophylaxis of affective disorders, increased precision of diagnostic classification, and the availability of reliable instruments for quantifying behavioral phenomena in these syndromes—all having obvious implications for the early diagnosis and secondary prevention of illness chronicity in child psychiatric populations.

Still, application of modern descriptive methods to the study of juvenile depression does not mitigate uncertainties which exist in connection with the utility and predictive value of the diagnosis in this age group. It remains unclear whether mechanisms of symptom production, treatment response, and prognosis in juvenile affective states are equivalent to those in adults. And insofar as depression represents an umbrella diagnostic concept, it can be assumed that young depressed patients will comprise a heterogeneous population varying considerably in long-term patterns of course and outcome. For this reason, a longitudinal perspective on the study of juvenile depression would seem especially pertinent to clarifying developmental continuities between pubertal and adult psychopathology and in identifying precursors and treatment needs of certain affective subtypes.

Of the various approaches to subtyping affectively disturbed pa-

© 1982, American Medical Association.
0-226-24056-8/82/0010-0022$01.00

tients, one that has benefited from substantial investigation in recent years and that may have significant application to longitudinal research on adolescent depression, particularly the early identification of premonitory signs of illness course and severity, is the unipolar-bipolar dichotomy. The practical importance of delimiting predictors of bipolar illness in adolescent depressives is underscored by several facts. First, epidemiological data (Loranger and Levine 1978; Perris 1966; Winokur, Clayton, and Reich 1969) indicate that as many as 35 percent of adult bipolars display initial episodes of illness during adolescence. Second, reports of significant depressive symptomatology foreshadowing the initial attack of mania in adolescents may be found consistently in the literature dealing with juvenile manic-depressive illness (Berg, Hullin, Allsopp, O'Brien, and MacDonald 1974; Campbell 1952; Hassanyeh and Davison 1980; Kasanin 1930; Landolt 1957; Olsen 1961; Warnecke 1975). And, last, certain follow-up data (Landolt 1957; Olsen 1961; Welner, Welner, and Fishman 1979) have suggested that onset of bipolar illness in early adolescence may portend an especially malignant outcome with a high prevalence of suicide and frequently recurring mood swings, presumably because uncontrollable fluctuations in the affective state have concomitant long-term effects on personality development.

In line with these considerations, we have completed a three- to four-year prospective follow-up study of sixty adolescents who ranged in age from thirteen to sixteen years at the time of their first hospitalization for a major depressive episode, twelve of whom (20 percent) developed mania during the follow-up period. This study is part of a larger program of research that is investigating, in adolescent depressives, the generality of relationships demonstrated in adults between clinical psychopathology, longitudinal course of symptoms, and family illness patterns. Because of the extreme psychological costs incurred by the emergence of bipolar illness during adolescence, and given the obvious relevance of early diagnosis to lithium prophylaxis, we have been especially interested in identifying precursor patterns of bipolar illness in this population. Having obtained extensive descriptive, family history, and treatment data on these sixty patients during the period of their index hospitalization, the question we address in this report is whether these variables bear any predictive relationship to the early development of bipolar illness. This statement of the problem coincides with recent work of Akiskal, Rosenthal, Rosenthal, Kashgarian, Khani, and Puzantian (1979) concerning the feasibility of differentiating primary from nonprimary affective disorder states on the basis of family history and pharmacologic variables, and which thus served as a useful guide for the present effort.

Methods

SUBJECTS

The sixty patients of the present study were consecutive admissions to the adolescent unit of the UCLA Neuropsychiatric Institute who satisfied research diagnostic criteria (RDC) (Spitzer, Endicott, and Robins 1978) for major depression and who were free of preexistent mania or other concurrent nonaffective major psychiatric disorders. All diagnoses represented the consensus judgment of two senior ward clinicians and were based on daily behavioral observations recorded during the initial two weeks of the patient's hospitalization; information concerning mental status on admission, preadmission social and academic functioning, maladaptive behavior and personality traits, and precipitating events relating to hospital admission, all recorded in standardized fashion at intake by the admitting physician and psychiatric nurse assigned to the patient; and an assessment of affective symptomatology using the Schedule for Affective Disorders and Schizophrenia (SADS) (Endicott and Spitzer 1978). Patients admitted with a presumptive diagnosis of major depression but who remitted spontaneously during the initial evaluation period were excluded from consideration in order to maximize homogeneity of the sample in terms of persistence and autonomy of the depressive episode.

At intake, a number of patients gave a history of intermittent periods of moodiness and irritability, generally originating in late childhood, although only two members of the cohort (3 percent) were actually judged to have had a previous episode of major depression fulfilling RDC standards; neither patient received psychopharmacologic treatment for the episode. Major demographic characteristics of the cohort are as follows: forty-seven (78 percent) were female and thirteen (22 percent) were male; the age distribution of the cohort at the time of hospitalization for the index is as follows: thirteen years, nine (15 percent); fourteen years, sixteen (27 percent); fifteen years, twenty-one (35 percent); sixteen years, fourteen (23 percent); full-scale IQ scores ranged from 92 to 144; all sixty patients were reared by one or both of their biological parents; the parents of sixteen (27 percent) were divorced.

EVALUATIVE PROCEDURES DURING INDEX
HOSPITALIZATION

As noted, the phenomenology of the index depressive episode was assessed using the SADS. We have previously shown this evaluative tool to yield highly reliable symptom ratings when applied to adolescent depressives (Strober, Green, and Carlson 1981). Each patient was interviewed toward the end of the first week of hospitalization by two experienced clinicians who made independent ratings of the presence and severity of twenty-seven signs and symptoms of depressive psychopathology and three items of nonaffective behavioral disturbance (alcohol use, drug use, and antisocial behavior). Administration of the SADS was intentionally delayed several days in order to use nursing observations of the patient's symptomatic behavior on the unit as an external check on the consistency and reliability of the information being reported by the patient in the interview. The patient's score on each of the thirty items was the average of the scores given by both raters, with the exception of one dichotomously rated item, psychotic features (mood-congruent delusions or hallucinations), which was scored positive only if both raters agreed on its presence. The percentage of agreement between the raters on the presence of psychotic features was 85 percent. The intraclass correlation coefficients of reliability between the two raters was deemed satisfactory ($r > .60$) for twenty-eight of the remaining twenty-nine items, the average coefficient being .77. One item, diurnal variation of mood, had low reliability ($r = .49$) and thus was deleted from the analysis.

Data concerning family psychiatric illness were ascertained from 200 first-degree (parents and siblings) and 422 second-degree (grandparents, uncles, aunts) relatives of the sixty patients by an experienced social worker specially trained in use of the SADS and RDC, who remained blind to the patients' hospital diagnosis. Direct interviews were carried out on 187 first-degree and 223 second-degree relatives using the lifetime version of the SADS; thirteen first-degree relatives were siblings below the age of twelve and were thus interviewed in the presence of a parent using a semistructured guide that probed major areas of affective disturbance. Diagnoses of first-degree relatives were made using the RDC. Information concerning the remaining 199 noninterviewed or deceased second-degree relatives was obtained from parents and collateral relatives of the patient using the family history method and associated research diagnostic criteria (Andreasen, Endicott, Spitzer, and Robins 1977).

Family history differences among the twelve bipolar and forty-eight nonbipolar outcome cases were assessed along the following dimensions:

1. Presence of a positive family history of affective illness of any type, of bipolar illness, and of suicide.

2. Multigenerational history of illness. In this analysis, fashioned along the lines outlined by Akiskal et al. (1979), the two outcome groups were contrasted in terms of the presence of affective illness spanning two ascendant generations.

3. Loaded pedigrees. Pedigrees were so designated if they contained three or more affected kin beyond the proband (Akiskal et al. 1979).

4. Familial morbidity risk. Morbid risks for affective disorder were calculated for both first- and second-degree relatives using the Weinberg Short Method (Rosenthal 1970) of age correction; the age risk employed was twelve to sixty-five. Risk estimates were determined separately for unipolar depression, bipolar illness, and combined affective disorder.

As a check on the reliability of the family diagnoses, a total of fifty interview protocols selected at random from relatives of bipolar and nonbipolar outcome cases were presented blindly to the senior author for secondary diagnosis using the categorizations affective disorder, other major psychiatric disorder, and no major psychiatric disorder. Agreement was reached in forty-six of the fifty cases (92 percent). The reliability of the unipolar-bipolar classification was also tested by submitting to the senior author for blind diagnosis the interview protocols of fifteen relatives diagnosed unipolar or bipolar by the social worker. Agreement on subtype classification was reached in fourteen of the fifteen cases (93 percent).

Fifty-six patients received an adequate trial of antidepressant therapy for the index depressive episode (two patients refused drug treatment and in two cases treatment was discontinued following the development of allergic symptoms). In each case, the choice of drug (amitriptyline or imiprimine) and dose level were determined by the treating physician. A trial was deemed adequate if a dosage of at least 150 mg was maintained for a minimum of two weeks. Eleven of the fifty-six patients also received initial treatment with antipsychotic agents to manage agitation and psychotic symptomatology. Treatment response in each patient was rated dichotomously (clear evidence of a decrement in affective symptom severity vs. no or minimal improvement) and was based on the treating physician's global evaluation of the patient's weekly progress following initiation of pharmacologic treatment. Also, since pharmacologically induced hypomania has been shown to predict the future spontaneous development of mania and is acknowledged to be more characteristic of bipolar depressives (Akiskal et al. 1979; Bunny 1978), a blind retrospective chart review of daily progress notes recorded on each patient receiving antidepressant therapy was carried out by two experienced psychiatric nurses using guidelines outlined by Akiskal et al. (1979) to assess evidence of this phenomenon. Hypomania was scored only if both raters agreed on its presence.

METHOD OF PROSPECTIVE FOLLOW-UP

All sixty patients were tracked successfully during the entire three- to four-year period of surveillance. During the index hospitalization, each patient and his or her parents had been asked to participate in postdischarge follow-up interviews that would be conducted periodically to assess general progress in social, academic, and affective functioning. It was also explained that if there was evidence of a recurrence of illness during the follow-up period, assistance would be provided, if needed, in assessing the patient's level of symptomatology and need for treatment. In actuality, all sixty patients received some form of psychosocial or pharmacologic treatment following discharge—some continuously, others on an intermittent basis. Eleven patients remained on antidepressant medication for brief periods following discharge; medication was subsequently instituted in one patient who experienced an immediate relapse and was maintained throughout the period of follow-up. Another six patients subsequently required additional antidepressant therapy during the period of follow-up for further depressive episodes, although pharmacologic intervention was not used in every patient who experienced relapses of depression.

Follow-up contacts were made at six-month intervals dating from the patient's discharge by a team consisting of a psychiatric nurse, social worker, and the senior author, all of whom had knowledge of the patient during his or her index hospitalization. To maintain as much consistency as possible with our baseline measures of the patient's affective state, a standardized follow-up interview form adapted from the SADS was employed to evaluate the occurrence of manic, hypomanic, and depressive symptoms, along with general school and interpersonal functioning, drug and alcohol use, and additional psychiatric treatment received during the interval since discharge or the prior follow-up contact. Information was obtained from both the patient and a parent, typically mother. Records of any outpatient and inpatient treatment received by the patient were also obtained by permission to provide a further external check on the validity of our follow-up diagnosis.

As noted, twelve of the sixty patients (eight females, four males) developed mania during the period of follow-up. The shift in polarity occurred an average of 28.42 weeks following index admission (range = 10–76; SD = 17.27). Two patients actually shifted during the index hospitalization following resolution of their depressive episodes. Of the remaining ten bipolar outcome cases, two were readmitted to our facility in an acute manic state prior to the first planned follow-up contact; one was judged to be hypomanic when seen at the six-month follow-up and was subsequently hospitalized at a state facility; and seven were hospitalized for their first manic attack at local community and private inpatient facilities at varying points after discharge from UCLA. In all instances, the follow-up diagnosis of mania was made in accordance with RDC guidelines. As it turned out, all ten of the twelve bipolar outcome patients whose switch in polarity came after their index hospitalization received an admitting diagnosis of mania when rehospitalized. Of the forty-eight nonbipolar outcome cases, one failed to recover completely from the index episode; ten had one or more further episodes of major depression; four had intermittent periods of dysphoria which failed to meet criteria for major depression; and thirty-three remained relatively asymptomatic throughout the follow-up.

The bipolar and nonbipolar outcome groups did not differ significantly in age at index hospitalization, IQ, incidence of parental divorce, the proportion of family members whose psychiatric history was ascertained via direct interview, or the proportion receiving completed trials of antidepressant therapy during index hospitalization.

DATA ANALYSIS

Analyses of the predictive association between symptomatologic family history, and treatment response data compiled during the patients' index hospitalization and eventual bipolar outcome, were conducted in two steps. First, the bipolar and nonbipolar outcome groups were compared to identify statistically significant ($P < .05$) differences on these variables. Comparison of symptom ratings was by the Student t-test; categorical data were analyzed by χ^2 tests corrected for continuity, or, when statistically indicated, the Fisher exact probability test. Second, differentiating variables were tested for their *sensitivity, specificity,* and *predictive* value in distinguishing bipolar outcomes in this cohort using formulae given by Vecchio (1966) and elaborated on by Akiskal et al. (1979). To summarize briefly, sensitivity refers to the proportion of bipolar outcomes exhibiting the characteristic in question; specificity refers to the proportion of nonbipolar outcomes not exhibiting the characteristic and thus indexes the accuracy of classifying patients in the cohort as nonbipolar outcomes; and predictive value, computed by dividing the number of bipolars with the characteristic by the total number of patients in the cohort with the characteristic, indexes the percentage of times that presence of the characteristic in question accurately depicts a bipolar outcome case.

Results

AFFECTIVE SYMPTOMATOLOGY AT INDEX EPISODE

A comparison of the bipolar and nonbipolar outcome groups on the thirty SADS items rated at the time of index hospitalization is presented in table 1. It may be seen that twelve items differentiated the groups at statistically significant levels. Compared to their nonbipolar counterparts, adolescents whose illness pursued a bipolar course exhibited a shorter duration of onset of symptoms ($t = 3.60, df = 58, P < .001$); received significantly higher ratings on depressed mood ($t = 2.38, df = 58, P < .02$), self-reproach ($t = 2.22, df = 58, P < .05$), bodily concerns ($t = 2.85, df = 58, P < .01$), diminished concentration ($t = 2.46, df = 58, P < .02$), and psychomotor retardation ($t = 3.28, df = 58, P < .01$); and were far more likely than nonbipolars to exhibit mood-congruent delusions or hallucinations (75 percent vs. 6 percent, Fisher exact $P < .000$). By contrast, nonbipolars received significantly higher severity ratings on five items: suicidal tendencies ($t = 2.27, df = 58, P < .05$); weight gain ($t = 2.21, df = 58, P < .05$); irritability ($t = 2.34, df = 58, P < .05$); self-pity ($t = 2.37, df = 58, P < .02$); and demandingness ($t = 2.87, df = 58, P < .01$). The data in table 1 also reveal considerable phenotypic overlap between the two outcome groups, both receiving relatively equivalent ratings for distinct quality of depressed mood, worry, self-negation, pessimism, sleep disturbance, anergia, appetite loss, withdrawal, loss of pleasure, nonreactivity of mood, and agitation. Thus, it is important to note that endogeneity per se was not a contributor in differentiating prospective bipolarity in the adolescents of this cohort; according to RDC rules of subtype classification, the

TABLE 1

SADS INTAKE RATINGS OF DEPRESSION AND ASSOCIATED CHARACTERISTICS IN BIPOLAR AND NONBIPOLAR OUTCOME GROUPS

	Group					
	Bipolar (*N*=12)		Nonbipolar (*N*=48)			
Item (Range)	*M*	SD	*M*	SD	*t*	*P**
Duration of onset (1 [acute]–9 [insidious])	4.94	.81	6.02	.96	3.60	.001
Depressed mood (1–7)	5.94	1.02	5.08	1.13	2.38	.02
Distinct quality of mood (1–4) ...	3.84	.43	3.62	.49	1.57	N.S.
Worry (1–6)	5.08	.86	5.21	.93	.43	N.S.
Self-reproach (1–6)	4.98	.99	4.18	1.13	2.22	.05
Worthlessness (1–6)	4.17	.94	4.68	.99	1.59	N.S.
Pessimism (1–6)	4.92	1.01	4.44	1.16	1.33	N.S.
Suicidal tendencies (1–7)	3.69	.91	4.37	.96	2.27	.05
Number of suicide attempts (1–9)	.50	.61	.91	.76	1.71	N.S.
Insomnia (1–6)	4.18	.79	4.32	.84	.54	N.S.
Excessive sleep (1–6)	3.51	.91	3.63	.78	.46	N.S.
Decreased energy (1–6)	4.80	.90	4.36	.97	1.38	N.S.
Decreased appetite (1–6)	4.42	.78	4.04	.81	1.46	N.S.
Weight loss (1–6)	2.18	.69	2.64	.74	1.92	N.S.
Increased appetite (1–6)	1.21	.61	1.67	.82	1.92	N.S.
Weight gain (1–6)	1.24	.46	1.77	.79	2.21	.05
Bodily concerns (1–6)	4.18	.94	3.24	1.06	2.85	.01
Diminished concentration (1–6) ..	4.67	.76	3.98	.88	2.46	.02
Loss of interest (1–6)	4.19	.85	4.09	.98	.33	N.S.
Irritability (1–6)	3.37	.92	4.12	1.12	2.34	.05
Social withdrawal (1–6)	4.64	.84	4.49	.98	.50	N.S.
Agitation (1–6)	2.97	.72	2.91	.93	.21	N.S.
Retardation (1–6)	4.44	.80	3.29	1.11	3.28	.01
Nonreactivity of mood (1–6)	4.29	.82	4.09	.92	.71	N.S.
Self-pity (1–6)	2.21	.68	2.78	.79	2.37	.02
Demandingness (1–6)	1.86	.67	2.55	.78	2.87	.01
Psychosis present (delusions or hallucinations)	(75%)	...	(6%)	...	...	.000†
Alcohol abuse (1–6)	2.11	.72	2.37	.84	1.00	N.S.
Drug abuse (1–6)	2.46	.79	2.82	.91	1.29	N.S.
Antisocial behavior (1–6)	1.36	.67	1.81	.78	1.88	N.S.

*Two-tailed probabilities.
†Fisher exact probability test, two-tailed.

index episodes of all twelve bipolar outcome patients were classifiable as endogenous compared to thirty-five of the forty-eight (73 percent) nonbipolars who were so classified (P = N.S.).

Because of the inherent unreliability of single items in predicting to an external criterion, we undertook a further analysis of these data to determine whether a clinically meaningful composite of SADS items could be identified in association with the bipolar group; if so, this syndrome description could then be tested for its generalizability in replication studies mounted by other investigators. From a methodological standpoint, a multivariate statistic would have been optimally suited for this exploration. However, reliable application of multivariate approaches to data reduction was precluded by the comparatively small and disproportionate sizes of the outcome groups. Instead, symptom profiles were constructed for each patient by considering a particular symptom present only if the patient received a severity rating of moderate or beyond for the item, reasoning that such a cutoff would serve to maximize differences between patients within the cohort (for most items this required a score of at least four on the SADS severity scale; for the duration of onset item, onset was considered precipitous if duration was rated as being less than two months).

Scrutinizing the data in this manner suggested a three-item cluster as offering the most face valid and heuristically meaningful discrimination of bipolar outcome, consisting, as seen in table 1, of those items with the greatest relative power in discriminating between the two outcome groups: precipitous onset of symptoms, psychomotor retardation, and psychotic features. This cluster characterized eight of the twelve (67 percent) patients with bipolar outcome compared to only two of forty-eight (4 percent) nonbipolar outcomes, a difference which is highly significant (Fisher exact P = .000015).

FAMILY HISTORY DIFFERENCES AMONG OUTCOME GROUPS

There was an extremely high percentage of patients in the total cohort with a family pedigree positive for affective disorder: altogether, forty-six patients (77 percent) had at least one affectively ill first- or second-degree relative (eleven of twelve bipolars, 92 percent vs. thirty-five of forty-eight nonbipolars, 73 percent; P = N.S.), while the percentage of bipolar and nonbipolar outcomes with an ill parent was 50 percent and 46 percent, respectively. As reported by others

(Mendelwicz 1974), family histories of suicide and alcoholism were both more common in the pedigrees of bipolars, but these differences were not significant. By contrast, family history takes on statistically significant predictive power when viewed from the standpoint of polarity of illness in relatives and the density and generational pattern of illness within the pedigree. First, the percentage of family pedigrees affected with bipolar illness is significantly higher in bipolar outcomes than in nonbipolar outcomes (50 percent vs. 10 percent respectively, Fisher exact P <.005). This is entirely consistent with accumulated evidence of contrasting patterns of inheritance in unipolar and bipolar depressives—specifically, the tendency for the more severe bipolar forms of illness to segregate in families. It is interesting to note that there is a preponderance of Bipolar Type I illness in the affected relatives: of the eighteen secondary cases of bipolar illness, thirteen were classifiable as Bipolar I and five as Bipolar II; there was no difference between outcome groups in the relative frequency of Type I versus Type II illness in affected kin. Fourteen of these eighteen secondary cases of bipolar illness were confirmed by personal interview—ten of the thirteen Bipolar I's and four of the five Bipolar II's. Second, the tendency for affective disorder to "load" in an individual pedigree was significantly more characteristic of patients with a bipolar outcome: six of twelve bipolar outcomes (50 percent) had pedigrees containing three or more ill relatives compared to seven of forty-eight (15 percent) of the nonbipolar group (Fisher exact P <.02). And third, the presence of a three-generational history of affective disorder was shown to be predictive of bipolarity, occuring in five of twelve (42 percent) bipolar outcomes compared to seven of forty-eight (15 percent) nonbipolar outcomes (Fisher exact P <.05).

These differences were amplified further by computing morbidity risks for affective disorder in the total group of relatives of patients in the two outcome groups. The overall risk for affective disorder in the combined group of first- and second-degree relatives of bipolar outcomes was 32.3 percent compared to 18.4 percent for nonbipolar outcomes, a statistically significant difference ($\chi^2 = 6.66$, P <.01). Separate morbid risks were also calculated for familial unipolar and bipolar illness in the outcome groups. This subanalysis revealed a significantly higher rate of bipolar illness in relatives of the bipolar outcomes (10.8 percent) compared to nonbipolar outcome relatives (2.2 percent; $\chi^2 = 10.31$, P<.005), as well as a nonsignificant excess of unipolar depression (21.6 percent vs. 16.2 percent, P = N.S.). Table 2 gives the sex

TABLE 2

SEX DISTRIBUTION OF SECONDARY CASES OF AFFECTIVE DISORDER AMONG RELATIVES OF BIPOLAR AND NONBIPOLAR OUTCOME GROUPS

Type of Illness in Relative	Group							
	Bipolar				Nonbipolar			
	Male Relatives		Female Relatives		Male Relatives		Female Relatives	
	Cases	BZ*	Morbid Risk (%)	Cases	BZ*	Morbid Risk (%)	Cases	BZ*	Morbid Risk (%)
Bipolar illness	4	43.0	9.3	5	40.5	12.3	5	158.5	3.2	4	156.0	2.6
Unipolar depression	4	43.0	9.3	14	40.5	34.6	7	158.5	4.4	44	156.0	28.2

*BZ = Age-adjusted number of relatives at risk.

distribution of secondary cases of unipolar and and bipolar illness among relatives of the two outcome groups.

TREATMENT RESPONSE

Twenty-four of forty-five nonbipolar outcomes (53 percent) were rated as showing an unequivocally positive response to antidepressant therapy compared to only two of eleven bipolars (18 percent; Fisher exact $P = .27$, two-tailed). In all likelihood, the comparatively lower rate of improvement in the bipolar group stems from the high incidence of psychosis in these patients, a clinical factor which is known to moderate antidepressant response in adult depressives. The groups were not found to differ significantly in the average maximum dose level of antidepressants attained during the course of treatment ($t = 1.06$, $df = 54$, $P = $ N.S.). However, the finding of greater predictive significance is that concerning pharmacologically precipitated hypomania. Two positive cases were found in the cohort, and both patients were from the bipolar outcome group (Fisher exact $P < .036$, one-tailed). The hypomanic state of one was recorded on the ninth day of treatment and was characterized by "motor acceleration, increased irritability, and intrusiveness with staff"; the episode was noted to subside on the twelfth day of treatment following a reduction in dose level. In the second case, the hypomanic symptoms of "elevated mood, frequent giggling, inappropriate physical contact with staff and peers" were recorded between the twelfth and fifteenth days of anti-depressant therapy and also decreased following a reduction in dose level. Thus, while the base rate of occurrence of pharmacologic hypomania in the cohort was low (4 percent), it has high discriminative power. This finding is in complete agreement with Akiskal et al.'s (1979) report that occurrence of transient hypomanic states during antidepressant therapy predicts a bipolar outcome with 100 percent confidence in adult depressives.

DISCRIMINATIVE VALUES OF DIFFERENTIATING VARIABLES

The sensitivity, specificity, and predictive value of the independent variables found to be associated with bipolar outcome are given in table 3. It may be seen that four of the five variables—symptom cluster, family history of bipolar illness, three-generation history of affective

TABLE 3

DISCRIMINATIVE VALUES OF CLINICAL, FAMILY HISTORY, AND PHARMACOLOGIC
VARIABLES ASSOCIATED WITH BIPOLAR OUTCOME

	Sensitivity (%)*	Specificity (%)†	Predictive Value (%)‡
Symptom cluster§	67	96	80
Bipolar illness in family pedigree	50	90	55
Affective disorder in three successive generations	42	85	42
Loaded pedigree	50	85	46
Pharmacologically induced hypomania‖	18	100	100

*Sensitivity is the proportion of bipolars exhibiting the characteristic.

†Specificity is the proportion of nonbipolars not exhibiting the characteristic. Thus, it represents the percentage of subjects accurately identified as nonbipolar.

‡Predictive value is the percentage of times that the characteristic will accurately detect a bipolar case. It is computed by dividing the number of bipolars with the characteristic by the total number of subjects with the characteristic.

§Acute onset of symptoms, psychotic features, and psychomotor retardation.

‖Successfully completed trials of antidepressant therapy (two weeks at 150 mg or more) were obtained on eleven bipolars and forty-five nonbipolars.

disorder, and loaded pedigree—possess moderately high sensitivity in the bipolar outcome group (range = 42–67 percent), while pharmacologically induced hypomania is the least sensitive (18 percent). However, given the relative infrequency of these five variables in the nonbipolar outcome patients, each possesses an extremely high specificity of association with bipolar outcome (over 85 percent), with pharmacologically induced hypomania emerging as the surest predictor. Accordingly, we may generalize from these figures that the presence of any of these variables in an individual patient takes on considerable prognostic significance.

Turning to the predictive value of each variable—the proportion of positive findings in the cohort that are true-positive for bipolar outcome—we see that the prediction of bipolarity can be made with virtual certainty in a patient exhibiting pharmacologic hypomania, and with a high degree of confidence (80 percent) in the case of a patient with acute onset of symptoms, severe psychomotor retardation, and psychosis. On the other hand, the family history variables yield only moderate degrees of confidence prediction (range = 42–55 percent). However, these figures are probably a bit conservative given the suppression of predictive value when specificity of a test find is less than 100 percent and the size of the criterion group is small. Moreover, considering the incidence of bipolar outcome in the cohort (20 percent), the family history variables still yield a prediction that is far better than chance alone.

In considering these data further, we wondered whether a more optimal prediction might be obtained by merely summing the number of variables present in the patient rather than considering each predictor individually and relating this summary index to outcome status. Examining the data in this fashion revealed the following: (1) Two of the five predictor variables were present together in seven of the twelve bipolar outcomes (58 percent) as compared to five of forty-eight non-bipolars (10 percent; Fisher exact $P = .001$; sensitivity, specificity, and predictive value = 85 percent, 90 percent, and 58 percent, respectively). (2) Six of the twelve bipolars (50 percent) were positive for three of the predictors compared to only two of the forty-eight non-bipolars (4 percent; Fisher exact $P = .0005$; sensitivity, specificity, and predictive value = 50 percent, 96 percent, and 75 percent, respectively). And last, three patients, all bipolar outcomes, were positive for four predictors (Fisher exact $P = .006$; sensitivity, specificity, and predictive value = 25 percent, 100 percent, and 100 percent, respectively). Thus, the discriminative power of a single composite index lies primarily in eliminating the risk of false-positive predictions of bipolar outcome. At the same time, it can be seen that neither the three-variable nor four-variable combination significantly improves upon the discriminative values obtained using the individual symptom cluster variable.

Comment

In considering the generality of the present results, several cautions must be borne in mind. First, the discriminative values of the predictor variables are necessarily sample-specific; from a statistical point of view, sample size, the base rate of bipolarity in the patients selected for study, and length of follow-up periods are all parameters which can significantly affect the magnitude and identity of variables found to predict outcome status. For this reason, utility of the clinical, genetic, and pharmacologic variables found to prognosticate bipolar illness in this cohort require further testing in replication studies carried out on comparably diagnosed cohorts of depressed adolescents. A second important qualification pertains to the relatively short duration of follow-up. Considering the lengthy period of risk for affective disorder

313

and the fact that bipolar illness peaks in onset between twenty and thirty years of age, it is conceivable that some of the patients presently classified as nonbipolar will ultimately experience a manic attack, thereby altering the discriminating power of the current predictor variables. Clearly, our findings would be strengthened had we employed a follow-up that was sufficiently extended into the period of maximum risk for the development of bipolar illness. However, while the actual risk of a manic attack in adolescents suffering a major depression remains unknown, the conversion to bipolar illness in 20 percent of our cohort is not inconsistent with existing literature on the incidence and timing of polarity switches in adolescent and adult depressives (Akiskal, Bitar, Puzantian, Rosenthal, and Walker 1978; Angst, Baastrup, Grof, Hippus, Poldinger, and Weis 1973; Welner et al. 1979). Still, it would perhaps be more appropriate to view the present data conservatively as being relevant to predicting the *early* development of mania in adolescents suffering major depression.

A third limitation arises in connection with the pharmacologic response data and concerns the lack of systematically controlled trials of antidepressant therapy or serum tricyclic level determinations. For this reason, it remains unknown whether more aggressive treatment with tricyclics or different choices of drug in the individual patient might have materially affected the observed incidence and specificity of pharmacologic hypomania in this cohort. Furthermore, given the inherent cyclicity of symptoms in bipolar patients, one cannot maintain with complete certainty that the abrupt transitory increases in social, motor, and verbal activity witnessed in the two bipolar outcome patients were truly drug-induced rather than short-lived, spontaneous switches that happened to coincide with antidepressant treatment. Nonetheless, we assume that former to be the case insofar as our observations are consistent with evidence that true pharmacologic hypomania tends to occur relatively soon after the initiation of drug treatment—often at low levels of tricyclics—and will often remit upon a lowering of dosage level (Bunney 1978).

And we acknowledge the absence of a blind follow-up and a possible underreporting of hypomania in some patients with a presumptive nonbipolar outcome to be justified methodologic criticisms. Yet these are not likely to have posed significant limitations since all predictor values were coded before determination of the patient's outcome status, and considerable care was taken to assess the presence of fluctuations in mood, verbal behavior, neurovegetative functions, and patterns of interpersonal relating via repeated follow-up contacts with both the patient and his or her parents.

The demonstrated utility of the symptom, genetic, and pharmacologically based variables as predictors of bipolar illness in adolescent depressives is very much in accord with reported differences among unipolar and bipolar subtypes in clinical phenomenology, inheritance patterns, and drug response. First, the validity of rapid symptom onset, psychomotor retardation, and psychoticism as predictors of bipolarity derives support from (a) the greater cyclicity of mood states documented in bipolar depressives (Angst et al. 1973); (b) evidence of more pronounced motor retardation in bipolar than unipolar depressives shown in comparative studies of symptom profile, psychometric test performance, and telemetrically monitored gross motor activity (Depue and Monroe 1978); and (c) mounting evidence that psychoticism is far more intrinsic to bipolar manic-depressive illness than previously believed (Pope and Lipinski 1978).

This latter point requires some elaboration, since the association between psychoticism during depression and liability to bipolar outcome in our cohort is inconsistent with studies (Beigel and Murphy 1971; Kathol and Winokur 1977) which fail to identify differences between unipolars and bipolars in the frequency of hallucinations and delusions during the depressed phase of illness. This apparent contradiction may be due to variations between studies with respect to sampling and data collection procedures, as well as the possible influence of age and maturational factors on symptom formation in the affective disorders. For instance, in the Beigel and Murphy study (1971), global ratings of psychosis were based on overt displays of symptomatic behavior during hospitalization rather than direct clinical interviewing of the patients. As a result, their data may suffer from significant underreporting of psychotic ideation, especially in more guarded or verbally withdrawn patients. Likewise, data summarized by Kathol and Winokur (1977) were largely retrospective in nature and averaged across several different cohorts of patients assessed by different investigators, thereby confounding interpretation by sampling biases and possible nonuniformity of assessment methods. Beyond these considerations, however, we believe it is the young age of our cohort that is the critical variable accounting for the predictive relationship between psychoticism and bipolarity. This hypothesis is suggested by recent threshold models of disease transmission which postulate the existence of a continuously distributed gradient of vulnerability underlying all forms of major affective disorder, wherein bipolar illness reflects the phenotypic outcome of a more extreme or deviant point on the liability curve (Reich, Cloninger, and Guze 1975). Granting the assumption that age of onset is under at least partial genetic control, a plausible extension of this model to our results might suggest that the unusually early onset of manifest illness in adolescence reflects transmittance of even greater combined liability (increased genetic load and adverse environment), which theoretically could account for a greater frequency of clinically morbid signs of illness severity (for example, psychosis) in adolescent bipolars compared to their adult counterparts. The additional possibility that developmental factors intrinsic to adolescence interact with genetically transmitted predispositions to produce a particularly severe clinical expression of depression in the latent bipolar outcome of patients is also worthy of consideration.

As summarized by Baron, Klotz, Mendelwicz, and Rainer (1981) and Taylor and Abrams (1980), the bulk of family history studies show adequate support for a partial genetic overlap of unipolar and bipolar illness, with bipolar families having a higher overall risk for affective disorder and a higher frequency of relatives exhibiting more severe bipolar form. Thus, the finding that inheritance patterns suggestive of greater genetic deviance (that is, loaded, multigenerational, and bipolar positive pedigrees) were predictive of bipolar outcome is compatible with existing family history data while lending support to a corollary of the liability threshold concept—namely, that much can be foretold of the subsequent course of illness in juvenile depressives from the degree of affective morbidity present in their family pedigree.

Last, the differential response to antidepressant therapy by the two outcome groups, specifically the exclusive association of drug-precipitated hypomania with eventual bipolar outcome, gains significance from available evidence, reviewed extensively by Bunney (1978), that bipolars are far more vulnerable than unipolars to switches into hypomania or mania. Accordingly, our data imply that biological differences between latent depressive subtypes are already present and detectable during the period of early adolescence and that pharmacologic challenge can serve as one reliable aid in delimiting specific affective syndromes in juveniles. Whether adolescent bipolars are actually more sensitive than adults to pharmacologic challenge is worthy of further consideration if the hypothesis of greater genetic load associated with an early age of onset is shown to be valid.

Conclusions

In summary, the present results support the need for further empirical investigation of the clinical and taxonomic properties of juvenile affective disorders. It seems clear enough that current descriptive and genetic approaches to adult psychopathology are also viable tools for investigating the prognostic significance of affective states developing in early and mid adolescence.

NOTES

We thank the patients and families for their cooperation, and the clinical staff of Ward A-South, especially Judy Prebble, R.N., and Jane Burroughs, M.S.W., for assisting with data collection and conducting the follow-up assessments.
1. This article originally appeared in *Archives of General Psychiatry* 39 (May 1982): 549–555, under the title, "Clinical, Genetic and Psychopharmacologic Predictors of Bipolar Illness in Adolescents with Major Depression: A Follow-up Investigation." We are grateful to the AMA for permission to reprint it here.

REFERENCES

Akiskal, H. S.; Bitar, A. H.; Puzantian, V. R., Rosenthal, T. L.; and Walker, P. W. 1978. The nosological status of neurotic depression: a prospective three-to-four-year follow-up examination in light of the primary-secondary and unipolar-bipolar dichotomies. *Archives of General Psychiatry* 35:756–767.
Akiskal, H. S.; Rosenthal, R. H.; Rosenthal, T.; Kashgarian, M.; Khani, M. K.; and Puzantian, V. R. 1979. Differentiation of primary affective illness from situational, symptomatic, and secondary depressions. *Archives of General Psychiatry* 36:635–643.
Andreasen, N. C.; Endicott, J.; Spitzer, R. L.; and Robins, E. 1977. The family history method using diagnostic criteria: reliability and validity. *Archives of General Psychiatry* 34:1229–1235.
Angst, J.; Baastrup, P.; Grof, P.; Hippus, H.; Poldinger, W.; and Weis, P. 1973. The course of monopolar depression and bipolar psychoses. *Psychiatrica, Neurologica, et Neurochirugia Psychological Bulletin* 76:489–500.
Baron, M.; Klotz, J.; Mendelwicz, J.; and Rainer, J. 1981. Multiple-

threshold transmission of affective disorders. *Archives of General Psychiatry* 38:79–84.

Beigel, A., and Murphy, D. L. 1971. Unipolar and bipolar affective illness. *Archives of General Psychiatry* 24:215–220.

Berg, I.; Hullin, R.; Allsopp, M.; O'Brien, P.; and MacDonald, R. 1974. Bipolar manic-depressive psychosis in early adolescence. *British Journal of Psychiatry* 125:416–417.

Bunney, W. E. 1978. Psychopharmacology of the switch process in affective illness. In M. A. Lipton, A. DiMascio, and K. F. Killam, eds. *Psychopharmacology: A Generation of Progress*. New York: Raven.

Campbell, J. D. 1952. Manic-depressive psychosis in children. *Journal of Nervous and Mental Disease* 116:424–439.

Depue, R. A., and Monroe, S. M. 1978. The unipolar-bipolar distinction in the depressive disorders. *Psychological Bulletin* 85:1001–1029.

Dunner, D. L.; Fleiss, J. L.; and Fieve, R. L. 1976. The course of development of mania in patients with recurrent depression. *American Journal of Psychiatry* 133:905–908.

Endicott, J., and Spitzer, R. L. 1978. A diagnostic interview: the Schedule for Affective Disorders and Schizophrenia. *Archives of General Psychiatry* 35:837–844.

Gittleman-Klein, R. 1977. Definitional and methodological issues concerning depressive illness in children. In J. G. Schulterbrandt and A. Raskin, eds. *Depression in Childhood: Diagnosis, Treatment and Conceptual Models*. New York: Raven.

Hassanyeh, F., and Davison, K. 1980. Bipolar affective psychosis with onset before 16 years: report of 10 cases. *British Journal of Psychiatry* 137:530–539.

Kasanin, J. 1930. Affective psychoses in children. *American Journal of Psychiatry* 10:897–926.

Kathol, R., and Winokur, G. 1977. "Organic" and "psychotic" symptoms in unipolar (UP) and bipolar (BP) depressions. *Comprehensive Psychiatry* 18:251–253.

Landolt, A. D. 1957. Follow-up studies on circular manic-depressive reactions occurring in the young. *Bulletin of the New York Academy of Medicine* 33:65–37.

Loranger, A. W., and Levine, P. M. 1978. Age of onset of bipolar affective illness. *Archives of General Psychiatry* 35:1345–1348.

Mendelwicz, J. 1974. A genetic contribution toward an understanding of affective equivalents. In S. Lesse, ed. *Masked Depression*. New York: Aronson.

Olsen, T. 1961. Follow-up study of manic-depressive patients whose first attack occurred before the age of 19. *Acta Psychiatrica Scandinavica* (suppl.) 162:45–51.

Perris, C. 1966. A study of bipolar (manic-depressive) and unipolar recurrent depressive psychoses. *Acta Psychiatrica Scandinavica* (suppl.) 194:9–189.

Pope, H. G., and Lipinski, J. P. 1978. Diagnosis in schizophrenia and manic-depressive illness: a reassessment of the specificity of "schizophrenic" symptoms in the light of current research. *Archives of General Psychiatry* 35:811–828.

Puig-Antich, J. 1980. Affective disorders in childhood: a review and perspective. *Psychiatric Clinics of North America* 3:403–424.

Reich, T.; Cloninger, R. C.; and Guze, S. B. 1975. The multifactorial model of disease transmission: description of the model and its use in psychiatry. *British Journal of Psychiatry* 127:1–19.

Rosenthal, D. 1970. *Genetic Theory and Abnormal Behavior*. New York: McGraw-Hill.

Spitzer, R. L.; Endicott, J.; and Robins, E. 1978. Research diagnostic criteria: rationale and reliability. *Archives of General Psychiatry* 34:136–141.

Strober, M.; Green, J.; and Carlson, G. 1981. Phenomenology and subtypes of major depressive disorder in adolescence. *Journal of Affective Disorders* 3:281–290.

Taylor, M. A., and Abrams, R. 1980. Reassessing the bipolar-unipolar dichotomy. *Journal of Affective Disorders* 2:195–217.

Vecchio, T. J. 1966. Predictive value of a single diagnostic test in unselected populations. *New England Journal of Medicine* 274:1171–1173.

Warnecke, L. 1975. A case of manic-depressive illness in childhood. *Journal of the Canadian Psychiatric Association* 20:195–200.

Welner, A.; Welner, Z.; and Fishman, R. 1979. Psychiatric adolescent inpatients: eight-to-ten-year follow-up. *Archives of General Psychiatry* 36:698–700.

Winokur, G.; Clayton, P. J.; and Reich, T. 1969. *Manic-Depressive Illness*. St. Louis: Mosby.

Winokur, G.; and Morrison, J. 1973. The Iowa 500: follow-up of 225 depressives. *British Journal of Psychiatry* 123:543–548.

23   FUNCTIONAL BRAIN ASYMMETRY AND AFFECTIVE DISORDERS

HAROLD A. SACKEIM, PAOLO DECINA, AND SIDNEY MALITZ

In this chapter we review much of the evidence suggesting that affective disorders are associated with right hemispheric dysfunction and/or overactivation. The possibility of differential hemispheric involvement in affective disorders necessarily raises for consideration the more general role of hemispheric specialization in the regulation of emotion.

It should be emphasized from the beginning that the clinical observations and experimental data that will be reviewed in reference to affective lateralization do not constitute a coherent and systematic body of evidence based on unequivocal findings. To date, there have been few attempts to measure brain activity directly and relate activation asymmetries to affective disorders. Because of the indirect nature of the evidence suggesting a relationship between cerebral laterality and pathophysiology of emotions, the conclusions to be presented should be considered preliminary and in need of further testing.

Anatomoclinical observations of differences in the sensorimotor and cognitive deficits secondary to unilateral brain damage originally led to the concept that the two sides of the brain differ in mediating various functions. Subsequent neuropsychological studies with normal populations as well as with patients who underwent surgical disconnection of hemispheres (commissurotomy) supported the characterization of the cognitive differences between the sides of the brain. Terms like cerebral laterality, cerebral dominance, functional hemispheric asymmetry, lateralization—all refer to these functional differences between hemispheres.

In the vast majority of right-handers (97 percent) and most likely a majority of left-handers (70 percent), the left hemisphere is superior to the right hemisphere in subserving verbal functions, that is, production of language and perception of sensory stimuli that follow in temporal sequence and that can be easily labeled with words. By contrast, the right hemisphere is mainly responsible for nonverbal, perceptual, and spatial functions (Hécaen and Albert 1978). Less than 4 percent of the general population, mainly left-handers, display an atypical pattern in direction and degree of hemispheric specialization for language functions. In this minority, the right hemisphere may be specialized for verbal functions usually subserved by the left. Another minority of individuals may show little or no difference in specialization between the hemispheres.

The nature of hemispheric specialization in cognition is still controversial. For some authors (for example, Milner 1968), the nature of the differences is a function of the material used in verbal and nonverbal testing, with the presumption that the hemispheres differ in the types of information they process most efficiently. For others (Hécaen and Albert 1978), the specialization relates to the different modes of information processing employed by the two hemispheres: logical-analytic processing associated with the left and synthetic-holistic processing associated with the right hemisphere. By this view, the functional differences are determined by the processing strategies imposed on information and not so much by the type of information, per se.

Affective Lateralization: Studies of Brain Damage

The serendipitous observation of a different emotional reaction following pharmacological inactivation of one or the other hemisphere originally formed the basis for the proposal that emotional states are linked to functional hemispheric differences (Terzian and Ceccotto 1959). Pharmacological inactivation of one side of the brain is a method particularly useful in the investigation of lateralization in brain functioning and is often used preoperatively to determine whether unilateral surgical insult will produce aphasia. This method was first used by Wada (1949), and it is known as the Wada technique. A rapid injection of sodium amytal into the internal carotid artery produces temporary inactivation of the ipsilateral hemisphere that results in marked alterations including, but not limited to, motoric and cognitive behavior. Following Terzian and Ceccotto (1959), a series of studies conducted in Italy (Alemà and Donini 1960; Rossi and Rosadini 1967;

Terzian 1964) found that pharmacological inactivation of the left side of the brain induced a "depressive-catastrophic" reaction, while right-side inactivation is characterized by the opposite "euphoric" reaction (Gainotti 1979). These findings have since been confirmed by other European investigators (Hommes and Panhuysen 1971; Rossi and Rosadini 1967).

Results obtained with the Wada technique prompted various clinical investigators to examine the relationship between side of insult and manifestations of mood change in patients with unilateral brain damage. Several studies of these patients were done with consistent results indicating that dysphoric reactions are more strongly associated with left rather than with right brain damage, while the reverse is found for euphoric-indifference reactions (Gainotti 1969, 1972; Hall, Hall, and Lavoie 1968; Hécaen 1962; Hommes 1965). The dysphoric reaction is a psychopathological state in which patients experience feelings of despair and hopelessness and may cry and express self-depreciatory ideation. The euphoric-indifference reaction is characterized by emotional placidity and/or social disinhibition with denial of symptoms and a tendency to joke. The phenomenology of these emotional reactions was very similar to the description of mood changes obtained with sodium amytal inactivation.

Overall, the sodium amytal and unilateral brain damage studies support the view that the two sides of the brain differ in subserving the experience of dysphoric and euphoric emotions. This support is qualified by the fact that both conditions produce a wide range of deficits, and it is conceivable that emotional disturbances are a secondary effect of other deficits and thereby only indirectly related to brain insult.

Evidence for a direct relationship between type of affective changes and side of unilateral insult has been recently presented by Sackeim, Greenberg, Weiman, Gur, Hungerbuhler, and Geschwind (1982). This group conducted three systematic reviews of the literature examining lateralization of destructive lesions in pathological laughing and crying, postoperative mood change following hemispherectomy, and lateralization of foci in gelastic (laughing) and dacrystic (crying) epilepsy. Alterations of affect often have been observed as ictal manifestations in epilepsy. More particularly, uncontrollable emotional outbursts of laughing and crying have been reported as components of all major forms of epileptic disorder. Ictal laughter has been termed gelastic epilepsy and ictal crying has been referred to as dacrystic epilepsy. The emotional outbursts may or may not be accompanied by corresponding mood changes that are random and/or inappropriate in regard to circumstances. Since the epileptic discharge is usually associated with increased electrical and metabolic activity and blood flow in epileptogenic neural tissues, associations between lateralization of foci and type of ictal emotional outbursts should most likely reflect the excitation of brain centers ipsilateral to foci. From more than 100 reports of gelastic and dacrystic epilepsy, in cases of gelastic epilepsy (uncontrollable laughing), foci were more than twice as likely to be predominantly left-sided. In a second study, this group reviewed fourteen cases of right hemispherectomy performed in adult patients. It was found that the majority of cases (twelve out of fourteen) became more euphoric after the operation, one case showed no mood change, and only one patient became dysphoric. This finding is consistent with the view that the left hemisphere subserves positive emotional states to a greater extent than the right hemisphere.

Studies of patients with destructive or silent lesions related left-side insult to dysphoric reactions and right-side insult to euphoric reactions. The work on ictal emotional outbursts, where there is hyperactivation in regions comprising foci, related left-sided foci to laughing outbursts. This suggested a particular view of the nature of affective lateralization. Destructive lesion may disinhibit emotional reactions subserved more by the contralateral side of the brain and these same affective changes, when observed as ictal manifestations, are due to release of regions ipsilateral to foci. By this view, in most people, the left side of the brain subserves positive or euphoric emotional states to a greater extent than the right side, whereas the reverse holds for negative emotional states.

Affective Lateralization: Studies of Normal Populations

The findings reviewed so far dealt with lateralization of brain damage in patients with altered mood or emotional expression. The affective states were often inappropriate and extreme. They did not share all the complexities of psychiatric affective disorders. They cannot be equated with normal variations of mood. In addition, damage to the brain may result in alterations and recovery in functioning not characteristic of normal brain activity (Hécaen and Albert 1978). These facts may limit the possible generalization from the above findings to the role of functional brain asymmetry in subserving mood fluctuations of normals and/or psychiatric patients.

A number of recent studies conducted on normal subjects have examined differences between the hemispheres in mediating emotional states, mainly the perception of and reaction to experimentally induced mood change. Before reviewing this area of research, the various methods used to study lateralized asymmetries should be mentioned.

Lateralized asymmetries can be investigated at a physiological level (hemispheric activation) and at a functional level (hemispheric competence or specialization). Hemispheric activation refers to asymmetric changes in neuronal activity (in the sense of hyperactivation or hypoactivation) as ascertained by measures that have been shown to be associated with changes in CNS arousal or stimulation (Butler and Glass 1976; Gur and Reivich 1980). Similarly, the level of functional competence of each hemisphere is often assessed by presenting information first to one side of the brain, by lateralizing the input of the information, as in dichotic listening and tachistoscopic split-field viewing tasks. Both activation and functional competence may show variations at a state level and/or a trait level. Generally, however, it is felt that hyper- or hypoactivation are transitory phenomena, while functional competence is thought to be related to often permanent structural differences between the hemispheres. Activation can be studied directly—for example, measuring regional cerebral blood flow or glucose metabolism—or indirectly, by assessing the direction of conjugate lateral eye movements (LEMs) in response to questions, measuring skin conductance, and/or using electrocortical measures like EEG and evoked potentials. However, the possible significance of most indirect measures of activation asymmetry is still a matter for controversy.

Direction of conjugate lateral deviation of the eyes has been used in several studies of cognitive lateralization as an index of contralateral hemispheric activation (see Erlichman and Weinberger [1978] for review). People who consistently move their eyes to the left (left movers) are said to manifest greater right than left hemispheric activation as a trait variable, while greater characteristic left-side activation holds for right movers. The amount or power in the α frequency wave band of the EEG traditionally has been associated to the level of hemispheric activity. The hemisphere displaying less α activity is typically interpreted as showing greater relative arousal. More controversial appears the significance of other indirect indices of overactivation. Skin conductance changes, for example, have been interpreted as reflecting changes in either contralateral or ipsilateral hemispheric activity (Gruzelier and Venables 1974; Myslobodsky and Horesch 1978). The significance of a number of electrocortical indices, such as mean integrated amplitude of total EEG and wave-form stability measures, is also problematic. Investigators have interpreted similar findings as indicating hemispheric dysfunction, hypoactivation on a particular side, or hyperaction on that side.

Hemispheric competence can be explored with tachistoscopic and dichotic techniques and neuropsychological tests. In tachistoscopic techniques, visual stimuli (of a verbal or nonverbal nature) are presented to each hemisphere. The limitation of stimulus presentation to a single hemisphere is accomplished with a very short (100–150 msec) exposure duration in the hemifield while the subject fixates on a central point. Right-handers typically better recognize verbal material when it is presented in the right field, corresponding to the left hemisphere, than in the left field, and vice versa for nonverbal material. In dichotic listening techniques, auditory stimuli (verbal and nonverbal, such as music) are presented simultaneously to the two ears. In this way, it is commonly thought the ipsilateral cortical projections of the ears are inhibited. With dichotic presentation of verbal stimuli, subjects show right ear/left hemisphere advantage and the opposite for nonverbal stimuli. Other types of neuropsychological testing involve use of standardized batteries such as the WAIS and the Halstead-Reitan. These batteries may reveal particular profiles related to relative hemispheric dysfunction.

To recapitulate, activation and functional competence are two dimensions related to manifestations of hemispheric asymmetries. The measures of activation are direct (e.g., regional cerebral blood flow) and indirect (e.g., LEMs, skin conductance, and electrophysiological indices). The measures of competence include processing of information lateralized in presentation (e.g., tachistoscopic and dichotic techniques) and neuropsychological testing.

Studies that have assessed the level of activation in normal subjects using indirect activation indices have consistently suggested a different involvement of the two hemispheres in the perception of and reaction to affectively charged stimuli. For instance, monitoring the LEMs, negatively charged emotional questions resulted in more deviations to the left and positively charged emotional questions resulted in more deviations to the right (Ahern and Schwartz 1979). A number of EEG studies found lateralized asymmetries in response to experimentally induced mood states. These asymmetries were sometimes interpreted

325

as indicating overactivation of the right hemisphere in response to experimentally induced dysphoric states and overactivation of the left in response to euphoric states (e.g., Davidson, Schwartz, Saron, Bennett, and Goleman 1978; Tucker, Stenslie, Roth, and Shearer 1981). At other times the interpretations were of hemispheric activation in opposite direction (Harman and Ray 1977; Ehrlichman and Wiener 1978).

Examining processing of emotional material, Dimond and Farrington (1977) compared heart-rate response of normal subjects viewing films in either the left or right visual field by fitting them with specially constructed contact lenses. Each subject saw three films, a humorous cartoon, a neutral travelogue, and a disconcerting movie about a surgical operation. While heart rate did not differ for the two groups when viewing the travelogue, it was higher in left- than in right-visual-field-viewing subjects when viewing the surgical operation, and higher in right- than in left-visual-field subjects when viewing the cartoon. If one considers the heart-rate change as an objective index of emotional response, this study suggests that the right hemisphere plays a more important role in mediating negatively charged emotions, while the reverse applies to the left hemisphere.

Other studies (Ley and Bryden 1979; Suberi and McKeever 1977) found that the left-visual-field advantage in face recognition was significantly increased when the stimulus faces were emotionally expressive. Likewise, dichotic studies (e.g., Carmon and Nachshon 1973) that have examined ear asymmetries in recognizing or identifying the emotional quality of sounds have found left ear advantage in this task. These last studies seem to indicate a right-side superiority in recognizing emotional contents. It is quite possible that the greater sensitivity of the right hemisphere in tasks requiring identification of emotion is an outcome of asymmetry in the cognitive strategies required for classification. On the other hand, Reuter-Lorenz and Davidson (1981) simultaneously presented normal subjects with a neutral face in one visual field and a happy or sad face in the other field. Subjects indicated which field contained the emotional face. Responses were more accurate and faster when the happy faces were in the right field and sad faces were in the left visual field.

Affective Lateralization: Studies of Psychiatric Patients

Given these findings of functional asymmetries in the regulation of mood in neurologically impaired patients and in normal subjects, disturbance or imbalance of cerebral laterality in affective disorders may not be unexpected. The first study to claim lateralized dysfunction in manic-depressive patients was conducted by Flor-Henry (1969). This author noted an overrepresentation of right-sided foci in epileptics who presented manic-depressive disorder. However, this claim was based on a small sample of patients, and the distribution of side of unilateral foci was not significantly different from that in a control group. The control group was unusual in that there was a two-to-one greater frequency of unilateral right-sided foci. Nevertheless, subsequent investigations have also suggested right-sided disturbances among bipolar patients.

The most robust evidence supporting hemispheric involvement in affective disorders has come from studies of electrocortical asymmetries in psychiatric patients. A set of limitations common to all these studies pertains to the diagnostic status of probands, not always adequately and/or reliably assessed, the possible confounding effect of psychotropic medications, and the interpretation of the significance of the abnormalities found. In most of the studies in this area the relations between psychophysiological indices and interpretation of differential hemispheric activation and/or dysfunction should be considered tentative.

Despite these limitations, the research has produced a relatively consistent set of findings. In virtually every investigation that has examined electrocortical measures in psychiatric patients comparing depressives with schizophrenics, the revealed lateral asymmetries in the two groups were generally opposite in direction (see Flor-Henry [1979] for review). Investigators consistently interpreted their findings as indicating greater involvement (overactivation and/or dysfunction) of the right relative to the left hemisphere of depressed patients, while the reverse was suggested for schizophrenics. Likewise, each of the four studies which compared patients with affective disorders (mostly depression) to normal controls (Flor-Henry 1976; Monakhov, Perris, Botskarev, von Knorring, and Nikiforov 1979; Myslobodsky and Horesch 1978; Roemer, Shagass, Straumanis, and Amadeo 1978) suggested greater right than left hemispheric involvement in depressed states.

To date there is only one study that has examined separate groups of manic and depressed patients during the acute phase of illness (Flor-Henry 1979). Temporal and parietal EEG were analyzed during resting conditions and during cognitive tasks. The results were complex, with some of the findings difficult to interpret. A few strong effects did emerge. During resting condition, the manic group showed left parietal activation along with bilateral temporal activation. The depressed group, on the other hand, showed evidence of relative right temporal activation. In response to the cognitive tasks, the manic group showed relative right parietal and temporal activation during the verbal task and bilateral parietal activation during the spatial task in comparison with a normal control group. The depressed group, while not quite resembling the control group, showed a pattern of response much more consistent with the findings obtained in normals.

One case report (Stepke, Harding, Jenner, and Mora 1979) examined EEG asymmetry in a patient being treated with lithium who exhibited a predictable shift between depressive and manic phases on a forty-eight-hour cycle. The elated states were associated with greater relative left hemisphere activation compared to the depressive states.

Two studies have found lateral asymmetries in skin conductance responses in depressed patients, although it was interpreted in one study (Gruzelier and Venables 1974) as evidence of right hemisphere dysfunction, and in the other study (Myslobodsky and Horesch 1978) as evidence of right hemisphere overactivation. In this latter study the depressed patients showed also more left LEMs than controls.

There have also been a few studies that have assessed the patterns of motoric and cognitive lateralization in psychiatric patients to investigate the possible relation between psychopathology and lateralized cognitive functions.

Two independent investigations (Flor-Henry 1979; Lishman and McMeekan 1976) found significant overrepresentation of sinistrality in endogenous psychoses. In both studies, the excess of sinistrality was particularly marked among manic-depressive patients. This fact would suggest that an abnormal pattern in degree and direction of cognitive lateralization may be present in psychiatric patients, since it is mainly in left-handers that this situation occurs. Such abnormalities may also reflect the superimposition of lateralized dysfunctions and/or lateralized abnormalities in activation upon a normally specialized brain.

Indications of right-side involvement in language functions in the depressed state is suggested by other studies. For instance, in one study (Hommes and Panhuysen 1971), unilateral inactivation by Wada technique was produced and it was found that a greater amount of dysphasic disturbances than expected followed right-side injection of sodium amytal in a sample of right-handed depressed patients. However, other studies found divergent patterns of results. No differences between patients and normal controls on verbal dichotic listening techniques was reported in one study (Lishman, Toone, Colbourn, McMeekan, and Mance 1978). In a second study (Bruder and Yozawitz 1979), two groups of depressed patients who met RDC criteria for bipolar or unipolar disorder were compared to a normal control group and two brain-damaged patients with right temporal lobe lesions. The bipolar depressed patients tended to show greater ear asymmetries than the unipolar and normal groups on the dichotic measures examined. The right-brain-damaged patients showed a performance similar to bipolar patients. Bruder and Yozawitz interpreted these findings as suggesting that right-side dysfunction was particular to bipolar disorder.

Another approach to examining cognitive lateralization in affective disorder is the evaluation of performance on neuropsychological test batteries which differentiate between left- and right-side impairment. All studies that have used this approach (Flor-Henry 1976; Goldstein, Filskov, Weaver, and Ives 1977; Kronfol, Hamsher, Digre, and Waziri 1978; Taylor, Greenspan, and Abrams 1979) suggested that depressed as well as manic patients evidence dysfunction for sensorimotor and/or cognitive skills subserved more by the right than the left side of the brain. Based on this evidence, it has been recently proposed that heightened activation of right-side centers interferes with ipsilateral information processing (Tucker, Stenslie, Roth, and Shearer 1981). The available data on this issue, however, do not allow us to draw any firm conclusion.

Electroconvulsive Therapy

Comparison of the therapeutic effects of electroconvulsive therapy (ECT) treatment modes provides another avenue for assessing the role of affective lateralization in psychiatric disorders. ECT has been administered bilaterally, with electrodes placement over regions on both sides of the brain, or unilaterally, to the left or right hemisphere.

Even though generalized seizures are elicited in all three forms of treatment, the effects of ECT are most pronounced on the side of the brain on which it is administered. Left ECT is associated with amnesic disturbance for verbal information, while right ECT produces greater disturbance for nonverbal information (d'Elia, Lorentzson, Raotma, and Widepalm 1976; Squire and Slater 1978). Bilateral ECT produces both types of amnesic disorder, perhaps to a more severe degree. EEG studies have shown that unilateral modes of treatment result in slowing of brain activity most on the side of administration (d'Elia and Perris 1970).

Six studies have compared the therapeutic efficacies of left and right ECT in major depressive disorders (Cohen, Penick, and Tarter 1974; Costello, Belton, Abra, and Dunn 1970; Cronin, Bodley, Potts, Mather, Gardner, and Tobin 1970; Deglin 1973; Fleminger, Horne, Nair, and Nott 1970; Halliday, Davison, Browne, and Kreeger 1968). When differences have been found, right ECT was associated with better outcome. This would also suggest that suppression of activity on the right side of the brain is associated with relief from depression.

Conclusions

Given the large body of findings suggesting functional asymmetry in the regulation of emotion, the indications of disturbance in lateralization of function among individuals with affective disorders may not be unexpected. Studies of motoric lateralization and electrocortical asymmetries have suggested disturbance or imbalance in lateralization, without necessarily specifying the nature of hemispheric involvement. With few exceptions, investigators consistently interpreted electrocortical findings as indicating overactivation and/or dysfunction of the right side in depressive states. The only study that examined patients during manic states reported findings consistent with left hemispheric activation. Investigations employing standardized neuropsychological batteries have provided initial suggestions that affective disorders may be characterized by right-side dysfunction in cognitive skills. Studies using dichotic listening techniques seem to indicate that right-side dysfunction is present in bipolar rather than unipolar disorder. It may be that right-side dysfunction, with possible structural abnormality, characterizes bipolar disorder. During depressed and manic phases, such patients may also manifest right-side and left-side hyperactivation, respectively. It appears that unipolar depressives may be characterized by right-side hyperactivation. This view seems to fit well with findings reviewed earlier, suggesting consistency in the role of functional brain asymmetry in the regulation of mood across brain-damaged, normal, and psychiatric populations.

REFERENCES

Ahern, G. L., and Schwartz, G. E. 1979. Differential lateralization for positive versus negative emotion. *Neuropsychologia* 17:693–698.

Alemà, G., and Donini, G. 1960. Sulle modificazioni cliniche ed elettroencefalografiche da introduzione intracarotidea di iso-amil-etil-barbiturato di sodio nell'uomo. *Bolletino della Società Italiana di Biologia Sperimentale* 36:900–904.

Bruder, G. E., and Yozawitz, A. 1979. Central auditory processing and lateralization in psychiatric patients. In J. Gruzelier and P. Flor-Henry, eds. *Hemisphere Asymmetries of Function in Psychopathology.* Amsterdam: Elsevier.

Butler, S. R., and Glass, A. 1976. EEG correlates of cerebral dominance. In A. H. Rissen and R. F. Thompson, eds. *Advances in Psychobiology.* Vol. 3. New York: Wiley.

Carmon, A., and Nachshon, I. 1973. Ear asymmetry in perception of emotional non-verbal stimuli. *Acta Psychologia* 37:351–357.

Cohen, B. D.; Penick, S. B.; and Tarter, R. E. 1974. Antidepressant effects of unilateral electric convulsive shock therapy. *Archives of General Psychiatry* 31:673–675.

Costello, C. G.; Belton, C. P.; Abra, J. C.; and Dunn, B. E. 1970. The amnesic and therapeutic effects of bilateral and unilateral ECT. *British Journal of Psychiatry* 116:69–78.

Cronin, D.; Bodley, P.; Potts, L.; Mather, M. D. ; Gardner, R. K.; and Tobin, J. C. 1970. Unilateral and bilateral ECT: a study of memory disturbance and relief from depression. *Journal of Neurology, Neurosurgery and Psychiatry* 33:705–713.

Cutting, J. 1978. Study of anosognosia. *Journal of Neurology, Neurosurgery, and Psychiatry* 41:548–555.

Davidson, R. J.; Schwartz, G. E.; Saron, C.; Bennett, J.; and Goleman, D. 1978. Frontal versus parietal EEG asymmetry during positive and negative affect. Paper presented at the meeting of the Society for Psychophysiological Research, September.

Deglin, V. L. 1973 A clinical study of unilateral electroconvulsive seizures. *Zhurnal Nevropatologii i Psikhiatrii* 73:1609–1621. [Russian.]

d'Elia, G.; Lorentzson, S.; Raotma, H.; and Widepalm, K. 1976. Comparison of unilateral dominant and non-dominant ECT on verbal and non-verbal memory. *Acta Psychiatrica Scandinavica* 53:85–94.

d'Elia, G., and Perris, C. 1970. Comparison of electroconvulsive therapy with unilateral and bilateral stimulation. I. Seizure and post-seizure electroencephalographic pattern. *Acta Psychiatrica Scandinavica* (suppl.) 215:9–29.

Dimond, S. J., and Farrington, I. 1977. Emotional response to films shown to the right or left hemisphere of the brain measured by heart rate. *Acta Psychologia* 41:255–260.

Ehrlichman, H., and Weinberger, A. 1978. Lateral eye movements and hemispheric asymmetry: a critical review. *Psychological Bulletin* 85:1080–1101.

Ehrlichman, H., and Wiener, M. J. 1978. Dimensions of EEG asymmetry during covert mental activity. Paper presented at the meeting of the American Psychological Association, Toronto.

Fleminger, J. J.; Horne, D. J. de L.; Nair, N. P. V.; and Nott, P. N. 1970. Differential effect of unilateral and bilateral ECT. *American Journal of Psychiatry* 127:430–436.

Flor-Henry, P. 1969. Schizophrenic-like reactions and affective psychoses associated with temporal lobe epilepsy: etiological factors. *American Journal of Psychiatry* 126:400–404.

Flor-Henry, P. 1976. Lateralized temporal-limbic dysfunction and psychopathology. *Annals of the New York Academy of Science* 280:777–795.

Flor-Henry, P. 1979. Laterality: shifts of cerebral dominance, sinistrality, and psychosis. In J. Gruzelier and P. Flor-Henry, eds. *Hemisphere Asymmetries of Function in Psychopathology*. Amsterdam: Elsevier.

Gainotti, G. 1969. Reactions catastrophiques et manifestations d'indifference au cours des atteintes cérébrales. *Neuropsychologia* 7:195–204.

Gainotti, G. 1972. Emotional behavior and hemisphere side of the lesion. *Cortex* 8:41–55.

Gainotti, G. 1979. The relationships between emotions and cerebral dominance: a review of clinical and experimental evidence. In J. Gruzelier and P. Flor-Henry, eds. *Hemisphere Asymmetries of Function in Psychopathology*. Amsterdam: Elsevier.

Goldstein, S. G.; Filskov, S. B.; Weaver, L. A.; and Ives, J. O. 1977. Neuropsychological effects of electroconvulsive therapy. *Journal of Clinical Psychology* 33:798–806.

Gruzelier, J. H., and Venables, P. H. 1974. Bimodality and lateral asymmetry of skin conductance orienting activity in schizophrenics:

replication and evidence of lateral asymmetry in patients with depression and disorders of personality. *Biological Psychiatry* 8:55–73.

Gur, R. C., and Reivich, M. 1980. Cognitive task effects on hemispheric blood flow in humans: evidence for individual differences in hemispheric activation. *Brain and Language* 9:78–92.

Hall, M. M.; Hall, G. C.; and Lavoie, P. 1968. Ideation in patients with unilateral or bilateral midline brain lesions. *Journal of Abnormal Psychology* 73:526–531.

Halliday, A. M.; Davison, K.; Browne, M. W.; and Kreeger, L. C. 1968. A comparison of the effects on depression and memory of bilateral ECT and unilateral ECT to the dominant and non-dominant hemispheres. *British Journal of Psychiatry* 114:997–1012.

Harmon, D. W., and Ray, W. J. 1977. Hemispheric activity during affective verbal stimuli: an EEG study. *Neuropsychologia* 15:457–460.

Hécaen, H. 1962. Clinical symptomatology in right and left hemispheric lesions. In V. B. Mountcastle, ed. *Interhemispheric Relations and Cerebral Dominance*. Baltimore: Johns Hopkins Press.

Hécaen, H., and Albert, M. L. 1978. *Human Neuropsychology*. New York: Wiley.

Hommes, O. R. 1965. Stemmingsanomalien als neurologisch symptoom. *Nederlands Tijdschrift voor Geneeskunde* 109:588–589.

Hommes, O. R., and Panhuysen, L. H. H. M. 1971. Depression and cerebral dominance: a study of bilateral intracarotid amytal in eleven depressed patients. *Psychiatrica, Neurologia, Neurochirurgia* (Amsterdam) 74:259–270.

Kronfol, A.; Hamsher, K. deS.; Digre, K.; and Waziri, R. 1978. Depression and hemispheric functions: changes associated with unilateral ECT. *British Journal of Psychiatry* 132:560–567.

Ley, R. G., and Bryden, M. P. 1979. Hemispheric differences in processing emotions and faces. *Brain and Language* 7:127–138.

Lishman, W. A., and McMeekan, E. R. L. 1976. Hand preference patterns in psychiatric patients. *British Journal of Psychiatry* 129:158–166.

Lishman, W. A.; Toone, B. K.; Colbourn, C. J.; McMeekan, E. R. L.; and Mance, R. M. 1978. Dichotic listening in psychotic patients. *British Journal of Psychiatry* 132:333–341.

Milner, B. 1968. Visual recognition and recall after right temporal-lobe excision in man. *Neuropsychologia* 6:191–209.

Monakhov, K.; Perris, C.; Botskarev, V. K.; von Knorring, L.; and Nikiforov, A. I. 1979. Functional interhemispheric differences in relation to various psychopathological components of the depressive syndromes. *Neuropsychobiology* 5:143–155.

Myslobodsky, M. S., and Horesch, N. 1978. Bilateral electrodermal activity in depressive patients. *Biological Psychology* 6:111–120.

Reuter-Lorenz, P., and Davidson, R. J. 1981. Differential contributions of the two cerebral hemispheres to the perception of happy and sad faces. *Neuropsychologia* 19:609–614.

Roemer, R. A.; Shagass, C.; Straumanis, J. J.; and Amadeo, M. 1978. Pattern evoked potential measurements suggesting lateralized hemispheric dysfunction in chronic schizophrenics. *Biological Psychiatry* 13:185–202.

Rossi, G. F., and Rosadini, G. 1967. Experimental analysis of cerebral dominance in man. In C. H. Millikan and F. L. Darley, eds. *Brain Mechanisms Underlying Speech and Language*. New York: Grune & Stratton.

Sackeim, H. A.; Greenberg, M. S.; Weiman, A. L.; Gur, R. C.; Hungerbuhler, J. P.; and Geschwind, N. 1982. Functional brain asymmetry in the expression of positive and negative emotions: neurological evidence. *Archives of Neurology* 39: 210–218.

Squire, L. R., and Slater, P. C. 1978. Bilateral and unilateral ECT: effects on verbal and non-verbal memory. *American Journal of Psychiatry* 135:1316–1320.

Stepke, F. L.; Harding, G. F.; Jenner, F. A.; and Mora, J. D. 1979. Studies of a changing laterality index in a patient treated with lithium. In J. Gruzelier and P. Flor-Henry, eds. *Hemisphere Asymmetries of Function in Psychopathology*. Amsterdam: Elsevier.

Suberi, M., and McKeever, W. F. 1977. Differential right hemispheric memory storage of emotional and non-emotional faces. *Neuropsychologia* 15:757–768.

Taylor, M. A.; Greenspan, B.; and Abrams, R. 1979. Lateralized neuropsychological dysfunction in affective disorder and schizophrenia. *American Journal of Psychiatry* 136:1031–1034.

Terzian, H. 1964. Behavioural and EEG effects of intracarotid sodium amytal injection. *Acta Neurochirurgica* 12:230–239.

Terzian, H., and Ceccotto, C. 1959. Determinazione e studio della dominanza emisferica mediante iniezione intracarotidea di Amytal sodico nell'uomo. I. Modificationi cliniche. *Bolletino della Società Italiana di Biologia Sperimentale* 35:1623–1626.

Tucker, D.; Stenslie, C. E.; Roth, R. S.; and Shearer, S. L. 1981. Right frontal lobe activation and right hemisphere performance decrement during a depressed mood. *Archives of General Psychiatry* 38:169–174.

Wada, J. 1949. A new method for the determination of the side of cerebral speech dominance: a preliminary report on the intracarotid injection of sodium amytal in man. *Medicine and Biology* (Japan) 14:221–222.

PART IV

THE ADOLESCENT, THE FAMILY, AND THE HOSPITAL

INTRODUCTION: THE ADOLESCENT, THE FAMILY, AND THE HOSPITAL

EDWARD R. SHAPIRO

The staff of a mental hospital develops a complex relationship with hospitalized adolescents and their families. This group of patients turns to the hospital at times of rage, despair, and hopelessness, searching for containment and a working space in which to address certain adolescent developmental issues. Resources of the hospital are sought when these issues cannot be managed in their families and communities because of a combination of internal developmental impasses and inadequate support from the interpersonal environment.

A central question that arises when an adolescent is hospitalized is, In what type of environment should his treatment be carried out? Should he be placed with younger children with attention paid to unresolved earlier latency conflicts? Should he be placed in all-adolescent groups utilizing the developmentally normative peer group interaction? Would the adolescent's need for adult models and the intense pressures of his impulsivity be better served on a generic unit with a mixture of adolescent and adult patients? And, in all of these settings, how should the family's necessary participation in the treatment be managed?

The authors in the following section attempt to represent some of the breadth of responses to these dilemmas. The issues that they raise, while not finally resolving these questions, do focus the discussion around three important dynamic themes: externalization, displacement, and regression. All of these defenses are characteristic of adolescent and family behavior as the adolescents enter the hospital, and the issues can be utilized in the construction of appropriate treatment milieus. In their descriptions of a wide variety of inpatient services, the authors reflect alternative approaches to the management of these phenomena.

Jacqueline Olds suggests that many of the younger hospitalized adolescents cannot tolerate the anxiety involved in the direct discussion of their conflicts in dynamic psychotherapy. She argues that these children have failed to develop both the necessary observing ego and the displacement defenses against drives that latency-aged children learn through constructive use of play. The environment she proposes is one in which adolescents are mixed with latency-aged children. Displacement and externalization are encouraged in this setting through the explicit use of projective figures in stories and games, in the encouragement of task mastery, and in the study of sibling relationships with younger children. The inference is that such an environment might be particularly useful for the younger, less mature, or more fragile adolescent.

Thomas Bond and Nancy Auger advocate a generic inpatient unit with a mixture of adults and adolescents. Their position is that the hospital environment should provide a close parallel to the community experience, with available "uncles and aunts" to serve as developmentally appropriate displacements for the more potentially conflicted relationships with parental figures. They note that a mixture of adults may have a calming effect on adolescents and suggest that grossly psychotic, organically impaired, or highly impulsive adolescents might do better in this setting. They offer clinical examples which illustrate the mutual benefits adult and adolescent patients might offer each other in a generic milieu.

Jonathan Kolb and Edward Shapiro describe an all-adolescent unit where the family is actively involved in sharing managerial responsibility with the staff. In this setting, there is an opportunity to study the regressive attempts on the part of both the adolescent and his family to externalize and displace aspects of both intrapsychic and intrafamilial conflict in their working relationships with staff members. The authors describe the ways in which the staff's efforts to model parental behavior and to set limits on and to confront both adolescent and parental acting out help illuminate the need for appropriate family responses to issues of separation and individuation. They describe how the staff's use of its authority allows peer group interaction and responsibility to be maximized and family behavior to be stabilized and contained. The inference here is that such a setting is useful for borderline, narcissistic, and antisocial adolescents where active family participation can be arranged.

Paul Rossman and Judith Freedman's chapter is a study of parent counseling groups for parents of hospitalized adolescents. In their view, parental dependency on the staff can usefully be exploited in the service of education, encouragement, generational boundary formation, and managing resistances to treatment (guilt, blame, separation anxiety, competitiveness). Supportive parent counseling groups offer direct gratification to people in need and facilitate the more active mobilization of their own resources in the treatment effort.

Richard Bonier describes an Adolescent Day Service where the major therapeutic interactions take place in an open setting without the security of office walls and limited time boundaries. His focus is on the manner in which specific developmental conflicts in the adolescent evoke group and individual countertransference responses in the highly exposed treatment staff that mirror tensions within the adolescent's family. The implication here is that both impulse-disordered and thought-disordered adolescents can be worked with in this more open setting with the intensive use of group process in both the adolescent peer group and the staff group.

In the final chapter, Joyce Shields and Peter Choras review the regression which affects the transition from the hospital to the community as the adolescent and family part from the various displacement figures in the hospital. They suggest the use of a new transitional figure—the aftercare specialist—whose task is to help all of the participants in this regression (the adolescent, the family, the staff, the therapist, and the community resource) acknowledge, bear, and put into perspective the disruptive tensions around this transition.

The spectrum of chapters in this section suggests that a variety of treatment milieus can be effective in the treatment of the hospitalized adolescent and his family. Although inferences can be made about which type of treatment might be appropriate for which adolescent and family, these decisions remain, unfortunately, at the level of clinical hunches or assertions. Too often, the type of treatment milieu an adolescent receives is determined by available resources, both financial and clinical, rather than by a specific match between psychopathology and program.

Given the broad spectrum of available programs and the increasing clarity about the specific underlying conceptualizations and programmatic choices relevant to each milieu, it may soon become possible to study in more detail the issue of matching adolescent to program. Since available research is weak in this area, it would seem wise to encourage this diversification so that ultimately samples of adolescents and families matched for demographic and psychopathological variables might be followed over time as they progress through these treatments into the community. Only then might there be substantial data to support the advocacy of particular hospital programs for these troubled adolescents and families.

24 MANAGEMENT OF SEPARATION ISSUES WITH THE FAMILY OF THE HOSPITALIZED ADOLESCENT

JONATHAN E. KOLB AND EDWARD R. SHAPIRO

Recent studies of hospitalized borderline adolescents and their families (Berkowitz, Shapiro, Zinner, and Shapiro 1974; Shapiro, Zinner, Shapiro, and Berkowitz 1975; Zinner and Shapiro 1972, 1974, 1975) illustrate the ways in which shared unconscious assumptions and the complementary use of projective identification within families may interfere with the separation and individuation of the disturbed adolescent. These unconscious processes deprive parents of a realistic view of their child and deprive the adolescent of needed family support at times of stress. Treatment plans for the hospitalized adolescent which include an attempt to work with these dynamic family interactions inevitably involve the treatment staff in the dynamics of the family process.

In an earlier study of staff-patient interactions on an adolescent and family treatment unit at McLean Hospital (Shapiro and Kolb 1979), we demonstrated how intrafamilial struggles become externalized in the relationships between family members and treatment staff. We suggested that these externalizations can be viewed, not merely as a resistance to treatment, but as an opportunity for treatment staff to help family members understand aspects of their family tension. In this chapter, we extend this earlier work to examine specifically how the treatment staff, through its exercise of authority, can increase the capacity of family members to take responsibility for these intrafamilial dynamics. By managing authority within a consistently structured program, the staff can provide a "safe" setting within which disavowed aspects of intrafamilial conflict can be mobilized for examination and integration. They allow family members to notice their differences from and their ties to one another. In the first section we consider the characteristics of hospitalized adolescents and their families and how the staff manages authority in relation to the salient issues facing them. In the second section we explore, in three case studies, specific ways the staff's exercise of administrative authority with families of border-lines enhances family members' capacity to support the separation and individuation of the troubled adolescent.

Adolescents and Their Families

THE ADOLESCENT

Low tolerance of anxiety and frustration and poor impulse control are characteristic of the adolescent with major character pathology. These ego deficits, in combination with the heightened drive pressures of adolescence, contribute to the rapid transformation of an adolescent's anxiety and frustration into actions, which result in tension relief for the patient but trouble for his environment. Members of their environment (family, schoolteachers, the community) experience anxiety and frustration with these adolescents and typically hospitalize in response to these affects.

These hospitalized adolescents are unable to sustain an integrated view of themselves and others. Serious ego weakness results in the continuing use of primitive defenses: splitting, projective identification, denial, and acting out. As a consequence of their reliance on these defenses, these patients have experienced difficulty in taking responsibility for their affects, their actions, and their lives. These adolescents feel that they are continually judged, exploited, victimized, and abandoned.

Their defensive position is accompanied by a syndrome of identity diffusion that is characterized by poorly defined self-representation and a lack of a stable and integrated concept of relationships of others with the self. They experience relationships in a polarized fashion as either all good or all bad. If they are frustrated in a "good" relationship, it becomes a "bad" one. Under the stress of frustration or anxiety, these patients experience a blurring of the boundaries around themselves and resort to primitive defenses in which superego functions and anger are projected. They experience helplessness and inordinately low self-esteem. They defend against these feelings by shallow claims of grandiosity and omnipotent fantasies and fail to develop a realistic sense of competence and achievement. They are impulsive. They have a chronic inability to neutralize instinctual drives (both sexual and aggressive) or to learn from experience, which often leads them into repetitive, fruitless encounters. They defend against their consequent shame, low self-esteem, and depression by distracting themselves with drugs, engaging in antisocial activities, and confronting their parents and other figures of authority.

In sum, these patients have failed to master the major tasks of adolescence. They are unable to separate intrapsychically from their original parental objects. This results in a continued and chaotic state of unacknowledged dependence on their family and permits only shallow relationships with peers and other adults.

THE FAMILY

Families of these adolescents have developed complementary defensive structures that are stabilized within the marriage. Like the adolescents, the families engage in continuous struggles over issues of autonomy and dependence. These struggles have their roots in shared unconscious fantasies and related defenses that derive from the parents' internalized childhood experiences in their respective families of origin. As a result the parents, rather than providing the necessary support to the developing adolescent, respond to aspects of his development with anxiety and tend to repudiate the changes that are occurring in their relationship with him. The splitting which is characteristic of adolescents is mirrored in family interactions when these issues of autonomy and independence arise (Zinner and Shapiro 1975). In many of these families the parent-child relationships are experienced in a polarized way. One parent is "good," insofar as he is purged of "bad" qualities which are projected onto the other parent, who is experienced unambivalently as ungiving and hateful. In other families, the whole family is experienced as "good" and the outside world is seen as hostile and dangerous. These distorted, polarized perceptions may not be characteristic of all family relationships at all times, but they appear to represent a pattern of family regression in the face of adolescent behaviors that touch on developmental issues of autonomy and separation. The family's anxiety over developmental issues and its pattern of splitting are intensified when these families respond to acute turmoil in the adolescent. For example, when the adolescent is admitted to the hospital, family members scapegoat him as the problem in the family and thereby deny all tension within the marriage or in the family at large. Many parents find themselves unable to agree on whether to hospitalize the child or not. They see such action as contrary to the wishes of their child and therefore potentially disruptive to the maintenance of a positive relationship with him.

THE HOSPITAL

The adolescent's continued need to act out and his profound, unacknowledged dependency, combined with the turmoil of the family and lack of adult support, suggest hospitalization as the preferable course of treatment. The way in which hospitalization provides the necessary support for the treatment of these adolescents is a subject of some disagreement.

Masterson (1972) argues that long-term hospitalization is a way to contain the borderline adolescent and provide the controls and limits that will allow him to become available for individual therapy and other mutative influences. He sees the hospital structure as providing the first phase of treatment. Here the adolescent can test his new environment (as an extension of the therapist) to see if it can contain him. Others, however, see the effect of structure as more than just a prelude to treatment. Miller (1973), for example, has described the function of hospital staff as role models with whom adolescents can identify. Rinsley and Inge (1961) have a still broader view of the role of the hospital environment as an empathic, confronting, interpretive agent in the treatment process. By its behavior, the staff responds to the behavioral communication of the patient, helps to quiet his current concerns, and fosters a relationship that upgrades the focus of the adolescents' communication from behavioral to verbal.

On the Adolescent and Family Treatment Unit (AFTU)[1] we add to the milieu an intensive focus on parents and siblings of the hospitalized adolescent. The structure affects not only the adolescent, but his family as well, and by filling in (at appropriate times) for deficient capacities of the adolescent and his parents, the structure provides a holding environment within which growth can occur (Winnicott 1969). As the parent observes the milieu struggle to contain his adolescent, he reexperiences some of the situations that have been overwhelming for

346

him and have called forth his most helpless responses. In this setting, the parent has the opportunity to observe the conflict in a staff member and can, through identification, explore it and learn about both the current situation and himself as well.

The reverse of this situation also occurs; the parent may engage in a struggle with the unit administration that recapitulates important family patterns, allowing the adolescent to observe from a distance, with a similar opportunity for learning. The milieu provides a holding environment, then, not just for the adolescent, but for parents as well, enabling them to face (in a relatively secure setting) the issues that have been reawakened by their child's troubled adolescence, issues which have in many cases been smoldering in an unresolved and pathogenic way since the parents' own adolescence.

THE ADOLESCENT AND FAMILY TREATMENT UNIT (AFTU)

The AFTU is a ten-bed, voluntary, unlocked unit. Therapeutic modalities include individual, family, couples, group, and multiple family therapy, in addition to school and various rehabilitation programs. A central element in the program is a highly structured sequence of privileges that the adolescents can obtain by demonstrating their ability to take responsibility for their own behavior.

Many interventions in this intensive program are designed to understand the use of projective identification and to interrupt both the adolescent and his family members' continual attempts to externalize conflict. The adolescents take responsibility for details of their day: cleaning their room, attending school, therapy appointments, and a variety of meetings. Evidence of their ability to manage these responsibilities, as well as input from their various therapists that indicates that they are thinking rather than acting out their difficulties, results in increasing privileges and freedom for the patient. Inability to handle these responsibilities results in restrictions and increased contact with nursing staff. This contact is thought of, not as punishment, but as an opportunity for them to consider the obstacles to more productive behavior. The adolescents come to regard their privilege status as the staff's most direct evaluation of where they stand at a given time.

In the career of an adolescent and family on the AFTU, situations repeatedly occur in which conflicts felt by the adolescent and/or his parent are externalized onto the treatment team. For example, externalization is seen in the interaction with staff concerning the unlocked

347

door. In the open-door setting, it is not the physical environment per se that acts as a restraint, but the relationship the patient has with the staff. The adolescent who is able to control his rage and frustration and not run out the door does so, not because of the physical presence of the door, but because he fears that in the process of running he will destroy a valued relationship with a staff member. In this way, the adolescent comes to control some impulses to action.

At times the adolescent's preferred defensive posture is to externalize a part of his conflict (whether to stay or go) onto the staff. He blames the staff member for keeping him on the unit and in this way relieves himself of the conflict he feels. The staff member may accept the projected part of the adolescent's conflict (in this case his dependency) and argue, persuade, or threaten to restrict him on the unit. In such an interaction, the staff member often finds gratification for his own unacknowledged wishes to flout authority or escape dependency in his unconscious identification with the adolescent. The resultant stereotyped interaction of two seemingly unambivalent people arguing about the impulses of the adolescent and the constraining wishes of the staff member often recapitulates pathogenic encounters from the adolescent's family.

If he avoids such an interaction, the staff member must also guard against a shift to the opposite pole of the stereotype, that is, to indicate that the door is open and that it is entirely up to the adolescent whether to stay or leave. To make this kind of invitation would be to abdicate the legitimate authority of the staff. It would similarly recapitulate a pattern of reversal typical in the families of disturbed adolescents.

The staff member's task is to tell the adolescent to stay without communicating either sadism or self-ridicule. When he does this he operates within the realistically limited relationship in a helpful way. Cognizant of his own conflicts about separation and dependency, the staff member can help the adolescent to acknowledge his conflict about his presence on the unit, including both his dependent yearnings and his often rageful responses to them. Such interactions constitute an important part of the treatment.

The struggles of treatment staff to master the vicissitudes of limit setting provide an opportunity for them to develop an empathic understanding of parental tension. The wish to remain in a positive relationship with the adolescent, combined with a sense of relative helplessness and guilt about one's own hostility, makes the setting of limits extraordinarily difficult. The tendency of these adolescent pa-

348

tients to split their object representations into all good and all bad aspects means that some staff members are singled out as good and understanding objects while others are seen as punitive. The staff members so delineated tend, as Main (1957) described, to see their differences as deep, philosophical, and not resolvable. This splitting thus contributes to the difficulties staff members experience both in setting limits and, perhaps more important, in supporting one another in the accomplishment of such acts. A major function of the complex of meeting and appointments is to keep the potential for staff splitting under scrutiny. In family therapy, the family is encouraged to explore the thinking behind decision making, particularly on the subject of weekend passes, where the disagreement in the family is similar to that experienced among the ward staff on the same issue. The development of a working alliance among staff, adolescent, and family through which these decisions can be realistically shared is one of the major tasks of the early part of treatment.

In couples therapy, the parents' hesitancy about limit setting can be explored in some privacy, with the support of their couples therapist who also participates in the family therapy. In the multiple family meeting the overlapping tensions on the part of all of the families in the unit around this issue can be shared and understood. The adolescents are aware that their individual therapists take an active part in decision making, so that therapy and administration are not split.

The administrative position does not merely represent an aspect of managing the adolescent that can conveniently be split off from the therapist to free him to be more exclusively therapeutic. Rather, because of the major themes that are of central concern to the adolescent and family, the crucial areas of treatment interaction almost always become administrative. There is an ongoing tension between the adolescent's need for enough autonomy to test his capacities for self-regulation, on the one hand, and his need for protection, on the other. His efforts to resolve these tensions are complicated by defective reality testing, poor judgment, inadequate internalized self-esteem regulation, and the results of traumatic prior experience. This tension is felt in the therapists as well as the parents. The parents have often dealt with this conflict in a stereotypical way by polarizing the possible responses among different family members (Zinner and Shapiro 1974). For the administrative staff, it is a crucial task in the face of such powerful tensions, often expressed in dramatic form, to avoid taking a polar position that would relieve the adolescent and family of the burden of tension and uncertainty. Cohen and Grinspoon (1963) advocate that the staff accept the role of protector which the self-destructive adolescent's behavior seems to solicit. On the unit, the staff's role is enlarged to include advocate for protection when this is needed, advocate for autonomy when this side of the issue needs to be spoken for, and, in either case, advocate for the development of awareness about the complexity of the conflict in both adolescent and parents, while attempting to maintain the autonomy of the family to manage its own decisions.

Clinical Observations

We have suggested that the exercise of authority in the interaction between staff to the adolescents and their families enhances the family's ability to manage issues of separation. We turn to case studies of three adolescents and their families in order to illustrate how the staff models appropriate parental behavior by providing firm boundaries within which separation can occur (case 1), how staff support for peer-group integration aids in the process of separation (case 2), and how staff promotes the integrity of the family structure (case 3). On an adolescent unit where the family is treated as a central element in the work with the adolescent, all three types of hospital interaction (modeling, setting limits, and confrontation) serve to demonstrate for family members the need for appropriate family responses to the adolescent's strivings for autonomy and dependency in the service of separation and individuation.

CASE 1: THE MIDHOSPITALIZATION RUNAWAY

The staff's use of authority to create a holding environment for the adolescent patient is seen quite clearly in the way runaways are managed. How staff handle runaways depends on how the runaway is viewed vis-à-vis the therapeutic environment. Although it may be true, as Rinsley and Inge (1961) argue, that "a runaway . . . terminates therapeutic contact between the patient and the treatment staff," we believe that this is an incomplete view of the process. In our experience, contact continues among the runaway adolescent, the family, and the treatment staff, often on an intensified level with long telephone calls and dramatic confrontations. Whether these interactions are therapeutic depends on whether they foster the integrity of the holding environment as a place within which the exaggerated struggle around separation can occur and be understood.

A runaway in a middle phase of hospitalization occurs in the context of a deepening attachment and dependence the adolescent feels toward the treatment situation and staff. The adolescent flees from this frightening development but concurrently expresses his wish for rapprochement through telephone contact with other patients, staff, and parents. What the borderline adolescent is often acting out in a runaway is the conflict he feels between unacknowledged and terrifying dependency longings and defensive, premature, and unrealistic strivings for autonomy.

The families of these children often become panicked by the adolescent's pseudoautonomous moves, because these are interpreted as evidence that the family is "bad" (Zinner and Shapiro 1975). The family's response to a runaway is to sacrifice the integrity of the family and to "get the adolescent back at all costs." This posture is one that meets the defensive needs of the parents but fails to acknowledge the conflicted state of the adolescent.

The runaway adolescent, in his phone contacts, tests the staff's (parental) authority and limits in several ways, one of which is a request for amnesty: "If I come back, will you promise not to take away my privileges?" Parents try to mediate a deal between runaway adolescent and staff by acting as go-between and making the request themselves. They are often angry and puzzled by a firm stance, taken by the treatment unit, that the adolescent must return without the promise of a "deal." The parents sometimes insist, "Just tell him he won't lose his privileges; of course you can change your mind after he's safely back." Requests such as these provide further indication of parental failure to provide a stable, reliable set of expectations and limits against which the adolescent can evaluate himself. The specific reenactment with the staff, with parents temporarily relieved of the primary parental responsibility, allows for learning to occur through identification.

CASE EXAMPLE

At about the midpoint of his year-long hospitalization, Billy ran away with another adolescent. The other youth returned the next day, while Billy remained in his own house with his mother in anxious attendance. Billy, a borderline adolescent, had been in emotional difficulty since age five, with encopresis, school failure, disruptive behavior, hyperactivity, and uncontrolled temper outbursts. His family life was complicated by father's alcoholism, with severe medical consequences, and mother's moralistic, masochistic detachment from her spouse. The parents had failed to engage in a variety of proposed treatments at earlier crisis points in Billy's life and had come to the unit, not in response to Billy's arrest for thirteen counts of breaking and entering, but on referral from an inpatient treatment program where father had been detoxified.

During a day-long siege, when Billy and his mother engaged in a struggle over a kitchen knife, they repeatedly interrupted their struggle to call the treatment staff and request a "deal" for Billy's return to the unit without a loss of privileges. After they heard firm and repeated refusals of such a deal, coupled with an offer to return to the relative safety and calm of the hospital, Billy and his mother were able to separate. They managed this by locating Billy's father (he had been out all night, intoxicated), who came home and to whom Billy willingly surrendered.

In this family, father's abdication of his parental role left Billy in the terrifying position of no protection against the tempting retreat into symbiotic confusion with mother. Mother's seductive offer ("I will bring you back with no limits or expectations") suggested to her son that he could be with her without any responsibility for his actions and impulses. The staff's firm response provided a model for Billy and his mother of respectful parental availability. The staff acknowledged their relative helplessness to control these dangerous events at a distance, but at the same time their continued availability suggested that what they could offer was security within realistic limits. The price of that security was that the adolescent take and maintain responsibility for his behavior.

Supported by this stance, the family could respond by father's temporary resumption of an active fathering role. This allowed mother and son to interrupt their entanglement long enough to return to the unit. The parents' identification with the staff's tolerance of their uncertainty and limitations provided a model of parental functioning which could gradually be internalized.

CASE 2: NEGOTIATING A WEEKEND HOME

In contrast to the runaway, when urgency and danger are the medium through which regressive wishes are expressed, there are circumstances in which a positive and hopeful ambient atmosphere conceals a regressive demand which similarly must be understood. One such situation takes place with regularity early in the hospitalization of many of the more schizoid adolescents, who, having complied with the rules and earned privileges, are ready to request a pass home for a weekend. The procedure for negotiating this request has several steps that utilize available treatment personnel and formats (individual and family therapy, discussions with nursing staff) in order to look at the issues and meanings of such a request from a variety of viewpoints. Even though there is room in the multistep process for the adolescent to express his ambivalence, he characteristically fails to do so during the early steps. Discussions of the first passes are pro forma until the final step, when the plan is to be presented to the Friday administrative group of adolescents and staff, the "privilege meeting."

CASE EXAMPLE

Daniel was the second of four children born to middle-class parents. He had difficulty almost from birth, when a minor deformity was experienced by his parents as a significant defect. His early feeding problems were eventually diagnosed as metabolic in origin, and these symptoms of milk allergy persisted and evolved into a long-standing pattern of binge drinking of milk (on family outings) followed by diarrhea, incontinence, and soiling. Daniel's close tie to his mother was accentuated during his early adolescence when father was away in military service. At that time, because of Daniel's schizoid withdrawal, hospitalization was recommended but refused by his mother, who proposed that she be hospitalized in his stead. By the time of this hospitalization at age fifteen, in addition to his chronic school failure, encopresis, and grandiose obsessions, the patient showed compulsive mannerisms and rituals, social isolation, stealing from his parents and siblings, and some mild drug abuse.

Initially Daniel responded calmly to hospitalization, complying easily with regulations and earning privileges rapidly. His first request for a weekend home came at the end of a busy privilege meeting. The general rowdiness of the group made it appear that Daniel's failure to assert himself earlier in the meeting and to insist on a fair hearing was a situation outside of his control. He was allowed to negotiate his pass in a one-to-one session with a nursing staff member.

353

The next week, the same situation was repeated, and again the group never addressed his request for a weekend pass. This time he was not allowed to circumvent the meeting; rather, he was told to wait until the following week and to try again to assert himself. Within five minutes, his mother was on the phone angrily confronting the administrator about his unreasonable stand. She reiterated a statement she had made at the time of admission, that the treatment on the unit must not interfere with the family's spending Christmas together. On the phone, she insisted that when Christmas came, Daniel would have to be granted an overnight pass home, no matter what his privilege status. The administrator informed her that weekend passes were Daniel's responsibility and would depend on his ability to earn and negotiate them, which meant that he would have to make sure that the adolescent group considered his needs during the privilege meeting. In this way a clear task was defined for the adolescent around which the conflict over separation from his family could be examined.

Daniel's vague requests for weekends and holidays at home were the only motivations he initially acknowledged. He denied any reluctance for a reunion with the family. He blamed his lack of a pass on the other adolescents, who were jealous of his better behavioral controls, and on the rigidity of the authority figures. In his individual therapy, however, Daniel began jokingly to discuss his anxiety about his closeness with his mother.

In the privilege meeting, where he was repeatedly confronted with his own responsibility to arrange his weekends, he continued to respond by passively failing to do so. This led to further angry phone calls from his mother. After repeated clarifications by the staff that Daniel was competent to use the privilege meeting and that his refusal to do so had meaning, the family began to consider the idea that Daniel was ambivalent about being at home with his mother.

For a time, the parents maintained that the other adolescents were a dangerous, uncontrollable, destructive group and that it was irresponsible of the hospital to subject Daniel to them or to expect him to influence them in any way, since he was so different. Daniel preferred the role of provoker within the group, taking interest in sadomasochistic exchanges between other boys and initially denying any impulses of his own. Over time, however, in the face of the staff's insistence that he was part of the group with a share in the responsibility for group themes, Daniel began to acknowledge and express both his ambivalence about home visits and his angry responses to group members. The staff's insistence that he take responsibility for these interactions provided him with the opportunity to negotiate an important piece of the developmental process. We affirmed his competence and supported the affirmation in action by not repeatedly rescuing him from the situations in which he expressed his conflict.

The major threat to Daniel's autonomy came from his mother, who developed a suspicious rage when she became threatened with prolonged separation from him. Daniel watched with interest as his mother tangled with the ward administrator. He would talk to her about the "unreasonable staff," provoke her to phone, and then eavesdrop to hear the results of his provocation. In his individual therapy he discussed the contrast between his own experience with his mother and the relative ease with which the administrator was able to handle her regressed, threatening calls. In this way he was able to develop some perspective on the crucial issue of separation from her, and over several months he became increasingly able to talk about his ambivalence about these visits. Similarly, his mother was able to use the separation provided by the administrator to work on her own feelings of guilt and responsibility for this "defective" child who had rejected her in infancy. She began to realize that she had overcompensated for her guilt about being a bad mother by becoming overly indulgent.

CASE 3: THE UNCOOPERATIVE PARENT

In the two preceding examples, as in most situations related to treatment of disturbed adolescents, the most noticeable "deviant" behavior is that of the adolescent. Often the parental contribution is covert or seems to be a response to situations created by the adolescent. Over time, however, especially as the adolescent begins to change, alterations in the family homeostasis evoke outbreaks of previously covert parental conflict. To the extent that parental turmoil surfaces and provides validation for the parents' fantasy that they will be exposed and blamed, it represents a crisis in treatment. Such crises may end by premature withdrawal from the program and another treatment failure added to the family's list. On the other hand, to the extent that the overt expression of parental psychopathology can be met with sensitivity and made part of the ongoing treatment process, it can relieve the focus on the adolescent and allow all family members to recognize their contributions to family strife.

CASE EXAMPLE

Maggie was a seventeen-year-old high school senior admitted after a drug overdose. Her recent history was characterized by depression, school avoidance, and impulsive sexual encounters followed by extreme guilt. It was after one such encounter with the husband of a friend that she returned home to an argument with father which she followed by a serious attempt at suicide. Throughout her life Maggie had been seen as a special, gifted, good child who would, through her success, compensate for the misfortunes and troubles experienced by both parents, but especially by her father. The oldest girl and second of four children, she had quickly assumed the role of confidante to both parents in their chronic marital struggles, a role she played with her coterie of friends as well.

From the beginning of her hospitalization, it was difficult for Maggie to focus on her own needs and concerns. Her parents' troubles preoccupied her, particularly her father's chronic depression. Her own suicidal potential and long-standing unhappiness were harder for her to acknowledge. She behaved well and dissociated herself from the acting out of the other adolescents. After three months of hospitalization, in the context of an increased focus on the marriage in couples therapy, her father suddenly announced that he would no longer participate in meetings because the meetings angered him. Maggie expressed moderate disapproval for this stand but went about her business as usual and continued with a previously discussed plan for a weekend home, for which she had anticipated approval.

In the next day's privilege meeting, her detached attitude toward her father's stand was explored. Compared to Maggie's quiet and low-keyed response, the outrage of the other adolescents at her father's behavior was striking. They recalled personal experiences of parents whose impulsivity jeopardized them. The adolescents swapped stories of speeding, reckless driving, arguments held on the highway that translated into errors in judgment, missed traffic lights, and car doors opened at high speeds. There was a high degree of anxiety and sadness in this discussion; their usual bravado was missing. At the close of the discussion the group recommended that Maggie not be penalized for her father's action and that she be allowed to have her weekend home. The staff pointed out the message in their stories and the feelings associated with them, that the adolescents were jeopardized at times by their parents' difficulties and that they needed to accept that fact. Maggie pleaded that her father could not respond, that he was too stubborn and unreasonable, and that her treatment would suffer if the staff did not overlook his lack of attendance.

The staff, however, insisted that weekends could not be granted without father's participation in the meetings. Her father responded by returning to the program "in Maggie's interest." In the couples therapy he raged at the rigidity of the staff but proceeded to discuss a subject that up until then had been only hinted at, his chronic sexual impotence. In response to the staff's insistence on the interdependence of all family members, Maggie was more able, in her own therapy, to acknowledge her needs for parental support as she moved out of the hospital and into her own apartment.

In this example, the adolescent had taken a parental role in a nurturant relationship with her father. Her clinical improvement and subsequent withdrawal from him precipitated a crisis in the marriage which revealed the parents' covert incompatibility, previously stabilized by Maggie. If father had been allowed to withdraw and Maggie had been sent home on weekends, it is likely that the pathological family equilibrium would have been re-established, with continued enmeshment of the adolescent in the marital conflict. The staff's insistence on the participation of all family members served to make explicit father's covert effort to capture his daughter for himself and allowed Maggie to recognize her need for both of her parents as they began to work on their marriage.

Conclusions

The chronic involvement of the characterologically disturbed adolescent in chaotic family pathology interferes both with his capacity to think for himself and with his ability to use individual psychotherapy (Shapiro 1978). A hospitalization experience which provides a firm

357

structure in which the entire family can observe its interactions avoids the panic of a premature and precipitous separation while allowing family members an opportunity to clarify their several contributions to the shared confusion. We have described an adolescent and family treatment unit on which staff members use their authority to uphold the integrity of the program and define its limits. The stability and integrity of the program and its boundaries, and the staff's capacity competently to exercise authority, provide models for parental behavior as well as defining a holding environment which protects the entire family from disruption as they proceed with the task of separation.

NOTE

1. From the Adolescent and Family Treatment and Study Center, McLean Hospital, Belmont, Massachusetts.

REFERENCES

Berkowitz, D.; Shapiro, R. L.; Zinner, J.; and Shapiro, E. R. 1974. Family contributions to narcissistic disturbances in adolescents. *International Review of Psycho-Analysis* 1:353–362.
Cohen, R. E., and Grinspoon, L. 1963. Limit setting as a corrective ego experience. *Archives of General Psychiatry* 8:90–96.
Main, T. F. 1957. The ailment. *British Journal of Medical Psychology* 30:129–145.
Masterson, J. F. 1972. *Treatment of the Borderline Adolescent: A Developmental Approach*. New York: Wiley-Interscience.
Miller, D. 1973. The development of psychiatric treatment services for adolescents. In J. D. Schoolar, ed. *Current Issues in Adolescent Psychiatry*. New York: Brunner/Mazel.
Rinsley, D. B., and Inge, G. P. 1961. Psychiatric hospital treatment of adolescents: verbal and nonverbal resistance to treatment. *Bulletin of the Menninger Clinic* 25:249–263.
Shapiro, E. R. 1978. Research on family dynamics: clinical implications for the family of the borderline adolescent. *Adolescent Psychiatry* 6:360–376.
Shapiro, E. R., and Kolb, J. E. 1979. Engaging the family of the hospitalized adolescent: the multiple family meeting. *Adolescent Psychiatry* 7:322–342.
Shapiro, E. R.; Zinner, J.; Shapiro, R. L.; and Berkowitz, D. 1975. The

influence of family experience on borderline personality development. *International Review of Psycho-Analysis* 2:399–411.

Winnicott, D. W. 1969. The use of an object. *International Journal of Psycho-Analysis* 50:711–717.

Zinner, J., and Shapiro, R. L. 1972. Projective identification as a mode of perception and behavior in families of adolescents. *International Journal of Psycho-Analysis* 53:523–530.

Zinner, J., and Shapiro, R. L. 1974. The family as a single psychic entity: implications for acting out in adolescents. *International Review of Psycho-Analysis* 1:179–186.

Zinner, J., and Shapiro, E. R. 1975. Splitting in families of borderline adolescents. In J. Mack, ed. *Borderline States in Psychiatry*. New York: Grune & Stratton.

THOMAS C. BOND AND NANCY AUGER

The hospitalization of adolescent patients for evaluation and treatment presents special problems for any institution. Their high level of energy, provocative behavior, bizarre modes of dress, sexual preoccupations, profane language, and musical tastes are disruptive to standard adult wards and have resulted in a reluctance to admit teenagers to the hospital; once admitted, they are often isolated on specialized adolescent units. Unfortunately, separating adolescent from adult patients creates as many problems as it attempts to solve. Inevitably, the adolescent becomes a scapegoat and is seen either as too needy, making unreasonable requests of the staff or the institution, or as too pampered, given special opportunities not afforded others by the staff. When an institution is committed to providing long-term treatment for the adolescent in a hospital setting, the need to address both adolescent and adult concerns becomes all the more necessary.

Records of the past twenty years have shown a fifteen-fold increase in the number of adolescent admissions to McLean Hospital, which has forced changes within the hospital structure and programs (Grob and Singer 1974). The current state of this evolution has in some ways come full circle. However, important changes have occurred, changes which we believe have created a richer and more realistic hospital experience for both the adult and the adolescent patient. Tracing these changes should help us understand better the current state of the generic or mixed-population units.

Twenty years ago, adolescent patients were admitted to adult units and hall-based individual treatment plans were developed. Schooling was ignored or special tutoring on a limited level was arranged through the local school system. Otherwise, the adolescent was expected to fit into existing adult programs. Given the adolescent's variable motivation, high energy, and lack of self-discipline, the programs proved inadequate. The adolescent would often spend long periods of time on the units with little to do but engage in restless inactivity and minor mischief—basically testing the patience of the staff and adult patients. The need for more structure in the adolescent's program was underscored by the fact that staff was forced to spend more time setting limits with the adolescents and less time with the adult patients, a situation resented by both adults and staff.

This system gave way to specialized adolescent units where the concepts of "peer pressure," "structure," and "group activity" were emphasized. While this move provided some relief to the adult units, the isolation of the adolescent patients by no means solved the problem of providing adequate hospital services to meet adolescent needs. To contain the increased turmoil on these adolescent units, patient programs became less individualized in the service of structure, groups, and peer pressure.

More important, this period ushered in the development of more extensive support services within the hospital which were tailored to reinforce adolescent strengths and interests. A fully accredited high school was established to provide the adolescent with a regular school exposure. This replaced the individual tutoring and enabled the student to increase schoolwork to five hours per day. The rehabilitation programs were expanded to provide classes in physical education, woodworking, crafts, music, art, and vocational training so that the students would gain academic credit in not strictly academic areas. The hours of the craft shop, music studio, gym, and art studio were extended to give the adolescent opportunities for extracurricular activity.

Several years ago, the decision was made to return to mixed adult and adolescent halls, with the exception of a small intensive treatment service for adolescents (ten beds) and a children's center for younger children and adolescents. The demise of the speciality units proved far less traumatic than anticipated because of the development of the ancillary support services in the interim period. Adolescents now spent a significant part of their day engaged in structured programs off the unit, which enabled the nursing staff to focus on other patient needs.

Reflecting on this history, one can see that the formation of an all-adolescent service arose from a lack of structured adolescent programs. Once programs were developed that allowed the channeling of excessive energy into constructive age-appropriate behaviors, the need for specialized adolescent units declined. Based on our experience, we think that this combination of mixed adult-adolescent halls and ancillary adolescent hospital programs is both a richer hospital experience for the adolescent and a benefit for adult patients and staff.

The Generic Milieu

The generic milieu recreates for the adolescent a community or family setting. Adolescents do not live in a vacuum or a world populated only by other adolescents; the presence of adults is of vital importance in helping them to achieve the independence necessary for further growth. Adolescents learn from adults and seek out safe, adult role models, often other adolescent's parents or extended family members (Beskind 1962; Schmiedeck 1961). Typically the adolescent's worst behaviors are saved for those on whom he or she is most dependent: his or her parents.

The unifying principle of the adolescent hospital program is to make the inpatient experience approximate the normal adolescent experience (Beskind 1962; Hartmann, Glasser, Greenblatt, Solomon, and Levinson 1968). This emphasizes the need to recognize the patient as an adolescent first and a patient second. The presentation of familiar experiences to the adolescent minimizes the problems of adjustment to and transition from the hospital. To accomplish this, one needs to provide opportunities for schooling, extracurricular activities, and peer socialization in addition to the more traditional therapies (Beavers and Blumberg 1968; Beckett 1965; Falstein, Feinstein, and Cohen 1960; Garber and Polsky 1970; Gossett, Lewis, Lewis, and Phillips 1973; Hendrickson, Holmes, and Waggoner 1959).

Two major criticisms of putting adult and adolescent patients together have been that adolescent patients are upsetting to adults because of their aggressive behavior and that disturbed adult patients present poor role models for the adolescent (Cohler 1973; Easson 1969; Suess and Hoshino 1961). Paradoxically, the attempt to remedy these issues through formation of adolescent units can create more problems.

Some measure of behavioral control is essential for any treatment to occur and be effective. It is widely reported that adults have a calming effect on adolescents and that all-adolescent units have a greater degree of turmoil (Beskind 1962; Falstein et al. 1960; Hartmann et al.

1968; Hendrickson et al. 1959; Miller 1957; Schmiedeck 1961; Suess and Hoshino 1961). The latter fact is confirmed by the higher staff-patient ratios and higher incidence of major ward disturbances on all-adolescent units compared with mixed adult-adolescent units. When adolescents are engaged in specific off-hall programs through the day, the annoyance to adults is greatly diminished, much as it is in normal families.

The issue of poor role models appears to be a gross oversimplification. No one is advocating that adolescents should be treated with only chronic regressed, back-ward patients. Many otherwise well-functioning adults enter the hospital because of acute crises and nonpsychotic behaviors which do not result in the massive regression seen in severe psychosis. These adult patients, having dealt with their own issues of adolescence, may be in a position to share this achievement in a nonthreatening way. The argument that enhancement of peer identification with emotionally disturbed adolescent peers is preferable to the presence of disturbed adults seems artificial. The positive role models of ward staff are present on all units regardless of population.

Several additional issues further highlight the shortcomings of the all-adolescent units, namely, exclusive patient selection, hospital isolation, and peer pressure. Selection of patients for inclusion on all-adolescent units is controversial in that many authors report that the severely disturbed adolescents—namely, the grossly psychotic, organically impaired, mentally retarded, or highly impulsive—fare better on adult halls (Beskind 1962; Hartmann et al. 1968; Hendrickson et al. 1959). Older adolescents, struggling with their own issues of autonomy, may tend to regress in a milieu with younger peers (Suess and Hoshino 1961).

The isolation of adolescent patients from the rest of the hospital community conveys an ambivalent message to the adolescent. The adolescent's rebellion and bravado mask an underlying insecurity and concerns over societal acceptance. Isolation of the adolescent from the rest of the hospital may transmit the message that the adolescent is a breed apart. The need for special treatment may be seen by the adolescent as a mark of denigration rather than as one of distinction and may be reinforced by the presence of specially trained staff. This runs counter to the underlying wish of most adolescents to become socially acceptable adults.

Peer pressure in the treatment of adolescents is inevitable. Unfortunately, adolescents are frequently rigid in their attitudes of appropriate behavior, which leads to scapegoating and ostracism of those who are unable to conform. For the more disturbed adolescent this is often a painful experience leading to further withdrawal and isolation (Hartmann et al. 1968). Adults are generally more tolerant and parental, being more supportive and sympathetic than impulsive adolescent peers.

Benefits to Staff and Patients

Inherent in the generic milieu approach are unique benefiits for the staff as well as adult and adolescent patients. As mentioned earlier, the degree of turmoil on mixed units is less than on adolescent units, and the need for constant limit setting and confrontation between staff members and adolescents is reduced. This decreases the potential antagonism of staff and patients and makes for the development of stronger treatment alliances.

For the adolescent, the presence of neutral adults affords several benefits. Much as they do in the community, adolescents turn to grandparents, aunts, uncles, cousins, and siblings for support and encouragement when parent-child tensions increase. Through this process, the adolescent often gains a greater understanding of the issues faced by parents in dealing with children and develops greater tolerance for his own parents. It is through this use of displacement that the adolescent is able to gain perspective on current dilemmas. Adults' comments of support and criticism have a greater impact on the adolescent than those of staff as they are viewed as more genuine and less easily dismissed as "therapeutic" (contrived) or controlling. The adult patient shares with the adolescent a sense of patienthood; as such, they are peers in the milieu. In this role, the adult becomes an ally for the adolescent, particularly concerning patient complaints. Staff is often more responsive to a suggestion when it represents the opinions of both older and younger patients (Falstein et al. 1960; Garber and Polsky 1970; Schmiedeck 1961).

The benefits for the adult patients are more subtle. Initially many adults complain of the noise and confusion generated by the adolescents, but with time the complaints subside. Adults are often sought out by adolescents for advice and comfort, which allows the opportunity for the adults to exercise their parenting skills and reexperience aspects of their own adolescence which they may have repressed. This opportunity for working through parenting issues using displacement in a controlled setting is invaluable toward restoring self-esteem. When the adolescent population on a unit decreases and the noise and activity diminish, adult patients often complain about the lack of life and zest.

Hospital Approach

The basic goal of hospitalization is the promotion or restoration of adequate daily functioning. Patients are hospitalized because their ability to function within the community is so impaired that outpatient programs prove ineffective. The task of the hospital is to restore sufficient stability in the patient's life so that he or she can return to the community for continued treatment.

The initial assessment of any patient is focused on identifying areas of inadequate functioning and determining an effective means of remedy. There are no simple prescriptions effective for all patients, a fact which is particularly clear on a generic unit. Once a treatment program has been agreed upon and established, the patient is given responsibility for following through and demonstrating competence and mastery to himself and the staff.

Individual, family, and group therapy; behavior modification; and psychopharmacology are seen as adjunctive services. These services aid the adolescent in overcoming those problem areas which led to his initial dysfunction. They are often valuable adjuncts to hospitalization in that their continuation outside the hospital after discharge allows a more gradual transition for the patient.

For the adolescent who has not completed a high school education, a school program becomes the central focus of his work; the rest of the treatment program is designed around the school. School is the one experience that all adolescents have in common; it provides a forum for peer relationships and a base for the future. Obtaining a high school diploma is an important milestone and serves as a source for self-esteem and a demonstration of competence. The school curriculum is sufficiently varied to allow the adolescent to elect courses which appeal to his or her interests. Most adolescents arrive at the hospital with a history of declining school performance and truancy and fear the return to school now that they are behind their peers. The school experience, which is a normal teenage activity, helps diffuse the identity of being a mental patient and facilitates rejoining former peer groups following discharge.

For the adolescent who has graduated from high school, the focus for the clinical program is on vocational training. Through the development of vocational skills, the adolescent acquires the ability to live independently from the family should this be appropriate.

Other parts of a patient's program are designed to appeal to specific interests such as music, art, crafts, and activities to develop greater abilities in these areas and to teach the adolescent how to structure free time.

Orientation

The generic units at McLean average twenty-three beds of patients of both sexes whose diagnoses include affective, psychotic, character, and behavior disorders. The population of the unit is one-third adolescents and two-thirds adults who range in age from twenty to fifty. Some control can be exercised over admissions by individual units. Adolescents' hospital stays vary from sixty days to two years.

Initially the adolescent is restricted to the unit to allow the staff to assess the youth's capability to handle certain aspects of the program, to facilitate integration into the patient group, and to establish a preliminary treatment alliance. The duration of the restriction is dependent on the degree of self-discipline and impulse control demonstrated by the patient. The adolescent begins a school evaluation as soon as possible and receives the privileges to do this. This gives the patient an initial opportunity to demonstrate personal responsibility and competence, which is necessary for obtaining additional privileges.

Patient Responsibilities and Role of Staff

The staff expectations for all patients stress personal responsibility for individual action, and patients receive privileges according to their ability to act responsibly. Those who demonstrate either an inability or resistance to meet minimal standards of behavior are presumed to lack the necessary internal discipline and structure. Therefore, the need for greater external structure provided by the staff and hospital becomes essential. Implicit within this process is the input of staff members, who make recommendations and provide information necessary to establish an adequate program. Adequate assessment of a patient's progress requires close coordination between unit staff and ancillary program directors for information about participation and performance.

Individual patient-staff conflicts arise most often around granting of privileges. While the staff views refusal of additional privileges as an opportunity to help the adolescent identify problem areas and invest greater energy in resolving them, the adolescent often views the refusal as a personal rejection. Such conflicts are approached through the use of contracts based on performance of the specified treatment program. Usually a staff member will negotiate a contract with the patient in which specific behaviors necessary to obtain a privilege are clearly defined. In order to maintain privileges the patient must continue to follow the assigned tasks. Use of a contract removes the focus for failure to make progress from an emotional personal struggle and places it directly on the patient and his inability to act responsibly.

Patient responsibilities on the unit include attendance at community meetings, mixed milieu groups, mandatory activities, and special adolescent and adult groups. In addition all patients are expected to demonstrate community responsibilities, including cleaning up after oneself, not interfering with another patient's treatment program, and dealing directly with patient-to-patient conflicts.

The staff is encouraged to provide advice and guidance but in large part to refrain from direct decision making for the patient. This approach conveys to the patients an expectation of competence and facilitates direct resolution of personal and family conflicts by enhancing self-esteem and decreasing excessive dependency on staff. When patient-to-patient conflicts arise, staff members seek to act as mediators by establishing boundaries and assuming limited responsibility for conflict resolution. The following illustrates this point.

CASE EXAMPLE 1

Sarah was a fifteen-year-old hospitalized for runaway behavior, declining school performance, and drug abuse. Her parents were unable to tolerate her anger when they tried to set limits.

Harry was a fifty-year-old, depressed, isolated patient with very set daily rituals, who generally interacted minimally with other patients. The patients either ignored him or took him for granted, rarely including him in discussions or activities.

One evening Sarah refused to clean the kitchen after using it, despite frequent staff encouragement. Patients appeared reluctant to confront her, fearing her wrath, and the staff elected to lock the kitchen until it was cleaned. The following morning Harry was unable to use the kitchen as usual. He angrily approached Sarah and directed her to "get off your ass and clean the kitchen."

Sarah's initial response was defiant, but she soon quietly complied. Harry's unexpected confrontation of Sarah surprised both patients and staff. Following this incident several patients made attempts to include Harry in informal discussions and activities. Even Sarah began to seek his advice concerning hall and personal issues. The interaction was one of a series of interactions between Sarah and Harry which offered her a new experience of limit setting outside of her family and allowed him to become integrated into the milieu.

As noted earlier, a school or vocational (for those with a high school diploma) program is the central focus of the adolescents' treatment program. Personal or family conflicts are frequently evidenced by resistance to school participation. The adolescent whose resistance to school participation persists, despite staff efforts, may be seen as needing greater structure in the form of increased staff supervision. For the psychotic patient this is reassuring. For the impulsive adolescent this increased attention may serve as an impetus toward overcoming the resistance to school attendance, as seen in the following example.

CASE EXAMPLE 2

Paul was a fifteen-year-old boy referred for unmanageable behavior, drug abuse, and truancy. On the unit he was extremely provocative, negativistic, and refused to participate in school or other programs. Since he was unable to structure his time productively, he was placed on a highly structured ward schedule. For two days he continued to refuse to attend school but changed his attitude with the consistent enforcement of the schedule by the staff and the increased concern and irritation directed toward him by his adult roommate with whom he had a generally good relationship. The consistent limit setting by the staff and their attention to him enabled Paul to develop an increased ability to talk with them. At a later point in his hospitalization, he again stopped attending school for a few days but returned to classes when his schedule was reinstituted.

Mixed Milieu Groups

The mixed milieu groups are limited to six to eight members of varying ages, which allows for more in-depth examination of personal problems and expression of mutual support. Patienthood and the hospital living situation are common issues for all patients and provide the initial cohesion for these groups. The task of the group is to develop a heightened sensitivity to one another's particular needs and expectations. This experience allows the adolescent to reach a greater understanding of adult concerns and the adult of adolescent concerns, as seen in the following example.

CASE EXAMPLE 3

Kathy was a sixteen-year-old girl, hospitalized for unmanageable behavior after discovering for the first time that she had been adopted as an infant. She was abusive toward her adoptive parents and refused to participate in family meetings.

Jane was a forty-year-old woman hospitalized for depression precipitated by her only daughter's move away to college. She had been unable to share directly with her daughter any negative feelings of loss surrounding the daughter's move.

In mixed group, the interaction between Kathy and Jane was initially hostile. With limits set by other group members on their lack of consideration for one another, they were eventually able to share their sense of rejection from opposite perspectives of adult and child. Kathy and Jane became more civil to one another and eventually began to seek one another's thoughts and feelings about personal issues. Kathy soon began to participate in family meetings. Jane was better able to discuss the hurt and anger she experienced when her daughter left home and reached a more realistic understanding of her daughter's need for increased independence.

Other group experiences can be tailored to the composition and needs of the population. Sexuality groups might be offered for women and men of varied ages. Groups restricted to adults or adolescents are useful to enhance discussion of age specific issues and concerns.

Adolescent Group

The adolescent group is one of the few structured groups which is designed specifically for adolescents. It provides a forum for peer discussion and support and encourages healthier peer relations. Adolescent participation is a privilege which implies shared responsibility for limit setting with one another. Issues such as clique formation, ostracism, and the sense of shame regarding hospitalization are best dealt with in this setting, as seen in the following examples.

CASE EXAMPLE 4

Eric, Tom, and Sharon were three adolescents who became inseparable on the unit. They encouraged one another's externalization of blame onto parents and staff, refusing personal responsibility for unpleasant experiences and creating havoc on the unit. Whenever Eric became angry with the staff or another patient, Tom and Sharon would come to his defense regardless of the circumstances. This issue was brought to the adolescent group by the staff. Eric was confronted about his refusal to take responsibility for his own personal problems, and Tom and Sharon were confronted about their inability to view Eric's actions impartially. They initially denied these accusations but subsequently showed greater independence from one another. Eric continued to struggle with staff but expressed his anger in more private areas to staff members. All three began spending more time with other patients.

CASE EXAMPLE 5

Bob, a fifteen-year-old schizophrenic, was generally avoided by his peers because of his bizarre behavior. Through the forum of the adolescent group, Bob was encouraged to share his experiences with other adolescents and to enter the discussion. Gradually he became better able to share his ideas and offer support to other group members. The other adolescents began to value his sensitivity and insight and would more often include him in activities on the unit. His self-esteem was greatly enhanced through this peer interaction, and his withdrawal and bizarre behavior declined.

Typically there are four phases these adolescent groups pass through in their evolution. First, the adolescents complain about their being in the hospital and the injustices done to them. This externalization provides the initial cohesion in the group. The focus then shifts from the hospital to their families, and the patients are encouraged to discuss their family experiences. The third phase is increased awareness of the role the patient played in the family struggles and a growing sense of responsibility for one's own behavior. The last phase is sharing concern for the future and dealing with the stigma of hospitalization.

Conclusions

Several decades ago, the hospitalization of adolescent patients on adult units was not by design but by necessity. Subsequent years have seen a trend toward development of specialized adolescent units and programs quite apart from hospitalized adults. It is our feeling that this trend has not been entirely favorable nor preferable.

The benefits of combining adult and adolescent patients are considerable for hospital staff and the patients themselves. Mixed units are more flexible with admission criteria and program development, provide a more stable treatment environment, and recognize openly the fact that adults and adolescents have much to learn from each other. Adolescents do have certain special needs which can be addressed as easily in a mixed setting as in an all-adolescent one.

REFERENCES

Beavers, W. R., and Blumberg, S. 1968. A follow-up study of adolescents treated in an inpatient setting. *Diseases of the Nervous System* 29:606–612.

Beckett, P. 1965. *Adolescents Out of Step: Their Treatment in a Psychiatric Hospital.* Detroit: Wayne State University Press.

Beskind, H. 1962. Psychiatric inpatient treatment of adolescents: a review of clinical experience. *Comprehensive Psychiatry* 3:354–369.

Cohler, B. 1973. New ways in the treatment of emotionally disturbed adolescents. *Adolescent Psychiatry* 2:305–323.

Easson, W. M. 1969. *The Severely Disturbed Adolescent.* New York: International Universities Press.

Falstein, E. I.; Feinstein, S. L.; and Cohen, W. P. 1960. An integrated adolescent care program in a general psychiatric hospital. *American Journal of Orthopsychiatry* 30:276–291.

Garber, B., and Polsky, R. 1970. Follow-up study of hospitalized adolescents. *Archives of General Psychiatry* 22:179–187.

Gossett, J. T.; Lewis, S. B.; Lewis, J. M.; and Phillips, V. A. 1973. Follow-up of adolescents treated in a psychiatric hospital: a review of studies. *American Journal of Orthopsychiatry* 43(4): 602–610.

Grob, M., and Singer, J. 1974. *Adolescent Patients in Transition*. New York: Behavioral Publications.

Hartmann, E.; Glasser, B. A.; Greenblatt, M.; Solomon, M. H.; and Levinson, D. J. 1968. *Adolescents in a Mental Hospital*. New York: Grune & Stratton.

Hendrickson, W. J.; Holmes, D. J.; and Waggoner, R. W. 1959. Psychotherapy of the hospitalized adolescent. *American Journal of Psychiatry* 116:527–532.

Miller, D. H. 1957. The treatment of adolescents in an adult hospital: a preliminary report. *Bulletin Menninger Clinic* 21:189–198.

Schmiedeck, R. A. 1961. A treatment program for adolescents on an adult ward. *Bulletin Menninger Clinic* 25:241–248.

Suess, J. F., and Hoshino, A. 1961. Therapeutic development and management of an adolescent in a state hospital. *American Journal of Psychiatry* 117:891–896.

26 THE INPATIENT TREATMENT OF ADOLESCENTS IN A MILIEU INCLUDING YOUNGER CHILDREN

JACQUELINE OLDS

Adolescents have been treated in combination with almost every other possible age group in the hope that their inherent difficulties might be decreased by some unpredictable ingredient in the milieu. In spite of the title of this chapter, let me say that we have found no way to stop adolescents from acting adolescent. Though we do have a population including ages three to sixteen, with 50–75 percent over twelve years old, we have not been able to stem the effects of adolescent patients in a unit with little people.

Our treatment philosophy[1] is based on a fundamental fact of child development, namely, that the use of play (as described by Peller [1954] and Sarnoff [1976]) in childhood (specifically latency) leads to growth and development of defenses against drives and overwhelming emotions such that an adolescent and later an adult will not be so vulnerable to their impulses and feelings. Although we accept a wide range of psychiatric diagnoses, we have found that the majority of the adolescents admitted to our unit could be diagnosed as immature personalities with impulse disorders. What this often means is that these adolescents did not adequately learn to use play during the latency period owing to deficits in their early ego development. Feelings affect them intensely, they have fewer ways to channel such feelings as anger, and they are apt to become angry and act directly on such feelings by trying to hurt themselves or others. Their counterparts, adolescents who have learned to use play in latency, show anger in a more modulated way, since they have other channels available to discharge their anger, such as fantasy or sports.

The Group for the Advancement of Psychiatry (1966) diagnostic list for children and adolescents includes the category "tension discharge disorder." This term describes a phenomenon that occurs in these adolescents, namely, that an increase of anxiety or tension within them will often result in some impulsive, often destructive discharge. Since we find that the majority of adolescents, especially the younger ones, admitted to our unit do fall into this category, and that their pathology often results from a deficit in their latency development, it has proved useful to have them exposed to a milieu partially designed for latency-age children to help them make up for this deficit. It should be mentioned that our patients also have prelatency deficits in their ego development, but often the latency deficits are easier to treat in the milieu.

I will illustrate this phenomenon as it emerges in actual practice and use examples, including privileges and privilege groups, community meetings, education, and therapy, to show that in a milieu including both latency-age children and adolescents ego building can occur to the benefit of both.

The privilege system is a central area of staff-patient interaction. Adolescents on our unit have to deal with different rules from those living on units with adults. For example, smoking cigarettes is forbidden except to those adolescents who have turned sixteen. Staff members often joke among themselves that we try to reform these adolescents from stealing, assault, and all sorts of other evil things by making smoking more alluring because we forbid it. Although this seems merely humorous, it does contain the important point that these rebellious, acting-out youngsters do not particularly care what rule they are acting out against. Therefore, if they are maintained in a safe environment and strict rules are enforced on more trivial subjects, the teenager's pattern of getting into trouble may continue but not with the same degree of serious self-destructiveness.

These adolescents are in a program in which they earn their privileges along with younger children, depending on their behavior and capabilities. The adolescents are able to earn privileges that are much more adult than the ones children can earn, but nevertheless they are often in a position of having to compare their freedom with that of much younger children. This often leads to great complaining and irritation on the teenagers' part because they feel their age should entitle them to greater freedom. But it gives us the advantage of seeing the ways in which these teenagers deal with stand-ins for their sibs or representations of their younger selves. Thus, important dynamic information emerges from this interaction.

On one unit, which has a majority of adolescent patients, we have a privilege group that meets weekly. In this group, each teenager makes a privilege request, hears a recommendation from a staff member on the request, and then can argue with the recommendation using peer and staff feedback as a means to understanding the final decision. The hope is that this kind of group will (1) allow the teenagers to see that the decisions have some rational and often protective basis and are not just arbitrary constraints; (2) allow them to feel some sense of authorship in the decision since a group of adolescents larger than the staff are both present and vocal, and decisions are based on a majority vote except when staff vetoes a decision for safety reasons; and (3) get each adolescent to emerge from self-preoccupation long enough to start observing what other teenagers on the unit are doing, since they will be involved in the privilege decisions for the others. Although these are goals by no means accomplished in every group, the group is the structure in which they can be accomplished by a skillful staff.

If we look at the community meetings held in the milieu, we can see another example in which the mixture of adolescents and latency-age children can be beneficial. First, the principle of helping the children and the adolescents to sublimate the feelings that overwhelm them rather than acting them out needs to be considered. With this in mind, we can look at an example from community meetings on a unit with both adolescent and latency-age boys. At the beginning of an academic year, when the patients were anxious and defensive because of the influx of new staff, there was often a barrage of insults aimed by the adolescents at the staff. Since many of the staff were new and relatively naive, they had little idea how to deal with these attacks and wanted to hand out restrictions quickly as a means of dealing with their anxiety. It was stressed in staff meetings that the adolescents were on the offensive because they expected to be put down by the large group of staff at community meetings. The leader of the meeting felt that, as the adolescents felt increasingly familiar and secure, staff would not be attacked and adolescent defensive insults would decrease and perhaps be sublimated into humor. This did in fact happen, with the help of one hypomanic adolescent boy who would spend time in the meetings making fun of everyone's shoes. The other patients followed suit, teasing each other and staff about oddities in each other's footwear. From the leader's point of view, this was definitely preferable to

375

character assassinations which really hurt staff members' feelings. Eventually the whole subject became a ward tradition, with staff and patients trying to outdo each other in wearing humorous shoes and boots. When new staff members would join the meetings in the middle of the year, they could not understand why we spent valuable therapeutic time laughing at each other's shoes. After a while they came to understand that the pursuit of this tradition was an indication of some group cohesion and a shared defense between children and staff—namely, humor. As play therapists, the staff could see that the joking was a sublimation of some of the defensive hostility patients used to protect their own sense of themselves as defective. Both adolescents and latency-age children were able to utilize this sublimation effectively.

The educational component of our program, like others including those of Bettelheim (1950) and Redl (1957), has a strong emphasis on mastery. Our theory is that many adolescents feel particularly inadequate and ineffective because they do not have many areas of sublimation into which their feelings can be channeled toward productive ends. Thus, our hope is that by teaching them how both to learn and to find areas in which they enjoy learning, we might reroute their energy from destructive to constructive ends. The school program on our unit is aimed at finding what gets in the children's way when they try to learn. Then the staff has various techniques for correcting the cognitive deficits they do find with the goal of making learning both possible and enjoyable. The techniques for teaching utilize the principles of play by presenting new skills in the form of games. The students at first tend to express skepticism that the hospital school could be a "real" school. On the other hand, in spite of their complaints that it is a "baby" school instead of a real one, they often experience the satisfaction of succeeding at schoolwork for the first time because the work is individually tailored to their cognitive capacities. The experience itself can give them some momentum to continue trying in the future.

There is also an after-school activities program including a spectrum from crafts to woodworking or art. At times more mature adolescents can get jobs in the hospital, such as working in the coffee shop, and this seems to have a very beneficial effect in terms of making them feel worthwhile and capable. This is a natural extension of the necessary emphasis on mastery in a program for latency-age children. This brings me to a crucial point in our philosophy.

Because many hospitalized adolescents are so vulnerable to affect that their symptomatology increases considerably when they experience any strong emotion, our task in a short-term intervention is to strengthen their existing defenses and help them to develop new ones rather than uncovering conflict and affect. This task means that staff and therapists need to unlearn their tendency to uncover affect-laden material as a first priority. They have to recognize that when they do indulge their wish to expose affect that they often make the adolescent so anxious that intolerable acting out within the hospital milieu is the result. We have discovered in our setting that those staff who work most skillfully with children and adolescents are not those who are confrontative and intrusive, but those who remain relatively neutral, helpful, and nonjudgmental.

Now, if the question were to be asked, "What has this to do with adolescents in a milieu with younger children?" we could answer that there is an intimate connection. The described techniques are those derived from applying some of the principles of play therapy for children to a milieu. All the parts of the program (except the privilege group) are those that one would design for a group of latency-age children knowing their developmental needs and limitations. In fact, latency-age children in our unit do rather well in the program as it stands because it caters to many of their developmental requirements.

Although our adolescents, because of their size, chronological age, and superficial maturity, seemed at first capable of insight-oriented therapy, we found that we had to use play therapy for them because their immature personalities kept them from having the capacity for an observing ego necessary for insight-oriented therapy (Geleerd 1957; Sarnoff 1976). Specifically, we have discovered that therapeutic work on issues and conflicts occurs best in displaced form since direct discussion of themselves makes these teenagers too anxious. Further, many of these issues and conflicts can be worked through in displacement. It should be noted, however, that we are dealing primarily with young adolescents and these generalizations do not necessarily apply to older adolescents.

The crucial difference between working with latency-age children and with young adolescents is that with the latter we do not use toys. Instead we listen to material about friends, other patients, heroes, or enemies with the knowledge that they are projective figures used by the patient the same way a child would use dolls or puppets. While many of these adolescents are often capable of using a direct interpretation or clarification, the more usual work with these teenagers is in displaced form. Ultimately we are trying to provide a nurturant and tranquil environment in which the adolescents are freed to go about their developmental task of completing latency and preadolescence. Our efforts are aimed at helping the teenagers to master skills, improving their ego function, building on their useful defenses, and helping them to understand and overcome any obstacles in their development.

The philosophy just described can be criticized in various ways. For example, some might say that it is threateningly regressive for an adolescent to be plunged into a milieu where he or she is not only surrounded by much younger children but also treated in many ways like one of them. Of course, each patient ought to be expected to function at his or her healthiest level. However, as I have described, many of these adolescents have never experienced the success of mastering skills during latency. If we can make this possible, they soon ignore the regressive pull of the younger children and bask in their frequent superiority in performing tasks. The challenge is for the staff not to be too threatened by some of the childlike provocative behavior on the teenagers' part (this is often a repeat of what went on between parents and teenagers); when the staff members get provoked, their own fear of regression may cause them to force the patient to look at the reasons for his or her behavior, which often has more of a punitive than a therapeutic effect.

Another criticism of our philosophy sometimes made by new staff members is that some teenagers are impossible to keep from insight-oriented therapy because they are overflowing with material about their family, themselves, and their intimate feelings. These intimate revelations often punctuate the most flamboyant and self-destructive periods of acting out. But the staff, nevertheless, may feel useful work is being done because these patients seem so candid and earnest when they are working in therapy and talking freely about their innermost feelings. Actually, this kind of behavior is often seen in extremely needy, hysterical patients who are able to comply unconsciously with the wishes of their audience. Their revelations often have little therapeutic effect except to keep staff attention on them, which is their greatest need. If they were to find that they could command the same amount of staff attention with small talk and sublimatory accomplishments, they would be just as satisfied. And since we feel that the latter are also useful for their future functioning in the real world, we would try to encourage the staff to reinforce the "small talk" rather than the sensational revelations. (As mentioned before, often the content of the small talk is quite revealing.) It should also be noted that it is age appropriate for adolescents to communicate more freely with their peers than with adults. Consequently our staff are trained to accept and work with the teenagers confiding more in each other than in staff.

The kind of ego building I am describing is long-term work that needs positive relationships between staff and patients in order to succeed. A large percentage of our patients, however, come to us only for an evaluation. This process may take eight weeks or more, and little time is available for developmental change. Often recommendations are made for the work to be continued on an outpatient basis (which is often difficult) or in a therapeutic residential school. The more turnover in staff or changes in program, the less likely it is that therapeutic change will occur since the work depends so heavily on consistent relationships built up over time. When we are able to work on a long-term basis with patients, we find that the turnover of short-term patients need not detract from the programs of the long-term patients because they get used to a part of the population being there for evaluation only. On the other hand, when we have some staff turnover, as for example at the end or beginning of the academic year, it is in fact a more confusing time and the work definitely proceeds on a slower basis.

It is noteworthy to consider instances when the mixture of age groups on our unit can be the most troublesome and problematical. Probably the most inflammable situation occurs when we have a unit on which there are some very young children (perhaps between four and seven) and some immature adolescents. At times the younger children may receive physical kinds of affection from staff (such as piggyback rides or goodnight hugs) that would be inappropriate for the adolescents. The adolescents, who may be fighting desperately against their infantile yearnings, often get very angry at and envious of the younger children who receive a kind of gratification they can no longer ask for. This often duplicates the situation in their family which led to their hospitalization. The staff need to work hard to speak to the adolescents' healthiest level and perhaps employ them in child care and role modeling. This gives the adolescents new routes into which they can channel their regressive feelings. At times the adolescents can vicariously satisfy their own wish for nurturance by caring for and teaching the younger children. We have also at times used gardening and live pets as channels for the adolescents' need for nurturance.

Conclusions

In working with a combination of adolescents and younger children, we find that both in the milieu and in individual therapy it is useful to employ the methods of play therapy without humiliating the adolescent with the use of actual toys. That is, we try to refrain from asking the adolescents directly to acknowledge their own feelings and explore their origins, as we might with an adult patient, because the anxiety provoked in the adolescent is often overwhelming. Instead, we often learn about the adolescent's feelings in displacement and use projective tools that will teach us about the adolescent's internal world without threatening him or her. The adolescent may often need help in solving problems but most likely will not be able to ask directly; thus argument and struggle may be the medium through which the adolescent receives instruction in adult methods of coping. These struggles often take place in the arena of hospital privilege requests. We also try to let the adolescents know that much can be learned from looking with them at their strengths rather than confirming their fears that their weaknesses will be exposed and dissected.

Our goal is to provide an environment where the adolescent feels he is in control of his emotions. This usually means a high degree of structure with clear limits about what behavior is acceptable and what behavior is not, since these teenagers usually have such meager internal controls. When the adolescent's feelings do overflow, the staff need to respond as consistently as possible without seeming too intimidated by the feelings or the accompanying impulses. Clearly, this is not easy and requires a sophisticated and well-trained staff. But as staff become accustomed to the adolescents' reactions, they will be able to retain some long-term perspective even when the adolescents are losing theirs. With luck and a lot of supervision, staff can learn not to take it personally even when adolescents direct their highly charged "transference" toward them. In conclusion, let me emphasize that my description has at times been a description of what we aspire to rather than what we always achieve. The adolescents described often have an uncanny way of distracting therapists from their goals because of their dramatic and self-destructive style.

JACQUELINE OLDS

NOTE

1. From the Hall-Mercer Children's Center, McLean Hospital, Belmont, Massachusetts.

REFERENCES

Bettelheim, B. 1950. *Love Is Not Enough: The Treatment of Emotionally Disturbed Children*. Glencoe, Ill.: Free Press.
Geleerd, E. R. 1957. Some aspects of psychoanalytic technique in adolescence. *Psychoanalytic Study of the Child* 12:263–283.
Group for the Advancement of Psychiatry. 1966. *Psychopathological Disorders in Childhood: Theoretical Considerations and a Proposed Classification*. New York: GAP.
Peller, L. E. 1954. Libidinal phases, ego development and play. *Psychoanalytic Study of the Child* 9:178–198.
Redl, F. 1957. *The Aggressive Child*. Glencoe, Ill.: Free Press.
Sarnoff, C. 1976. *Latency*. New York: Aronson.

27 STAFF COUNTERTRANSFERENCE IN AN ADOLESCENT MILIEU TREATMENT SETTING

RICHARD J. BONIER

Countertransference has been defined as "arousal of the analyst's repressed feelings by the analytic situation: especially (but not always)
the transference by the analyst of his repressed feelings upon the
analysand" (English and English 1958). In this chapter the term will be
somewhat broadened to include patient-staff relationships in the adolescent milieu treatment setting. While I will be concerned with the
arousal in the treatment staff of repressed or unresolved feelings as a
function of treatment interactions with a given population, I will not be
positing transference of these feelings onto the adolescent patients.
Rather, my focus will be on the manner in which repressed and unresolved staff conflict may be elicited by contact with the patient
population and subsequently transferred and acted on in staff relationships. The developmental characteristics of this particular patient
population will be seen as the stimulus which evokes staff countertransferential behavior.

Treatment Program

The Adolescent Day Service (ADS)[1] is an adolescent day-treatment
facility which operates in conjunction with a day school for disturbed
adolescents. The ADS serves approximately thirty adolescents between the ages of fourteen and twenty-one, approximately two-thirds
of whom manifest severe problems in impulse control. The group is
made up largely of character disordered and borderline adolescents.

About one-third of the total group manifests psychosis, primarily process schizophrenia. The character disordered and borderline patients are characterized by boisterousness, frequent abrogation of rules and limits, aggressiveness, and periods of rage-filled defiance and contempt alternating with periods of warmth and engaging humor. The schizophrenic patients are less variable, more quiet, tractable, passive, frightened, and upset by disturbances in scheduling and the antics of their peers, and consistently adult oriented in their asking for structure and protection. The average length of stay is about two years; most graduate from school in the program, though a few will return to their public high school before graduation, and many will continue in attenuated ADS programs following graduation.

Treatment programs are distributed among three approaches. First, a full range of the more traditional approaches are available—individual, group, and family psychotherapy. Second, there are interventions subsumed under the term "street corner social work." All staff members spend a part of their time in the dayroom and other places preferred by the adolescents, interacting more or less at leisure and with no explicit agenda on their part or the patient's. Third, all staff members are available throughout the day for crisis intervention as acute problems develop in the school or elsewhere. A substantial portion of staff members' time is devoted to interventions that may involve calling a variety of significant figures together on the spot. The latter two types of intervention are similar to Redl's (1966) "life space interview." While professionals value the more traditional, scheduled types of intervention, the adolescents often do not; however, they do present themselves for the more informal approaches.

Research cited by Grob[2] indicates that in inpatient and day treatment, the variable most clearly associated with positive outcome in follow-ups is not time spent with the therapist but, rather, time spent with the mental health worker. For adolescents, particularly, the mental health worker is on the ward, has a great deal of unstructured time available, observes the patient in a variety of social contexts, and can interact with the adolescent according to the patient's rhythms rather than in schedules usually determined by adults.

Countertransference

Countertransference is a significant element in transactions between adults and adolescents in the family, school, and treatment setting.

Benedek (1959) and others have addressed the manner in which parenting involves reexperiencing, with each child, one's own developmental successes and failures. She describes characteristic crises occurring when developmental struggles coincide with poorly resolved conflicts of the parent's past. At these points a high probability of distortions of both perception and response by the parents exists, further complicating the child's adaptive efforts.

Schools represent another area where adult and child meet. In the schools, however, the adult (teacher) is generally alone, confronted with a substantial number of children, all roughly the same age and all struggling with the same developmental concerns. The adolescents' perceptions of themselves and their teacher are determined and biased in many respects by the life issues which are paramount to them at that point. Their view of the adult is colored by their own narrowed world view and personal preoccupations. Their response to the teacher's personality will be similarly heightened and strained. For the teacher, the situation may function as a remarkably powerful conditioner determining his or her approach to the children and his view of himself and others.

Countertransferential responses will vary according to each staff person's individual life history. There is another level of countertransference, however, with a high probability of expression across all staff members. It is this latter form which is more likely to be shared but unexamined by the staff since it constitutes a set of postulates about their immediate world and the issues important within it.

In working with parents, especially during periods of stress, one becomes aware of the remarkable degree to which staff approaches to the adolescent are similar if not identical to modal parental responses. These congruences may be more the rule than the exception in staff patterns of dealing with adolescents. In inpatient settings, when one observes these recapitulations unfolding, one can, with a certain amount of patronizing, ascribe their occurrence to youth, relative lack of experience, and lack of specialized graduate education. But, when one begins to observe the same behavior in oneself, one becomes more ready to examine the situation as an important and intrinsic aspect of the whole treatment process.

The staff's response to the adolescent's intensity may serve as a paradigm for all staff countertransferential responses within the somewhat altered definition represented in this chapter. When the staff responds, the effect on the adolescent is either to add whatever power the patient attributes to the treating adult, to further confirm the sense of urgency experienced by the adolescent, or, in the response to many schizophrenic youngsters, to disconfirm the meaning of an internal state of being. Clearly not all staff members automatically respond to these situations as described. However, such responses do seem common enough to reflect some important and modal categories of countertransference.

In the response to the impulse-disordered adolescent's demand for action, staff members may report feeling that to offer alternatives to a relatively immediate demand is to risk dangerous adolescent wrath which would jeopardize a developing alliance. Thus, the staff tends to give in, to make excuses, or to refuse on the basis of past experiences. It is a rarity for the staff to respond with some cognitive recognition of the powerful imperative driving the adolescent at that moment. Yet it is at these moments that central characterological difficulties are being enacted in microcosm, in the here and now, that can ideally begin to be attached to new ways of self- and world-perception. Here the clinicians can utilize their own personal distance from the shared sense of felt immediacy.

The converse problem is often met in exchanges with chronic schizophrenic adolescents, who may present themselves as unduly agitated and upset about some aspect of their personal world which is out of order or sequence, for example, a change of school schedule or confusion about transportation. A not-uncommon staff response is a good-natured, ostensibly supportive reassurance that they need not worry, that the procedures for assuring predictability are simple enough, and that even if things should go awry, corrective procedures could easily enough be instituted. While the observations are generally valid and in one sense supportive, they do not acknowledge or legitimize the current experience of the patient. Instead, these responses suggest that the patient's perceptions are distorted, unreal, and invalid. One unfortunate product of this kind of intervention is to confirm exactly what has been so problematic for the schizophrenic patient, namely, the difficulty in experiencing and understanding internal cues, as well as in receiving any affirmation of their meaning to him.

It is my primary contention that most severely disordered individuals, and particularly adolescents because of the greater age-appropriate intensity and confusion, evoke in significant others exactly those responses which serve to confirm their disordered views of self and others, of causality and predictability. As Redl (1966) and others observed, interventions around naturally occurring behaviors in the here and now may be the best way to treat a disturbed adolescent. It may also be that it is the rule rather than the exception for these classes of countertransference to occur.

Clinicians will often verbalize some consciousness of the dimensions which they failed to acknowledge during the exchange, often feeling that to make such a clarification at the time interfered with a developing alliance. Even that assumption may be seen as countertransferential, mirroring the adolescent's conviction, acted rather than verbal, that to step in the way of the felt imperative would result in disaster. Clinicians tend to feel at the time of the encounter that any exchange which recognized the process would be cumbersome, unwieldy, verbose, and warded off by the adolescent. Words and action seem hopelessly separated—one awkward, unwieldy, and offensive and the other commanding and real. To attempt a wedding of the two at best would be clumsy and artificial and at worst would destroy a bond felt at that moment as tenuous and unstable.

Secondarily, the intensity and immediacy of the situation and the feelings being acted out by the adolescent rekindle those never fully resolved themes in all of us, that is, the sense of a greater legitimacy in action than in reflection. This rekindling and subsequent acting out on the part of the staff member occurs in a situational context exquisitely designed for it—the clinician's positioning on adolescent terrain, not in his or her own office. It happens in the midst of a living situation rather than a situation in which one is dealing with memory derivatives and reduced affect as the aliveness of the situation decays. Granted that a dichotomy between office and milieu may be exaggerated; yet the features of an office visit certainly offer greater containment of adolescent expression than does an open milieu. Small wonder that those of us who have been trained to flex our observing egos experience a sense of failure and exhaustion in the midst of milieu work. Small wonder that the inevitable progression of well-trained milieu clinicians is away from the milieu and into the office, their own treatment philosophy often notwithstanding. The notion of staff burnout must represent a more differentiated phenomenon than merely fatigue related to constant control struggles with adolescents.

Utilization of countertransference feelings and enactments helps in a most powerful way to develop further awareness of the critical matters with which the adolescent is struggling. Structures enabling the staff to recognize and use their individual and shared reactions seem an absolute necessity in a milieu treatment setting. A common initial sense among staff members examining their own process is a sense of failure that they have not been able to relate to the adolescent's imperatives more dispassionately during an encounter, which is, in its own way, an expression of hubris. In the fluid, intense, and often conflictual immediacies of milieu exchanges, only islands of observing ego may be available at any one time. Fortunately, the issues acted out by adolescents are characterized by both chronicity and stereotypy. Once identified, they can be assured of many repeated performances.

Impact of Adolescent Behavior on Mental Health Staff

One of the tragedies of disturbed adolescents is that they enter the demands of this period with many of the prior developmental tasks poorly resolved. The chronic schizophrenic adolescent, in particular, manifests early developmental task failure to such an extent that age-appropriate adolescent issues are often difficult to recognize.

With the majority of impulse-disordered adolescents, most staff-patient interactions are concerned with control battles which involve the setting and resetting of limits. Not infrequently the exchanges are best measured in decibels rather than in substance. Our adolescents tend to engage in violating conventional boundaries and limits usually set around such issues as pot smoking, alcohol consumption, petty vandalism, physical threats, scapegoating of the more passive patients, skipping classes, and intrusion into staff offices during scheduled sessions. Almost all of the adolescents who engage in these activities are very active, likable, and noisy, combining what Horney (1945) called the "moving toward" and "moving against" types of interaction.

Many of these infractions are expressed clearly and immediately to a staff person. There can be no doubt that Dan just left big boot prints on the wall only moments ago, but no one actually saw him. No one ever sees him. In no time a sizable number of staff members are aware: Dan doesn't fully deny the action but he demands proof of his guilt. If pressed, he becomes rather jovially defiant and contemptuous, indicating that while it cannot be proved that he did it, there is no way that anyone is going to limit his freedom to replicate it exactly, at whatever time he should choose.

When a substantial subgroup of adolescents is engaged in sustained defiance and rule breaking, staff tolerance becomes stretched, morale is very much in jeopardy, and concerns are voiced that things are in danger of becoming totally out of control. What further lack of control would entail is usually not spelled out; the potential outcome is ineffable and menacing. Sense of humor, otherwise much in evidence, begins to disappear and becomes, in fact, impermissible (a sign that the bearer is not taking the crisis seriously enough). Something must be done and done decisively. Fears of violence against staff members begin to be voiced, and various splits begin to appear between male and female staff: "The men aren't around enough, aren't there when needed, don't act decisively enough." Something is very wrong within the staff organization, someone is at fault. Staff members suggest that the director failed to anticipate the current siege. Invidious comparisons are made suggesting that one of the other staff members could have handled the situation better. Mutual trust and support among staff members are found to be in short supply. Staff members spend less time chatting together, either about patient issues or just passing the time of day.

During these periods, the male staff seems impotent, while the female staff may be more concerned about being physically assaulted. Male staff must act decisively, preferably in a bellicose manner with stentorian roar, imposing draconian consequences on the troublemakers. Any clinician who finds him or herself confronting the boot marks on the wall with a leering, testing, provocative adolescent is not a free agent. The immediate situation is embedded, for both adolescent and staff member, in a larger situation which may embody a wide variety of the elements inherent in the adolescent's intrapsychic and familial developmental experience.

In one sense, there exists an exploratory probe on the part of the adolescent assessing the current power balance between father and son. While the probe itself may be seen as an acting out of a real question for the adolescent, it is expressed here in the form of provocation, a challenge. Furthermore, the adolescent's experience is likely to be dichotomous, that is, one person controls the other and has power while the other is weak, emasculated, shamed. A concept involving graduated shifts in the power relationship is unavailable either intellectually or as a guide to action.

With respect to time orientation, the "now" exists apart. It is not embedded in a context reflecting prior experience, nor does it carry with it future consequences. All the investment is in what happens in the now, and, as such, there is a tremendous pressure for a personalized type of closure. Either the other person, the adult, exercises a compelling power at that moment, or the adolescent "wins" and the adult is humiliated. Both outcomes may be desired at some level of consciousness. That is, there is a wish for father to reinstate his former reassuring quality of total power, thus also addressing the depression associated with a catastrophic deidealization.

The conflict around new power balances also serves as a medium in which concerns about management of impulse are met. To many of our adolescents, the concept of self-regulation of impulses is new and foreign and is not connected with much information about the self or the real world which assists in this struggle. As it feels toxic for the adolescent to be directed to examine his or her experiencing of the self during periods of impulsive pressure, so also can whole staffs resonate in a similar manner so that "action must be taken." At these times countervailing pressure from any staff member to "slow down" and consider the situation becomes easily equated with "giving in" to the adolescent and "encouraging" the adolescent to continue acting out. On an action-reflection continuum, the adolescents feel that self-respect lies in action; often their adult helpers share this perspective. Kernels of reality usually exist in most of the dialogues among the staff members and between staff and adolescent, even in the midst of such stress periods. What appears countertransferential are the elevated and personalized feelings; the imperative to act and eschew reflection; and the sense that action and reflection are incompatible, personal, and group processes that potentiate imperatives to act. The degree to which staff does act without reflection at these times serves to confirm the adolescent's restricted view of causation and available choice. In other words, the adolescent is presented with a learning situation similar to that with which he has grown up.

Conclusions

The special stresses in adolescent milieu treatment warrant supportive staff structures for containing and correcting countertransferential situations. Regular staff processing of work interactions seems essential, perhaps more during quiet intervals than during periods of stress. One approach found to be useful is the staff-process session in which staff members discuss the experience of working together that week. Periodically such meetings may be led by an outside person skilled in regulating confrontative group meetings.

A philosophy acknowledging the inevitability of countertransference may relieve some of the pressure felt by staff members to be more professional. An orientation which focuses on the interplay between specific developmental concerns and their impact on the adults present should sharpen staff awareness of critical issues in the milieu. Such sensitization may then be used diagnostically. Powerfully felt imperatives to act are often an indication of matters which need to be relocated in the adolescent rather than acted out by the adult.

NOTES

1. From the Adolescent and Family Treatment and Study Center, McLean Hospital, Belmont, Massachusetts.
2. M. Grob, personal communication, 1975.

REFERENCES

Benedek, T. 1959. Parenthood as a developmental phase. *Journal of the American Psychoanalytic Association* 7:389–417.

English, H. B., and English, A. C. 1958. *Dictionary of Psychological Terms*. New York: Norton.

Horney, K. 1945. *Our Inner Conflicts*. New York: Norton.

Redl, F. 1966. *When We Deal with Children*. New York: Free Press.

28   HOSPITAL TREATMENT FOR DISTURBED ADOLESCENTS: THE ROLE OF PARENT COUNSELING GROUPS

PAUL G. ROSSMAN AND JUDITH A. FREEDMAN

The clinical axiom that psychiatric treatment for disturbed adolescents requires parental support and involvement is widely accepted. Whether treatment is initiated on an outpatient or inpatient basis, the clinician's ability to engage both the adolescent and the family seems crucial (Davids, Ryan, and Salvatore 1968). Without significant parental involvement, the treatment of early and mid-stage adolescents, who manifest serious behavioral difficulties, is almost always compromised (Miller 1974; Sperling 1979; Stone 1979). The importance of positive parental involvement is particularly evident in hospital and residential treatment of disturbed adolescents. In these settings, failure to engage the family often results in a variety of disturbed behaviors expressed both by the adolescent and the parents—sometimes with an unfortunate outcome—in which the teenager is prematurely removed from treatment (Miller 1958).

Functions and Problems of Parent Groups

When children and adolescents present with disturbed behavior, the family treatment approach is an attempt, in part, to free the identified patient from the role of scapegoat (Zinner and Shapiro 1972). There is a rich literature detailing the collusion of family members to maintain symptoms of disturbed behavior in the identified patient so that family homeostasis is not disrupted (Stierlin 1975). Family treatment approaches require considerable parental involvement, beyond eliciting

391

cooperation and support for the adolescent's treatment, and conjoint family and marital interviews are frequent components of residential treatment programs (Masterson 1972; Orvin 1974; Shapiro and Kolb 1979). Many treatment facilities will not admit a disturbed adolescent without parental willingness to support, cooperate with, and participate in the treatment process.

This shift of treatment focus, away from the individual adolescent and toward examination of interaction between the teenager and the family, may prove psychologically painful for parents. In addition, parents of adolescents in residential or hospital treatment must cope with both the stress of the resultant separation and the burden of parenting a child now identified as severely disturbed. Common negative parental reactions include intensification of ambivalence about the treatment process, self-doubt and guilt about parenting abilities, and shame over perceived exposure of personal liabilities.

To cope with this perceived stress, many residential facilities offer group meetings for parents. Nevertheless, there is a limited literature regarding the purpose and function of these groups, treatment goals, techniques employed, and the impact of the counseling group on the overall treatment process (Adler 1968; Irwin and Lloyd-Still 1974; Robinson 1974). This chapter considers the background and development of a parent counseling group on an adolescent inpatient service, reviews objectives and goals for the meetings, considers recurrent themes in the group process, and discusses the role of parent meetings as a component in the hospital treatment program.

The Setting

The West Unit, a twenty-four-bed, semiclosed unit at a university teaching facility,[1] provides treatment for both adolescents and adults. The average length of stay for the teenagers is about six months. The treatment program emphasizes a psychodynamic understanding of the adolescent's behavioral and verbal communication, the impact of a milieu treatment program on patient behavior, and the importance of family participation in the treatment process. The program offers individual, group, and family therapy and attempts to meet the teenager's need for recreational, educational, and creative outlets.

The unit relies primarily on controls and limits derived from interpersonal relationships and, in particular, utilizes group restriction when one or more of the teenagers engages in serious disruptive behavior. With this approach, each adolescent is held responsible for his behavior to the adolescent group; the group itself is held responsible for the behavior of each teenager (Lewis, Gossett, King, and Carson 1973). Thus, when one or more of the patients engages in disruptive behavior—that is, runaways, drug usage, violence—the adolescent group is restricted until events leading to the disruptive action are reviewed and the teenagers consider their active or passive collusive roles in the outbreak of the disturbed behavior. During a group restriction, the teenagers are not allowed phone or visiting privileges, so that previously scheduled contact with parents may be interrupted.

The Evolution of the Group for Parents

As the treatment program developed in our setting, there was no provision for group counseling for parents. Areas of resistance in work with families soon emerged, initially observed in sessions alone with parents. Establishing collaborative treatment relationships with one or both parents proved a formidable task. The caseworker was often the object of parental criticism, blame, or anger as the parent(s) externalized feelings of badness or helplessness or displaced disappointment and annoyance away from the adolescent or spouse. Often, the parents became distressed after a stressful family meeting, when the teenager behaved disruptively in the hospital, or following a group restriction and interruption of scheduled visits.

With a number of families, an atmosphere of ongoing crisis arose in both family and marital sessions requiring frequent supplementary interviews or ongoing telephone contact with distressed parents. In the face of this explicit threat to the collaborative treatment relationship, the teenagers often behaved in disturbed ways—especially by running away—thereby testing parental resolve and commitment to the treatment program. A number of premature discharges then resulted as parents removed their children from the hospital against medical advice. During the course of a twelve-month period, approximately 15 percent of the adolescents admitted were prematurely discharged as relations between families and hospital staff simply broke down.

A review of these treatment failures revealed several recurrent themes: (1) the parents felt extremely ambivalent about the treatment program, apparently concerned that the hospital staff would view them as bad, rejecting, or responsible for the adolescent's disturbance; (2) despite attempts to establish a supportive and nonjudgmental setting in both marital and family interviews, some parents nevertheless felt isolated and alone—apparently convinced that problems encountered with their teenager reflected unique and shameful family circumstances; (3) some parents seemed continuously perplexed about the nature of the hospital treatment program, skeptical of the rationale, and experienced events in the treatment process as unpredictable; and (4) the teenager's disruptive behavior apparently expressed, in part, parental ambivalence toward hospital treatment and resultant loyalty dilemmas—reinforcing the adolescent's own ambivalence about engaging in therapeutic relationships.

Formation of the Parent Group

In the face of these treatment obstacles, a weekly meeting for parents was initiated. The meeting was scheduled for the early evening to avoid conflict with parental work schedules. Most parents attended on a regular basis, although sometimes one parent would participate more actively and regularly than the spouse. The meetings lasted approximately seventy-five to ninety minutes, coffee and snacks were provided, and the group atmosphere was deliberately structured as informal. As many parents felt estranged from the inpatient treatment program, meetings were led by a cotherapy team: a staff social worker and a nurse or mental health worker from the inpatient unit.

The Structure of the Group Meetings and Treatment Goals

A central treatment problem with a parent group in a hospital or residential setting is the absence of selection criteria for admission to the group. Thus parents with varying levels of emotional disturbance, motivation, and verbal or empathic ability are encouraged to participate. Disturbed families are known to request help for an adolescent as a means to obtain treatment for a disturbed parent or to secure help for a troubled marriage. Thus the presence of parents with significant personal problems is anticipated, and the goals and format of the group meeting accommodate to this reality. The parent counseling group is structured to provide a task-oriented, supportive educational setting focused on the shared experience of parenting a disturbed adolescent, now admitted to a hospital treatment program.

The group leaders seek to elicit parental reactions to the experience of separation within the family: feelings of loss or rejection, anticipated criticism for failure to solve family problems, or guilty relief over the departure of a disturbed adolescent. Parents are encouraged to verbalize anticipated feelings of demoralization, guilt, and ambivalence arising from both past and current problems in parenting a disturbed child. The group also provides a setting in which parents may ventilate feelings of anger, anxiety, and exposure arising from family therapy sessions. In addition, the leaders seek to elicit, accept, and absorb parental reactions of anger or disappointment about the treatment program—particularly when the teenager's progress is gradual or marked by regression.

An important treatment objective is to establish cohesiveness within the group, as parents share their common experiences, to alleviate feelings of isolation, guilt, or painful uniqueness. The leaders maintain an extremely active stance, prompting the expression of responses that increase cohesiveness within the group.

Many interventions by the leaders are similarly designed to minimize or reduce the level of anxiety in the group. Parents are not encouraged to express feelings related to personal past experience, and the expression of ambivalent feelings concerning the marital relationship is redirected toward conjoint marital sessions. The rationale for aspects of the hospital treatment program is frequently reviewed, particularly use of group restriction when the adolescents behave in disturbed ways. Sometimes didactic explanations are offered regarding common family problems or to illuminate the meaning of adolescent acting-out behaviors.

Finally, an important goal is to establish a setting in which each parent felt cared about, the object of interest and concern rather than criticism. In a framework of benevolent concern, parental reactions and behaviors are often relabeled to support the fragile self-esteem of the group members, that is, when a parent angrily overreacts either to the behavior of the teenager or to another group member, the presence of underlying parental understanding, concern, interest, and affection is assumed and stressed in the group meeting. As many parents appear secretly envious of the adolescents' intensive treatment experience, the leaders encourage the parents to view the group setting as "a special time for parents alone." Feeling cared about, the parents will hopefully nurture one another, and the more experienced group members are encouraged to orient and nurture newcomers to the parent meetings.

Recurrent Themes in the Group Process

SEPARATION ISSUES

An early theme in the group meetings is the expression of parental anxiety and anger as a result of separation from the hospitalized adolescent. During the initial phase of hospital treatment, the parents often express concern about how the teenager will get along on the unit, whether treatment will be successful, or what will happen if the teenager runs away. Sometimes rather thinly disguised reunion fantasies with the adolescent are encapsulated in these apparent worries and anxieties.

CASE EXAMPLE 1

The parents of a newly admitted teenager came to a group meeting, tense and irritable following several phone calls from the youngster, in which the latter complained about treatment in the hospital. Father voiced doubts about whether treatment would be helpful; mother worried about the teenager's capacity to cope in the hospital. The group leaders acknowledged the parental concern for the welfare of the teenager and their understandable worry about whether the teenager was "in good hands." The leaders then suggested that many parents missed their problem children, despite the previous anger and upset in the family, yet felt relieved with the troubled teenager's departure from the home. At that point, several experienced group members recalled missing their children during the early phase of hospital treatment; one mother remembered that she experienced the family as a "bit empty" after the teenager left. The group leaders then indicated that the adolescents probably felt some relief to be hospitalized, yet also missed their parents, and complaints about the hospital were one way of expressing their ambivalence.

Unresolved separation issues are a common problem for disturbed adolescents and their families. In the group meeting, parental feelings of anxiety, anger, grief, and guilt, as a result of the separation experience, are accepted and examined in a framework of benevolent concern for the child. The teenager's complaints are reinterpreted as requests for the parents to allow the teenager to engage in the hospital treatment program. At times, the discussion deliberately centers on the adolescent's problem with separation so that parental anxieties are not intensified through examination of their unresolved ties. A discussion of the teenager's problem in learning how to grow up and leave home—viewing the hospital separation as practice for a later separation—enables parents to come together, encouraged (by the leaders) to help the teenager cope with the separation problem.

GUILT AND BLAME

Parents typically enter the group with common feelings of guilt, self-blame, and demoralization. Sometimes the parents report dramatic overreactions to the teenager's behavior; the resultant sense of guilt is not necessarily discouraged in the group. In these instances, the leaders simply accept parental expressions of guilt and anxiety, while indicating that the meetings can help parents to learn new behaviors that will leave them feeling less helpless and unhappy.

More often, parental guilt feelings serve varying defensive functions. Parents often experience a guilt-laden relief with the departure of the disturbed adolescent from the home. Parental self-criticism could then be understood as a way of forestalling anticipated critical comments from the leaders or other group members. Guilt feelings sometimes conceal underlying anger toward the adolescent—the result of the latter's behavior—or reflect parental ambivalence in providing realistic behavioral limits. Frequently, the expression of guilt feelings seems related to separation problems in the family. Parental self-blame for the teenager's action encapsulated a belief that the parents could (or should) effectively control the teenager's behavior, as if the latter were still a latency-age youngster. Underlying parental feelings of separateness and helplessness could thereby be avoided. In these instances, the parents' ability to be helpful to one another, with more experienced group members empathizing with the newcomers' feeling of guilt and helplessness, seems particularly helpful.

CASE EXAMPLE 2

In one group, several parents expressed disapproval of their teenager's choice of friends. The parents suggested that other teenagers had led the adolescent astray, encouraging truancy and drug use. One parent spoke of the struggle with her spouse about this issue, each blaming the other for allowing the adolescent to associate with "bad friends." Another parent recalled frustrating debates with the teenager about the latter's right to choose friends. The leaders suggested that the parents could, of course, spend hours trying to unravel the roots of the teenager's problem. Perhaps the parents simply felt an angry helplessness when the teenager defiantly insisted on choosing "bad friends." An experienced group member then recalled her inability to express irritation in response to the teenager's behavior. This mother indicated, "The group meetings have helped me to accept the feelings without so much guilt, and in time I felt o.k. about expressing my anger in family sessions, when we discussed problems during the home visits."

As the counseling group enables the parents to feel less burdened with guilt, an underlying anger with the spouse or with the teenager may then emerge. The expression of anger between the spouses is, however, actively discouraged in the group—and redirected toward marital interviews (where indicated). The group leaders assume the position that the parents must relinquish (understandable) wishes to find someone or something to blame for previous family predicaments. The parents are directly encouraged to come together, agree to establish behavioral guidelines for the adolescent, and prepare for anticipated problems on home visits so that they both may help the teenager to learn to behave more responsibly. Parents are encouraged to view the adolescent's disruptive behavior as misguided and irresponsible, while appreciating that it does reflect the teenager's maladaptive attempt to establish autonomy and independence.

The leaders facilitate the expression of parental anger and disappointment (short of scapegoating) regarding the adolescent's "irresponsible behavior." The open expression of anger seems to augment the process of separation within the family. Buried resentment, expressed through parental complaints about the teenager's disturbed behavior, often conceals underlying unresolved ties as parents blame the adolescent for "making us feel bad."

EDUCATION

A recurrent theme in the meetings is the effort to strengthen the collaborative working relationship between the hospital staff and the parents. Offering a rationale for aspects of the hospital program is particularly helpful for newly admitted parent members. Explanations may be offered either by the group leader or by more experienced group members. There are frequent discussions regarding the objectives of individual, group, or family therapy and explanations regarding the hospital program. The issues requiring discussion will, of course, vary with the particular treatment program; in this setting, the parents often discuss the use of group restrictions.

CASE EXAMPLE 3

Following a group restriction with interruption in anticipated weekend passes, several parents complained about the restriction, which was the result of a suicide gesture by one of the teenagers. One parent particularly insisted that her daughter would never stand by while another teenager behaved self-destructively; to restrict this adolescent seemed unreasonable punishment and a disruption for the entire family. The leaders then reviewed the rationale for group restriction: disruptive behavior in the hospital usually reflected covert involvement of all members of the adolescent group. The leaders further indicated that the restriction was not intended as punishment but to lessen the isolation of the teenagers, to push them toward some degree of involvement with one another—surely a change the parents hoped the teenagers could effect prior to returning home. The parent still insisted that her daughter did not know of the suicide gesture. The leaders acknowledged that this was a possibility, indicating that errors were sometimes made. Unlike experienced detectives, both hospital staff and parents could not presume expertise in determining innocence or guilt. The leaders then inquired whether some of the parents recalled similar dilemmas with their children. At length, a father recalled a series of bitter quarrels between his daughter (now hospitalized) and her brothers. However, this parent's effort to decide who was really responsible for the struggle led only to frustration and further disagreement. This father now understood that the fights probably had to do both with his daughter's disturbance and with tension and upset in all family members. The leaders then agreed that the hospital staff sometimes unwittingly contributed to the outbreak of disturbed behavior—and this would be reviewed with the teenagers.

A second broad educational focus centers on the meaning of the teenager's behavior, especially those behaviors to which the parents react with helplessness, uncertainty, or anger. For example, when the teenagers run away, the parents' upset is often expressed as criticism of the hospital staff for apparent negligence. Alternatively, some parents shake their heads and express bewilderment about the "senseless runaways." Sometimes the group leaders simply discuss the meaning of the runaway behavior and the varied motivations for the action: the adolescent's need to avoid helplessness, to arouse concern and interest, to punish both parents and staff for perceived disappointment, and so on. This review also allows parents to obtain some distance and, as a result, to feel less helpless and reactively angry.

Underlying the educational approach regarding the hospital program and meaning of the teenager's behavior is an implicit effort to encourage group members to think over and reflect on parenting issues with disturbed adolescents as an alternative to more immediate emotional responses. For parents who have been embroiled in self-defeating struggles with their teenager, the leaders' flexibility and willingness to offer suitable explanations provide a more rational model for parent-adolescent interaction.

ENVY AND COMPETITIVENESS

Many members of the parent group have experienced varying degrees of emotional deprivation; thus there are times when guilt about hospitalizing a youngster reflects undisclosed envy for the adolescent's intense emotional experience in the hospital. The envy, and resultant competitiveness, is sometimes expressed through anxiety about the adolescent's attachment to the hospital staff or concern that the staff offers a more gratifying parental model to the teenager. The parents' resultant need to castigate and devalue the staff "for letting the kids run away" can be understood in this framework.

CASE EXAMPLE 4

One father stated his concern that "so many things are discussed by the staff and the teenagers in the hospital. When my kid comes home, he will have a real dependency on constant discussion." Another parent spoke of her teenager's recent home visit

PAUL G. ROSSMAN AND JUDITH A. FREEDMAN

when the adolescent suddenly became depressed and "could not wait to get back to the hospital." The first parent then said, "When I was young and had troubles, there weren't five or six people waiting around to speak with me."

In these instances, the treatment approach is to offer the parents a supportive, gratifying, and nonjudgmental group setting to lessen feelings of envy of the teenager. Increments in the parents' self-esteem, reflecting the supportive group process, enable members to feel less deficient and thus less competitive with hospital staff. The leaders encourage parents to view the meetings as a time for them alone—to feel a sense of specialness about belonging to the group.

CASE EXAMPLE 5

One parent mentioned that her son asked whether she liked the group and she replied affirmatively. Another parent recalled that their daughter asked about the parents' meeting; the teenager doubted that the parents would have much to say in the group and so would remain silent with one another. The parent replied that she often spoke in the meetings and that the conversations were enjoyable and useful. One of the leaders then said that it was important for parents to keep the content of the meetings confidential and not to review these matters with the adolescents. After all, parents were not encouraged to ask the teenagers about the content of their sessions. The parents responded with vigorous agreement, and one member added, "I just say to the kid, listen kid, you've got your sessions, and we've got ours."

COHESIVENESS AND HOPE

The parents frequently enter the group with feelings of defeat, anxiety about perceived criticism, and a sense of demoralization. These reactions, cemented through a history of family conflict and previous unsuccessful treatment efforts, pose powerful resistances when marital or family therapy sessions are initiated. Despite the common parental reactions, many members enter the group with a sense of profound isolation. The leaders deliberately structure sessions to encourage collaboration among parents, underlining shared reactions in coping with a disturbed adolescent and emphasizing similarities rather than differences among parents, to foster an atmosphere of peer support and cohesion. While many sessions focus on the parental experience of despair, frustration, or helplessness with the teenager, encouraging parents to feel some hopefulness was crucial.

CASE EXAMPLE 6

At the midpoint of one meeting, a father said that he wished to talk about the family therapy sessions. He then complained about the content of the sessions, particularly upset that the therapist had asked about the parents' family of origin. "What does this have to do with my son staying out all night or flunking out of school?" One of the leaders said this was, in fact, a common reaction and perhaps some of the other parents could respond. Two parents, both experienced group members, recalled initial reactions to the family meetings: a feeling of personal exposure and disbelief when the caseworker indicated that no one was to blame for the teenager's difficulty. One parent recalled a series of difficult casework sessions prior to her daughter's first home visit. "The social worker insisted that my husband and I had to agree about rules when Sue came home and what we would do if she misbehaved. The sessions were a real pain in the neck, but they did help us to lay down the law." The first parent continued to complain and seemed unconvinced, but several of the parents persisted, encouraging him to adopt a "wait and see" attitude. Significantly, the meeting lasted twenty minutes beyond the usual closing time, and many of the parents lingered together afterward, drinking coffee and chatting informally together.

The group leaders make efforts to structure a supportive network for the parents beyond the group sessions. Parents are routinely encouraged to speak to one another between meetings or to call one another when difficulties arise with the teenager. Some parents socialize together after the group sessions or following visits to the hospital. With the adolescent's discharge from the hospital, a stressful period for the family, departing parents are encouraged to return to the sessions and to remain in contact with group members whom they had previously befriended.

SELF-ESTEEM

Finally, a central element in the counseling group is an attempt to create a setting in which the parents experience increments in self-esteem. Encouraging peer support or alleviating guilt and self-criticism provides a useful beginning, but the parents need to experience gratifying interaction with the teenager to nourish feelings of competence and resultant hope. Although the teenager may continue to behave provocatively, feelings of competence emerge as the parents learn to react more adaptively. Parental reports of altered interaction with the teenager are encouraged to foster an atmosphere wherein parents learn from the success of other group members. In addition, the parents are encouraged to feel that they have good things to offer one another, instead of having to rely on experts alone for advice and directives.

CASE EXAMPLE 7

Mrs. T, a single parent, told the group about her daughter's recent pass home. On the second day of the pass, the adolescent insisted on seeing some old friends with whom she had engaged in many delinquent activities. Mrs. T refused and explained her position. Nevertheless, her daughter became belligerent and said she would go anyway. Mrs. T indicated that her daughter could leave, but she said she would call the police and have her picked up and returned to the hospital straightaway. The teenager became furious but did not leave the house and went to her room for several hours. The adolescent then requested to be returned to the hospital, but Mrs. T reminded her that the pass extended until evening and saw no reason to change the schedule. The mother suggested that they have dinner together, watch some television, and she would then take her back. The teenager moodily acquiesced but seemed in better spirits when she returned to the hospital at the end of the day.

More experienced group members are encouraged to be supportive and empathic with less experienced parents as frustrations, disappointments, and worries are shared. An informal subsystem of "senior parents" usually evolves within the group. The underlying group theme is that the senior parents often have good things to offer to the less experienced group members.

Conclusions

This report summarizes a two-year experience with a counseling group for parents in a hospital treatment program for disturbed adolescents. A measure of success for the parent group is that premature discharge from the hospital did not occur during the two-year interval. At the end of hospital treatment, almost all the parents interviewed expressed positive feelings for the group experience, agreed to continue with outpatient treatment, and felt more confident about providing their adolescent with realistic behavioral guidelines. While it may be argued that premature discharge ceased following the selection (at intake) of families motivated for treatment, the expressed degree of parental satisfaction suggests that the result reflects more than selection factors alone.

It is particularly important to determine whether the presence or absence of a parent group significantly affects treatment outcome for some of the patients (Gossett, Barnhart, Lewis, and Phillips 1977). Some correlations with successful treatment outcome might be anticipated. For example, a common characteristic of families with a behaviorally disturbed adolescent is a breakdown in the family hierarchical structure. The parents often feel helpless, frustrated, and reactively angry, while the teenager dominates family interactions through the expression of disruptive behavior (Madanes 1980). If the adolescent is to return home following hospital or residential treatment, it seems crucial to alter the structure of these families and to aid parents to exercise responsible executive leadership roles. Regardless of the particular family treatment approach, parent counseling groups seem especially helpful in providing isolated, demoralized parents with an opportunity to experience gradual increments in self-esteem within a supportive treatment setting. The group offers a network of helping relationships within which the parents unburden themselves, obtain guidance and advice from both other parents and the leaders, and in turn experience the gratification of having something to offer to others.

Data from this clinical report suggest that a parent counseling group provides an important therapeutic ingredient in the hospital or residential treatment of disturbed adolescents. The group appears to offer a useful treatment modality to increase parental feelings of self-esteem, competence, and hope; to aid parents to cope with ambivalent feelings about hospital treatment; and to strengthen collaborative relationships between parents and professional staff, one hopes expressed through parental support for both hospital treatment and subsequent aftercare. Further research in treatment outcome is required to validate these clinical observations.

NOTE

1. From the New Mexico Children's Psychiatric Center, Albuquerque, New Mexico.

REFERENCES

Alder, G. 1968. A parent therapy group. In E. Hartmann, ed. *Adolescents in a Mental Hospital*. New York: Grune & Stratton.

Davids, A.; Ryan, R.; and Salvatore, P. D. 1968. The effectiveness of residential treatment for psychotic and other disturbed children. *American Journal of Orthopsychiatry* 38:469–475.

Gossett, J. T.; Barnhart, D.; Lewis, J. M.; and Phillips, V. A. 1977. Follow-up of adolescents treated in a psychiatric hospital. *Archives of General Psychiatry* 34:1037–1042.

Irwin, S., and Lloyd-Stil, D. 1974. The use of groups to mobilize parental strengths during hospitalization of children. *Child Welfare* 8:305–312.

Lewis, J. M.; Gossett, J.; King, J. W.; and Carson, D. 1973. The development of a protreatment group process among hospitalized adolescents. *Adolescent Psychiatry* 2:351–362.

Madanes, C. 1980. Protection, paradox, and pretending. *Family Process* 9:73–86.

Masterson, J. 1972. *The Treatment of the Borderline Adolescent*. New York: Wiley.

Miller, D. 1958. Family interaction in the therapy of adolescent patients. *Psychiatry* 21:277–284.

Miller, D. 1974. *Adolescence: Psychology, Psychopathology, and Psychotherapy*. New York: Aronson.

Orvin, G. H. 1974. Intensive treatment of the adolescent and his family. *Archives of General Psychiatry* 31:801–807.

Robinson, L. H. 1974. Group work with parents of retarded adolescents. *American Journal of Psychotherapy* 28:297–409.

Shapiro, E., and Kolb, J. 1979. Engaging the family of the hospitalized adolescent. *Adolescent Psychiatry* 7:322–343.

Sperling, E. 1979. Parent counseling and therapy. *Basic Handbook of Child Psychiatry* 3:136–149.

Stierlin, H. 1975. Family theory: an introduction. In A. Burton, ed. *Operational Theories of Personalities*. New York: Brunner/Mazel.

Stone, L. 1979. Residential treatment. *Basic Handbook of Child Psychiatry* 3:236–263.

Zinner, J., and Shapiro, R. 1972. Projective identification as a mode of perception and behavior in families of adolescents. *International Journal of Psycho-Analysis* 53:523–529.

29 TREATMENT OF THE HOSPITALIZED ADOLESCENT: MANAGEMENT OF REGRESSION DURING DISCHARGE

JOYCE D. SHIELDS AND PETER T. CHORAS

Discharge planning and aftercare phases in the treatment of a hospitalized adolescent signal the beginning of separation from the inpatient milieu and staff. This stage of treatment can be compared to a departure and separation from home and family. Despite the adolescent's perception of the value of the hospitalization as positive or negative, impending discharge is felt as a stressful event. In the turmoil surrounding the discharge, anxiety and consequent regression can reflexively occur in the adolescent, the family, the staff, the therapist, and the community resource to which the adolescent is being referred. Recognition and interpretation of these regressions can stimulate continued mastery and ego development for all concerned, as well as enhance the possibility of a successful treatment outcome. If the regressions are misinterpreted, those involved are deprived of an opportunity to gain a useful perspective on their understanding of separation and its meaning in their lives.

The Regression of the Adolescent

Regression in a psychoanalytic sense refers to an earlier, more primitive form of mental activity (Freud 1933). It is motivated by a flight from pain and danger (Greenson 1972) and is set in motion by an instinctual frustration on a given level which impels the drives to seek outlets in a backward direction (Fenichel 1945).

The regression of an adolescent during the aftercare phase of treatment can be precipitated by the stress of impending discharge and separation from the surrogate inpatient family. With the more severely disturbed adolescent, the regression may be heralded by a return to psychotic functioning as seen upon admission or it may consist of old characterological defenses aimed at actively impeding the aftercare process (Jacobs and Slakter 1974).

CASE EXAMPLE 1

A sixteen-year-old schizophrenic girl was informed by her treatment team that she should begin discharge planning. Shortly thereafter she became withdrawn and developed delusions about decay in her body. As transfer to a halfway house became imminent, she began to have paranoid thoughts about the halfway house staff. She turned to marijuana to cover her intense affects and ultimately became progressively psychotic and deluded. Prior to discharge planning, she had achieved a more advanced level of functioning which became unstable in the face of the stress of separation. She had a strong alliance with her psychotherapist. In the milieu she had developed relationships in which she could tolerate both negative and positive affects. Graduation from an on-grounds school program was followed by a three-day-per-week cashiering job in a local restaurant. Her decompensation to an earlier level of functioning represented a regression and flight from the pain of separation from the inpatient milieu and staff.

In another form, regression serves to hide separation affects; the adolescent utilizes reaction formation and denial. The regression is characterized by a lack of genuine active participation in the aftercare process. The treatment team is confronted with an adolescent who agrees blandly to all the aftercare recommendations but denies any anxiety regarding discharge. Characteristically, the denial gives way to the stress of the transition and some action on the part of the adolescent sabotages the final implementation of the plan.

CASE EXAMPLE 2

A fifteen-year-old adolescent willingly reviewed her history in the first aftercare interview. She agreed to research residential schools without protest. A return home to live with her mother, who was often psychotic, was contraindicated. Her inpatient treatment had begun thirteen months earlier. Several months prior to discharge planning, she had emerged from a psychotic episode to become an active milieu leader and an excellent student in the on-grounds school program.

In a subsequent interview, she reported feeling agitated and depressed. She was resistant to exploring why this was so. She reluctantly admitted, however, that the source of the agitation was the fact that she lied to the inpatient staff about a recent overnight visit to a residential school. In fact, she had not gone to the school but had visited with her mother at home. Further discussion with her was punctuated by her concern that she was unable to separate from her mother, as we had suggested. In addition she feared that staff would be angry and disappointed with her and that her entire discharge would be jeopardized.

Active participation by the adolescent is important in all phases of the discharge process (Colvin 1978). The hospital staff function as a surrogate family, and separation from them is complex. Of great significance is the loss of support that must be sacrificed by the adolescent as discharged becomes imminent, with the coincident need to become more active on his own behalf. As in a normal separation from one's family, the adolescent must be active in several ways: (a) The individual must begin to give up entitlement and decrease the expectation for passively received support and gratification from the treaters. There will be a need to seek staff advice about aftercare plans and to say goodbye to people who have provided support, structure, and meaningful relationships. (b) The adolescent must begin to evaluate the outcome of the treatment and confront the illness with all its ramifications. Denial, distortion, projection, and acting out become less effective disguises as one is prevailed upon to develop a discharge plan. The adolescent must look realistically at his or her personal style of relating to people and evaluate what homework remains in that area. No longer can deficits be concealed by illusions maintained with peer patients in the treatment milieu. (c) The adolescent must be aware of personality strengths and decide how they can be integrated into an aftercare plan. The treatment is focused on long-standing character problems such as a chronic inability to relate to peers or to sustain a school program, rather than on the admission crisis. In short the adolescent must evaluate what has been learned in the hospital. What has been internalized from the milieu now becomes evident. Even if what has been internalized has been considerable, we will still normally see some regression (Freud 1958). The discharge phase provides an opportunity for the staff to assess realistically the outcome of the treatment thus far. We see precisely what we have succeeded in teaching the adolescent about his illness. It is a chance to evaluate whether an adolescent has learned that transition can be perceived as a separation, a natural phenomenon analogous to a departure from home instead of a death or loss in which people who have provided substitive relationships simply disappear (Mahler 1965). (*d*) Finally, the adolescent must address all of these issues within a finite period of time and develop a plan in light of this knowledge. If the adolescent chooses to avoid this process, a sense of ownership of the plan is missing and, generally, the plan then becomes inoperative.

The individual who can discuss transition as a process that cannot be stopped, but rather anticipated, examined, and understood, is more likely to have had a productive hospital course. Specifically, the adolescent has developed ego strengths with an ability to test reality and a capacity to tolerate anxiety. It is the process of examining and understanding the separation from the hospital, not the details of the plan, that constitute the real work of transition. It is clear that an adolescent who can discuss transition in this way has also confronted his illness and has developed ways of managing it, however difficult.

The majority of hospitalized adolescents avoid an active approach to discharge as well as deny their affects of sadness and helplessness. Most adolescents we have observed endeavor to sabotage their discharge. Acting-out behavior and somatic complaints mask the anxiety regarding separation. Drugs and alcohol help to relieve the tensions of transition. Unauthorized departures from the hospital by adolescents obstruct aftercare progress and are utilized during this period to deal with their feelings of helplessness.

CASE EXAMPLE 3

A sixteen-year-old adolescent willingly made several overnight visits to a residental school. While she was ambivalent about the school, she did relatively well with the initial visits. On the third overnight, she called the nursing staff and requested that a staff member come and get her. She reported that the other adolescents at the school were "too young for her," the staff was "unfriendly and a bunch of idiots," the other young women there were "uptight squares," and her room was "too small and crowded." She had decided that a job and a return home to live with her parent would be best. Anxiety about the transition was also expressed somatically; she sprained her ankle and had several allergic episodes following her first aftercare interview.

Approaches to Adolescent Regression

The goal of aftercare treatment is to encourage all participants to move away from a passive, reactive, obstructionist position toward an active collaborative role that enhances, for the adolescent, a sense of mastery and increased self-esteem. This process begins with a request that the adolescent take responsibility for making an appointment with the clinical specialist. Generally there is some obstruction in this initial step in which the adolescent declines or delays making the first appointment. At this point the clinical specialist recommends to the staff a discussion with the adolescent about possible sources of resistance: resistance to termination of staff relationships, reluctance to examine problem areas such as communication with parents and the development of peer relationships, and reticence to accept the limitations of finite time. Discussion of these issues at this phase puts the adolescent and staff into a dialogue. A collaborative process begins and the adolescent's struggles about the transition generally emerge.

In the next phase of the process, the adolescent is asked to outline an ideal aftercare plan irrespective of financial concerns, specific discharge date, and staff or family expectations. The adolescent is then encouraged to research all aftercare options by visiting various community resources. In subsequent meetings the clinical specialist and adolescent together review the adolescent's evaluation of the visits. Invariably the adolescent finds the halfway houses or residential school to be unsatisfactory. Discussion of these resistances leads to the uncovering of ambivalence and fear regarding discharge.

These approaches have as their goal the development of an active participation by the adolescent in the process. It is made clear to the adolescent that unless one designs one's own plan in one's own interest, the plan is likely to be unsuccessful. The adolescent hears, however, that one must take into consideration the concerns of the staff, therapist, and family. A plan must be developed that furthers the adolescent's own goals yet is compatible with the reasonable issues presented by the collaborators in the treatment process.

A study of the process of termination is initiated by the clinical

411

specialist with the adolescent. Previous termination and aftercare experiences are reviewed. The adolescent is encouraged to reflect about one's own patterns of dealing with separation and termination. If the individual interrupts the actual process with regressive mechanisms, the adolescent is encouraged to view the obstruction as a struggle designed to deal with separation stress. The regression is identified as old nonproductive behavior. The adolescent is encouraged to draw upon the new coping patterns learned in the milieu and psychotherapy to deal with the crisis of transition.

These particular approaches help the adolescent to see termination as a positive process which can be anticipated, examined, and understood as opposed to a crisis to be feared, denied, and avoided. This is most productive when the therapist also explores these issues in the individual treatment.

Regression of the Family

The family and the adolescent are buffered from each other by the hospital as long as the adolescent remains an inpatient and there is not stress, tension, or anxiety of constant interaction because of this support and distance (Stein and Test 1976). Family members function better with each other while the inpatient treatment lasts. Often when discharge planning starts, the family's high expectations, guilt, and needs for control again become focused.

The family's use of projective identification intensifies at the time of discharge. The way these families interact with the aftercare specialist and outpatient facility often resembles their interactions with the adolescent.

CASE EXAMPLE 4

A residential placement is recommended for an adolescent. The parents immediately contact the clinical specialist and suggest a residential school near the parents' home despite its clinical inappropriateness for their son. Mother suggests that since no immediate openings are available, she will contact a senator and bring political pressure to bear on the school. If that is not effective, they will donate a large sum of money to the residential school as they have heard that a second residence would be opened if finances were available. This would in effect make an opening available for their son. They neglect to elicit their son's opinion about his preferences or plans. Their controlling, manipulating style with the clinical specialist typifies a long-standing interactive pattern with their son.

Financial Stress

Insurance companies often cover inpatient psychiatric hospitalization but usually do not pay for psychiatric day-care treatment or halfway houses. Families therefore are expected to pay out of pocket or collaborate with social agencies for funding. Financial stress at time of discharge often causes families to react in a way typical of pre-hospitalized behavior and rarely seen by inpatient staffs.

The anxiety evoked by financial stress often precipitates resistance to logical aftercare planning. Primitive defenses such as denial, projection, and distortion often control the families' ability to plan.

CASE EXAMPLE 5

The mother of a recently diagnosed sixteen-year-old schizophrenic declined to allow her son's records to be forwarded to the local school system evaluation team, the Department of Public Welfare, or the State Office for Children. This family had good inpatient insurance coverage for a short period of time, but they had no outpatient insurance coverage and little family money. They needed the cooperation of the public sector to get the proper treatment for their son. The family was cooperative while their son was an inpatient, but at time of discharge, mother regressed and started to project and distort as she faced the financial stress of outpatient treatment. She suggested that the local school system was responsible for her son's illness because it did not diagnose his condition earlier. Ultimately her son returned home, which was mother's wish in the first place. She had used her lack of financial resources and noncooperation with the public sector to sabotage any separation.

Denial as a Defense at Time of Discharge

Families who have had good social work treatment and have matured in many ways while their adolescent was an inpatient often pre-

413

sent to the outpatient treater in a different way. Families often cannot understand why their adolescent does not leave inpatient care cured. The outpatient caretaker, when reviewing the adolescent's diagnosis and outpatient treatment program and its costs with the family, frequently finds the family surprised. They claim that they have never before been told that their offspring was seriously ill and that they did not realize the cost, time, or personal involvement needed for the outpatient treatment. (These were all issues taken up and explained by the inpatient treater many times before discharge.)

The family has temporarily regressed. There is evidence of the use of a shared defense, denial, which is precipitated by the anxiety of their own separation from the hospital caretakers. Immediate staff involvement is needed to stop destructive interaction with the adolescent's aftercare treatment.

These families are often very involved in the inpatient treatment of the adolescent, but initially push away outpatient involvement. They become anxious and try to control the outpatient treaters as they controlled their adolescent. They have not taken seriously their anxiety at losing the inpatient staff and facing their adolescent more intimately again. They question the outpatient treaters' competency (as they do their adolescent's abilities and their own). The real issue is who controls whom and what the treatment means. These interactions between outpatient caretakers and families often mimic the adolescent-family interactions.

It is essential to respond to the family's anxiety and control quickly. An important aspect of this anxiety is their feelings of incompetence and inadequacy, which are best approached by providing them with necessary data and support. Going over again with them what the inpatient staff recommended and trying to replace the loss of the inpatient staff with support are often helpful. Such cognitive support can include careful explanations of plans, explanations of diagnosis, prognosis treatment goals, and strategies.

This type of regression in the family is a natural process in the discharge planning. It should be understood as such and as much as possible be anticipated and processed prior to discharge to facilitate attachment and alliance with the outpatient treaters.

Termination with Inpatient Staff

There may be anxiety in the family over termination with the hospital staff itself which has provided support for the family during times of crisis. The termination experience may elicit a powerful exacerabation of dependent needs directed toward the hospital.

CASE EXAMPLE 6

The sister of a young adult patient in transition initially agrees to provide financial support for her sibling's aftercare plan. She relates that she will consult with her seven other brothers and sisters as well as her parents, who all live approximately 3,000 miles away from the hospital. She feels certain that they will agree to share equally the expenses of sister's continued treatment. Inpatient treatment has been completely covered by insurance for one-and-one-half years. As the discharge date approaches, sister becomes elusive and vague about closure on financing. She begins to distort conversations and statements made by the halfway house managers and hospital staff. As the aftercare specialist carefully confronts her behaviors, she begins to experience her own affects regarding her family. In fact, they will not agree to support the patient's continued treatment and their old patterns of irresponsibility and narcissism come again into her awareness. They are satisfied to allow her to remain the principal support of their sister both emotionally and financially. When she is able to articulate her angry feelings and recurrent disappointment in her family, she ultimately is able to mobilize to renew aftercare planning for her sister.

The regression in the family during this phase may relate to the family's need to use denial, projection, and distortion about its own difficulties and a reluctance to expose its vulnerabilities. The active participation of the family in the aftercare planning is essential. The task of designing an aftercare plan for an adolescent requires an assessment of resources available for emotional and financial support as well as defining future structure for family interactions. This planning cannot be successful without family involvement. The family's regression may relate to difficulties in interpersonal collaboration and trust. There may be ambivalence and guilt toward the patient which might lead to either a pattern of overprotectiveness or underinvolvement or both.

In the following example, we see a family that uses financial limitations, projective identification, denial, and projection as maneuvers to ward off their sense of inadequacy and anxiety over their son's illness. They are reacting to losing the hospital support and structure but cannot look at their dependency.

CASE EXAMPLE 7

The parents of an adolescent with a history of a previous admission to our facility were informed that their son is to begin aftercare planning and were asked to join this process. Their son was an A student through eleven years of school, a good athlete, and popular in a quiet way. He never had difficulty and they expected great things of him in college. Patient had a schizophrenic break in his senior year of high school before graduation. He was discharged, graduated from high school, and was rehospitalized a month before college admission.

The previous admission had uncovered a family pattern of initially collaborating in aftercare planning, but ultimately sabotaging any plan. We suspected that the family became anxious at the time of discharge out of their fears of losing the hospital structure. They could deny their son's illness as long as he was in the hospital. Their anger at him was assuaged by the support they got from the inpatient staff. They were compliant about discharge planning, never taking it seriously until almost the date of discharge. Then their sense of incompetency and inadequacy, which they denied, was projected.

On this admission (the second), their ambivalence about their son came to the fore almost immediately in the joint aftercare planning when we suggested a program (halfway house and day care) close to the hospital. They raised financial issues, although they could well afford the program. They wanted him to live at home and commute to the day-care program at the hospital. We tried and got a consensus around this plan. As a date for discharge was set, the family took the position that any program in which the patient had to be transported was out of the question. This implies his day care, his psychotherapy, and his transitional group will all terminate at the hospital.

The adolescent was initially angry, but the staff were surprised that their patient got better and ready to leave the hospital. The patient became slightly depressed and passively agreed to visit "an affordable day-care center" close to home. Another discharge date was set, but the parents became surprised and furious. They began to project their inadequacy onto the psychotherapist and blame him for the patient's continued illness. They increasingly demanded family meetings. The patient responded by abandoning plans to move to a day-care center. He indicated, however, that he was frightened and reluctant to leave the hospital. He eventually decided with mother to live at home, get a job, and prepare himself for college, dropping out of all treatment. This patient remained at home for two months getting into increasing social difficulties. Finally he had a hypomanic episode that embarrassed mother and led to another hospitalization.

As outlined in our example, during the period of aftercare planning, the family's style of dealing with stress and conflict became clearer than at any other time in the hospitalization. How families set goals, what their hidden agendas are, how a family negotiates difficult issues, and how its members relate to each other and the outside world under stress become clearer. The aftercare planning phase of hospitalization spotlights those areas of difficulty and may reveal patterns which previously remained concealed or unacknowledged.

The family's ability to regress at the time of discharge is striking. Outpatient treaters and discharge planners must be ready to handle regressive maneuvers and not overreact to the family's pathology. The regression should be seen as a resistance to handling the problems the adolescent poses as an outpatient and should be taken up as such. Often the regression is temporary and resolves itself as the family's anxiety is lowered.

Staff Regression

Until the aftercare phase of treatment begins, the staff as surrogate parents and the adolescent are united in a single task of understanding and developing ways of managing the adolescent's illness. A new task now emerges; the development of a discharge plan and a mutual sharing of affects about an imminent good-bye. There is often shared difficulty in accepting and working through the discharge. Feelings of sadness and helplessness about the separation can be expressed by staff in a regressive fashion by withdrawal from the adolescent. As the adolescent sabotages the discharge, a heightened sense of pessimism within staff can emerge. A feeling that the work done with the adolescent has been fruitless sometimes occurs. Consideration then is given to cancelling the discharge.

Several factors can emerge which may contribute to a regressive or nonproductive resolution of the separation.

1. *The staff's need to see a positive treatment outcome.* The resolution of an acute crisis or a psychotic process is tedious and draining for both staff and adolescent. In addition, the development of a positive alliance with an adolescent requires intensive study and constant reassessment. The discharge planning phase requires staff to shift the focus from the treatment of the acute illness to the management of long-standing character problems (Semrad, Grinspoon, and Feinberg 1973). It is difficult for staff to uncover still more problem areas which remain in the adolescent's character and which can emerge as the transition proceeds. Staff members often have unreasonable expectations about how the adolescent should be functioning at the time of discharge. In fact, at time of separation, it is normal to expect struggle and ambivalence. If this expectation is discussed, both staff and adolescent can develop some perspective about the separation (Mahler 1965). Adolescents, however, often attempt to conceal their loneliness and fears of failure as they do not wish to disappoint staff who have invested energy in their treatment. Both staff and the adolescent need to recognize that a positive treatment outcome entails authentic expression of both positive and negative affects which the stress of separation precipitates.

2. *The lack of treatment goals.* The extent to which specific treatment goals in the individual and milieu therapy have been achieved must be evaluated before discharge planning can proceed. Evidence of lack of treatment goals can emerge in several ways. Conferences can occur without a discussion of aftercare options. Aftercare appointments can be forgotten by the adolescent or staff.

3. *Faulty communication and collaboration among staff members.* Patient and staff regression are heightened when there is a lack of cohesion in the staff group. Power struggles, competitions, and alliances can emerge during the discharge phase of treatment because aftercare planning requires that the treatment team collaborate in the development of a single plan. As in the adolescent's biological family, the surrogate family must examine their tensions and conflicts and develop realistic resolutions of their differences.

4. *Lack of a focus on staff initiative, planning, and understanding of the discharge process.* A unit which rewards staff for their participation in the discharge process is likely to have less difficulty engaging in productive interactions and planning with an adolescent in transition.

Staff emerges from the turmoil of the transition with a sense of gratification and accomplishment. Units which devalue or simply avoid acknowledging staff activity in the discharge process find the discharge process frustrating and chaotic. The adolescent is then left alone to master the separation process.

5. *Reluctance of staff to process the termination with the adolescent.* The recognition and discussion of the end point of a relationship with an adolescent precipitate turmoil and anxiety within the staff group. The adolescent and staff often respond to the anxiety in a number of ways. There can be an extensive focus on the details of the aftercare plan or on the adolescent's sabotage maneuvers. Staff also anticipate the adolescent's failure in the aftercare plan much like normal parents dealing with separation from their children. They can become too preoccupied with the level of sophistication of the community resources. Withdrawal from the adolescent by staff also represents an unconscious attempt to avoid examination of the task at hand, that is, to process the separation.

6. *Approaches to assist staff in the aftercare process.* To help staff confront their own anxiety about separation, it is essential to encourage their involvement in the aftercare planning early. Asking for assessment of the adolescent's treatment progress and aftercare recommendations is essential. Staff participation in a dialogue with community resources and the family during discharge planning also promotes a continued sense of involvement and ownership of the plan. The termination phase should be highlighted as a process to be studied and examined thoroughly. As staff resistances become manifest, an opportunity is given to assess its meaning and develop approaches to its resolution. When discharge is imminent, more frequent staff talks are encouraged to summarize and bring closure to the relationship between the adolescent and staff.

Regression of the Therapist

The therapist of an adolescent is vulnerable to regression when the patient is close to discharge. When the patient is in the hospital, the alliance with the therapist is supported by the therapeutic milieu. When the adolescent is discharged, the therapist assumes the role of the primary treater with more responsibility and less support from others. Therefore, at the time of discharge, the therapist becomes increasingly concerned with how much of the treatment has been internalized and how much of "how well" the adolescent looks has been an illusion supported by the hall structure.

A positive patient-therapist relationship and alliance is an important ingredient in helping patient to leave the hospital and to remain community based (Singer and Grob 1975). The therapist probably has the most information on how well the adolescent is at the time of discharge. If the therapist is anxious about the discharge plan, something is probably wrong. It is imperative to include the therapist in the aftercare plan for the following reasons: you get vital information on the patient's ability to be discharged, and working with the therapist around a discharge plan should decrease any chance of the therapist regressing at the time of discharge and should increase the chances of the patient's acceptance of the plan.

Therapist-Family Regression

When the adolescent is out of the hospital, the therapist is more inclined to get involved with the patient's family either because of the increased stress the family puts on the adolescent or because the family begins to treat the therapist in the same manner as the adolescent. The easiest way a regressed family has of intruding on the therapy is through control of the therapist's fee. If a family is angry or anxious, payment is often delayed. The therapist's fee can be used, therefore, in an attempt to make him feel helpless and devalued.

Our approach is to view these experiences as part of a process of family regression. We try to take these issues up actively and objectively.

The Adolescent-Therapist Regression

At the time of the adolescent's discharge, communications issues with the hall, disagreements on treatment, trouble with the parents, and transference-countertransference issues often are magnified and played out as part of the scenario of discharge. According to Jacobs and Slakter (1974), therapists often get more interesting and regressive psychotherapy material from their patients at the time of discharge, which may argue against discharge. They often hear more problematic issues and become more concerned about the adolescent during this period. The therapist's anxiety and regression at the time of discharge are usually proportionate to the adolescent's denial of illness. The more projective identification in the adolescent, the more anxious the therapist. The more the adolescent denies his illness, the more the therapist feels discharge is premature and the hospital is needed as a base for therapy.

The therapist at this time often expresses the adolescent's anxiety, which the adolescent cannot directly feel or express for himself. This occurs in two ways: one response is to resist any discharge plan as premature, and a more covert resistance is expressed through nonverbal compliance and a submersion of the therapist's ambivalence. It is important to be active in aftercare if you are the therapist of a hospitalized adolescent.

Inpatient Hall and Halfway House Problems

Therapists tend to support utilization of aftercare structures when dealing with adolescent patients but may develop either patterns of overprotectiveness or selective inattention if their ambivalence goes unrecognized. In this type of regression, the therapist may initially overidentify with the adolescent and then project feelings about the hall treatment onto the patient.

CASE EXAMPLE 8

A therapist contacted the aftercare specialist to complain that a halfway house had threatened that her patient might be asked to leave. The patient had failed to maintain her contract in regard to acceptable parameters of behavior. The therapist complained that the hospital had never been interested in the treatment of this particular patient and had therefore selected a poor halfway house for the long-term management of the patient who has a history of chronic failure in community settings. The patient was required to keep her contract—the therapist's assumption that the halfway house was unsophisticated was erroneous.

CASE EXAMPLE 9

A nineteen-year-old borderline patient, who has been an inpatient for two years, heard from her clinical team that she was to begin to develop an aftercare plan as she was to be discharged in two to three months. Several weeks later an error in the calculation of the inpatient coverage was discovered and the patient had to leave the hospital within a week.

The family was unable to afford an aftercare plan and a catchment area treatment program was recommended. The therapist heard that the aftercare would be based in the local mental health center where adequate long-term programming was available on a sliding scale. The patient concurred with this plan, as it afforded her the opportunity to be financially independent of her parents. The therapist, however, insisted that individual therapy continue but refused to do so without a hospital connection. He also declined to refer the patient to the clinic for a new therapist and gave the patient a reduced therapy fee. The patient, due to the therapist's regression, was prohibited from involving herself in a long-term treatment system upon which she will eventually have to depend. A split again occurs in the treatment of the adolescent patient.

Again, early planning for aftercare offers an opportunity in an optimal setting for review and processing of treatment issues in the adolescent that are often hidden in a hospital setting.

Regression of the Community Resource

Similar to the stress individuals feel as new parents, the resource staff following an adolescent referral may experience tension and anxiety about the prospect of accepting a new member into the program. Uncertainty within the resource about its own internal equilibrium heightens the tension and anxiety. Resources undergoing change in staffing patterns, programs, or methods of collaboration are likely to hesitate to accept complex adolescent referrals. The combination of a stressed community resource and an adolescent who is ambivalent about being transferred to the resource enhances the likelihood of a premature rejection of the adolescent by the facility.

CASE EXAMPLE 10

A residential school with whom the clinical specialist had a strong liaison rejected in sequence three adolescent referrals. The manifest reason for the rejections was that the adolescents seemed incapable of resolving their ambivalence about a transition to the school. Upon further inquiry by the clinical specialist, it was discovered that the staff did not wish to discourage admissions openly. However, they were grieving the recent death of their

JOYCE D. SHIELDS AND PETER T. CHORAS

director. This diminished their available energies to encourage and process adequately these complex adolescent referrals.

Approaches to Community Resource Regression

Several approaches have proved to be productive. The development over time of a trusting, respectful liaison with community agencies provides a firm foundation for all referrals. When a referral is initiated, resource staff will then feel free to discuss the issues within their system that limit their capacity to respond to the referral. This avoids a reactive, nonproductive outcome with most referrals and creates an atmosphere of collaboration among agencies. Inclusion of community resource staff in the early phases of discharge planning for the adolescent averts a nonproductive, resistant response to referrals. By inviting agency staff to discharge planning conferences and seeking their suggestions regarding the implementation of the details of the plan, a sense of ownership of the adolescent's aftercare program is achieved by the community resource staff. Describing the adolescent's behavior accurately rather than deceptively at the time of referral increases the likelihood of a positive response from the resource. In particular, the resource staff will seek data about what treatment goals have been attained. Specific approaches in the milieu treatment and therapy which have been growth producing for the adolescent are also useful data to the resource staff. Areas in which no progress has been made should also be mentioned. This captures for the community resource staff a sense of what struggles are likely to emerge with the adolescent as he enters their program.

Conclusions

The discharge phase in the treatment of the hospitalized adolescent is seen as a stressful event which can precipitate regressive responses by all concerned. The adolescent unwillingly struggles to separate from his surrogate hospital family and often deploys old nonproductive defensive maneuvers to fend off the tensions of loss and grief. Family members deflect the focus from the turmoil of separation to a continuous struggle with hospital staff about community resources or money. The hospital staff, therapist, and community resource attempt to contend with their anxieties about the transition but often unwittingly collude in the regressive behavior of both the adolescent and his family. Recognition and examination of this shared phenomenon of regression

423

as a response to separation-individuation can enhance for all concerned a productive treatment outcome.

REFERENCES

Byer, S.; Cohen, S.; and Harshbarger, D. 1978. Impact of aftercare services on the recidivism of mental hospital patients. *Community Mental Health Journal* 14:26–34.
Colvin, S. M. 1978. The cycle of hospitalization from the patient's viewpoint. *Hospital and Community Psychiatry* 29:396–397.
Freud, A. 1958. Adolescence. *Psychoanalytic Study of the Child* 13:255–278.
Freud, S. 1933. *New Introductory Lectures on Psychoanalysis*. New York: Norton.
Fenichel, O. 1945. *The Psychoanalytic Theory of Neurosis*. New York: Norton.
Greenson, R. 1972. *The Technique and Practice of Psychoanalysis*. New York: International Universities Press.
Jacobs, B., and Slakter, E. 1974. Some considerations of aftercare problems of therapy, training and preceptions. *International Journal of Psychoanalytic Psychotherapy* 3:116–123.
Leavitt, M. 1975. The discharge crisis: the experience of psychiatric patients. *Nursing Research* 24(1):33–39.
Mahler, M. S. 1965. *On the Significance of the Normal Separation-Individuation Phase*. In M. Schur, ed. *Drives, Affects, Behavior*. New York: International Universities Press.
Semrad, E. V.; Grinspoon, L.; and Feinberg, S. 1973. Development of an ego profile scale. *Archives of General Psychiatry* 28:70–77.
Shapiro, E.; Shapiro, R.; Zinner, J.; and Berkowitz, D. 1977. The borderline ego and the working alliance: indications for individual and family treatment in adolescence. *International Journal of Psycho-Analysis* 58:77–87.
Singer, J. E., and Grob, M. 1975. Short-term versus long-term hospitalization in a private psychiatric facility: a follow-up study. *Hospital and Community Psychiatry* 26(1):745–748.
Stein, L. I., and Test, M. A. 1976. Training in community living: a follow-up look at a gold award program. *Hospital and Community Psychiatry* 27:193–194.
Zinner, J., and Shapiro, R. 1972. Projective identification as a mode of perception and behavior in families of adolescents. *International Journal of Psycho-Analysis* 53:523–530.

PART V

PSYCHOTHERAPEUTIC ISSUES IN ADOLESCENT PSYCHIATRY

EDITORS' INTRODUCTION

Clinical, genetic, and developmental considerations of adolescents are linked in a final common pathway centering on the psychotherapeutic approach to adolescent psychopathology. The chapters in this part range from a sequential treatment approach to anorexia nervosa to follow-up studies of treatment approaches to the developmental arrest associated with borderline and acting-out adolescents. Several chapters deal with the dilemmas confronting clinicians not only in making predictive judgments about the effects of separation in college-bound youth but also in utilizing closeness and peer relationships as a predictor of outcome subsequent to psychiatric hospitalization.

Regina C. Casper writes that anorexia nervosa is the product of an interplay of constitutional, biological, and psychological forces. Food has lost its primary function of nourishment and is usurped for the regulation of feelings and intrapsychic tension states. The lack of a stable self-concept and secure self-regard predisposes patients to use thinness in a misguided striving for individuation. Casper reviews past treatment approaches and presents a sequential treatment plan based on a conceptual model. She discusses engaging the patient as a collaborator, recognizing and correcting the physical and psychological sequelae of starvation, acknowledging adolescent developmental lag, weight gain and the psychosomatic aspects of anorexia, and family therapy. The treatment approach to anorexia nervosa consists of the initial evaluation, the recommendation session, treatment in the starvation phase, restoration of body weight and normalization of the body image, and the psychotherapeutic approach to the specific disorder. The most important treatment issue is seen as improvement of the patient's self-concept through expressing and integrating previously unacceptable wishes and feelings in renewed, meaningful, interpersonal relationships.

Paul G. Rossman considers psychotherapeutic issues with depressed, acting-out adolescents in the initial stages of outpatient therapy. The immediate goal is to engage the adolescent in a treatment relationship so that he might relinquish the gratification obtained through disruptive behavior and find socially acceptable means to express underlying feelings and impulses. Treatment strategies discussed include dealing with the original resistance, interfering with acting-out behavior, resolving negative transference, using acceptance and reassurance, establishing a flexible ego ideal, utilizing humor, and preserving the adolescent's sense of autonomy.

Eugene H. Kaplan deals with psychiatric decision making with the college-bound high school senior. He describes the dilemmas of disposition in making predictive judgments about the effect of separation from the family, the influence of the university setting on the present psychopathology and continuing development of the adolescent, and treatment planning and strategies. Recommendations that an adolescent remain at home or go away to college should be based on the therapist's informed grasp of the distinction and complex interaction between intrapsychic and external reality. Kaplan illustrates how the impending deadline of departure may motivate the adolescent to seek therapy, the therapeutic effect of removal from destructive family influences, and the efficacy of intermittent or episodic psychoanalysis.

William S. Logan, David Barnhart, and John T. Gossett study the quality of peer relationships as a predictor of outcome during psychiatric hospitalizations of a group of adolescents. The researchers focus on the development of a practical technique for measuring perceptions of closeness. Reporting the results of the adolescents' evaluation of their closeness to peers and staff, and staff rankings of their feelings of closeness to the adolescents, the authors find that certain measures appear to have predictive value for future functioning and recommend increased staff sensitivity to adolescent patients' perceptions of each other.

James F. Masterson, William V. Lulow, and Jacinta Lu Costello theorize that the borderline syndrome is a stable diagnostic entity owing to a failure in separation-individuation and is related to the mother's libidinal unavailability. The authors present the results of a follow-up study that demonstrates their therapeutic approach has a wide range of effectiveness—from relief of symptoms and improvement in functioning to profound and enduring change in intrapsychic structure. Masterson, Lulow, and Costello conclude that, in borderline adolescents, the inpatient hospital part of the long course of psychoanalytic psychotherapy was crucial to final recovery.

Stuart Rosenthal and Perihan A. Rosenthal describe a case of koro, a rare syndrome found historically among the south Chinese, in an adolescent. Koro is characterized by acute, severe anxiety associated with the conviction that his penis is shrinking and will eventually disappear, leading to death. The authors document the unrealistic interpretations leading to the fear of having a serious disease. The authors discuss the cultural aspects of this syndrome and its relationship to hypochondriasis.

REGINA C. CASPER

Inasmuch as extreme emaciation is the most conspicuous sign in
anorexia nervosa, treatment approaches in the past have concentrated
on ways to return the body weight to normal. The assumption of an
organic etiology for anorexia nervosa has led to a variety of pharmacological treatments according to the spirit of the time. The endocrine regimes of the 1940s and 1950s (Greenblatt, Barfield, and Clark
1951; Rahman, Richardson, and Ripley 1939) were eventually discarded when antipsychotic agents (Dally 1969) became available in the
1960s, and these were later superseded by newer psychotropic drugs
(Needleman and Waber 1976; Plantey 1977).

The rationale for using hormones was rooted in an understanding of
anorexia as an endocrine deficiency state, but etiological considerations were not decisive for the introduction of psychotropic drugs.
If at all effective, the accessory or side effects of the psychotropic
drugs were found more expedient in promoting weight gain than were
their antipsychotic, antidepressant, and antianxiety properties in re-
mitting the psychological disorder, although the notion lingers that
anorexia nervosa represents a special form of psychosis, depression, or
phobia (Cantwell, Sturzenberger, Burroughs, Salkin, and Green 1977;
Crisp 1980). None of these drugs or their combination has shown a
convincingly specific or effective treatment effect to justify their general application.

The psychologic treatment advocated by proponents of a purely
psychogenic origin for anorexia nervosa has suffered a similar fate. The
expectation that psychotherapy or psychoanalysis with the emaciated

patient would lead to a resolution of the psychologic problems, which then would bring about automatic weight gain and recovery, was not confirmed by actual experience (Selvini-Palazzoli 1978). In some cases prolonged psychotherapy with the enfeebled patient proved dangerous. Current treatment practice has tended to leave etiological considerations aside and instead has turned to an informed pragmatic-symptomatic approach with good short-term and as yet undefined long-term results. Several groups who specialize in anorexia nervosa have previously described their treatment programs (Crisp 1980; Dally, Gomez, and Isaacs 1979; Groen and Feldman-Toledano 1966; Halmi, Powers, and Cunningham 1975; Moldofsky and Garfinkel 1974; Rollins and Blackwell 1968; Russell 1977; Swann VanBuskirk 1977) but generally, with the exception of Minuchin, Baker, Rosman, Liebman, Milman, and Todd (1975), have refrained from basing treatment on a conceptual model of the illness.

In this chapter I will present a tentative conceptual model of anorexia nervosa which I believe can serve as a guideline for treatment. I intend to show how the circumstances and the dynamics of the illness suggest a sequential treatment approach and to describe some of the practical steps in setting up a treatment program.

My conceptualization of the psychological structure in anorexia nervosa was shaped by treating seriously ill anorectics and thus is more easily recognized in such patients. While I confine myself to discussing the treatment along psychological lines, I do not want to give the impression that there is no evidence for a biological and perhaps a constitutional contribution to this illness; quite the contrary. For example, the perceptual disturbance in the experience and integration of the body image, such as body-size overestimation and the failure to "feel" emaciated and bony, may be biologically rooted. Without this distortion, it would be virtually impossible for emaciated patients to assert that they feel "just right." Similarly, the unusual capacity to maintain a high energy level and remain active and fit when normal individuals would give in to their fatigue and rest not only forcefully promotes the illness but also raises questions about organicity. We know too little about the presumptive organic factors to make proper use of them in treatment. Some physiological correlates of anorexia nervosa, such as the psychological behavioral and physical concomitants of the starvation state, have been identified previously (Casper and Davis 1977; Keys, Brozek, Henschel, Mickelsen, and Taylor 1950; Rahman et al. 1939; Schiele and Brozek 1948) and are highly relevant for treatment.

Anorexia nervosa is an illness of adolescent girls, although it occurs rarely in boys (Falstein, Feinstein, and Judas 1956) typically during prepuberty or early puberty. Some of the psychological issues are remarkably similar, but there are certain differences, for instance, gender identity problems are common in boys but not in girls.

As in any other illness, the psychological disturbance in anorexia nervosa can range from mild to severe. The mild form, being not more than oscillations of an adolescent adjustment reaction, is usually easily treatable with sympathetic attention and vigorous refeeding, whereupon normal growth is resumed with the support of mature parents. Most moderately ill patients fit fairly well into the picture which I am going to describe. The severely afflicted group undergoes a profound pathological regression and often remains irreversibly entrapped in an anorectic life-style.

Anorexia Nervosa: A Misguided Striving for Individuality

Anorexia nervosa occupies a unique position among the psychiatric disorders by virtue of the fact that the patient herself has a stake in propagating the illness. The patient believes her thinness to be her own accomplishment, borne through prolonged deprivation, hunger, sacrifice, and against her parents' protests. For many months, sometimes years, all other activities, pleasures, and even moral values have become subjugated to the one goal. The patient comes to value the process of thinning as a way of life which makes her feel unique and gives her a sense of purpose that was absent before. Patients refuse to accept that scrawniness is not a value in itself, in the erroneous belief that they have attained a state of exquisite, enviable slenderness.

Initially, patients give the impression that they are merely dieting to lose some weight. It is less obvious that they have discovered that they can use dieting to relieve psychic pain in order to master feelings of abandonment, inadequacy, and being victimized—all implicating helplessness—produced sometimes by a trifle and sometimes by a traumatic event. The patient is convinced that her successful weight loss is a matter of willpower and is unaware of the biological facilitory factors. She mitigates her irrational fear of becoming "fat" or overweight upon eating even a negligible amount of food through guaranteeing further weight loss. When weight gain is required in treatment, this fear again seizes the patient with full force.

433

What are the elements that promote and support such exclusive attention to body shape? Anorexia nervosa typically sets in around puberty or during middle to late adolescence. That it occurs in a physically and physiologically immature organism suggests that the increased vulnerability of psychophysiological and psychoendocrine structures during the maturational flux has some role in the illness. Psychophysiological dysfunctions are perhaps also influential in the not infrequent persistence of a disorganized eating pattern after weight recovery and in bulimia, but their precise impact is not known. Experimental evidence shows that virtually all endocrine abnormalities return to normal with recovery. The present social climate which culturally sanctions the adolescent girl's attention to and sensitivity about the shape and form of her body is favorable to the development of anorexia nervosa. Confronted with an excess and an infinite variety of food rather than the scarcity of times gone by, the issue of how to resist its enticement has crossed almost every girl's mind at one time or another. Strictly speaking, there is rarely one clear-cut precipitating event which leads to the decision to restrict food intake. A variety of events or experiences in successive interaction sets off the dieting and then feeds an ever more entrenched anorectic defensive constellation which serves to counterbalance a progressively severe internal disorganization.

Initially, dieting might have started when friends talked about weight reduction or on the occasion of selecting swim suits for the summer. The selection of dieting can be reinforced by weight regulation problems in the family. Initial weight loss is not self-induced in every case. On occasion, an illness leads to true anorexia and weight loss, but usually a decision is made at some point to maintain a low weight. With the discovery that her venture can be successful and induce weight loss, which makes her feel more adequate and self-contained, the girl detects that the process can be used to dispel emotional distress. The satisfaction derived from losing weight is greater than one might expect because it serves the secondary purpose of improving the patient's self-concept. This along with relative physical well-being— unbeknownst to the patient, probably biologically determined— produces the desire for ever greater weight loss. What makes anorexia nervosa distinct is that the patient emotionally appropriates the process.

Once the fear of overeating sets in, anorexia nervosa has developed. All psychological forces are from then on directed vigorously toward the goal of slimming down and are worth any sacrifice in youngsters accustomed to sacrificing their own needs. When this happens, inner tumult by and large subsides. Patients feel in charge, more adequate, less dissatisfied with themselves, and, moreover, often engender admiring comments. Slimming down is a solution to their misery, albeit a temporary and pathological one. In a concrete way, they are in control and have differentiated themselves.

For the outside observer, it is obvious that this attempt at self-determination through self-starvation has interrupted normal adolescent growth, including sexual maturation. Physiologically starvation induces a regression of the cyclic secretion pattern of luteinizing hormones to prepubertal levels, resulting in a decline of estradiol to very low levels and a virtual disappearance of progesterone in plasma. When some emaciated patients express the wish for a Barbie-like bustline, they want to attract attention and admiration; its narcissistic motivation should not be interpreted as sexual. The psychological catastrophe imminent in every case of acute anorexia nervosa, in conjunction with reduction in the hormonal substrate during the starvation state, has reduced the conflicts about femininity and heterosexuality to insignificance. Not until the psychological and physiological issues are largely corrected do sexual issues regain import.

The Personality as Antecedent

When I propose that the lack of a stable self-concept and secure self-regard predisposes patients to use thinness in a misguided striving for individuation, I want to connect this to one of Bruch's (1980, 1981) most recent propositions that serious developmental deviations make patients ill-prepared for the responsibilities of adulthood. From her psychotherapeutic work Bruch (1981) identified certain personality features: "One can recognize a paralyzing sense of ineffectiveness which pervades all their thinking and actions. People suffering from eating disorders experience themselves as acting only in response to demands coming from others, and as not doing anything because they want to." These features are easily recognized in treatment. As part of the patient's character, they are interrelated and cannot be dissociated from the patient's hypercritical attitude toward herself being responsible for her poor self-esteem (Casper, Offer, and Ostrov 1981).

One of the repeatedly mentioned characteristics of patients obtained from parents' reports is their good, sometimes perfect, behavior as children. Patients remember themselves in a different light. Their goodness, they say, was a disguise; it was not happy contentment but, rather, shyness and refrainment from creating trouble through action. What was interpreted as "goodness" by their parents, was experienced by patients as compliance and yielding submission motivated by the wish to please their parents and to feel accepted in a world they thought was critical toward them. This wish to conform to the expectations of others and to mold themselves according to their demands into an illusionary ideal of perfection was supported by a conviction that this was the only way they would be acceptable to their parents and, in turn, to themselves. Such early tendency toward reaction rather than action (Bruch 1974) and the other-directedness and dependence on others for self-regulation would make an excessive use of denial of inner sensations, feelings, thoughts, and volition necessary and thereby inhibit self-expression and initiative. The inordinate use of denial as a defense mechanism, so plain during the illness, may have its origin in these dynamics. Giving into the demands of others in a yearning for approval and recognition eventually would lead to an increased sensitivity to other people and make patients excessively dependent on other's opinions.

We have shown in investigations of the self-image in anorexia nervosa (Casper et al. 1981) that young girls with acute anorexia nervosa as compared with their normal peers are highly critical of themselves and therefore assume that others view them with the same severe criticism. Even though most are well-proportioned, pretty children, anorectics usually have extended this critical view of themselves to their body and physical appearance and have thought about improving it. Most patients date the disparaging self-image back to early childhood. Such critical self-evaluation probably accounts for their premature seriousness and perhaps lies at the heart of the wish for approval. Without sharing their inner world, their pleasures and pains, and by placing the well-being of others before their own, most patients have lived since childhood in relative emotional isolation (Stonehill and Crisp 1977) and often carry a cynical, pessimistic attitude toward human relationships. Being overly dependent on others for approval, direction, and acceptance leads these girls to view themselves—as is uncovered in treatment—as incapable and deficient in preserving an emotional equilibrium on their own and thus different from other children. They feel slighted by and envious of children who are at ease with themselves and assertive in expressing their wishes and feelings. It can be argued that feelings and wishes become part of the self and eventually the personality through being acknowledged and expressed. Only through the observation and experience of self-expression in an emotional interaction can attitudes, feelings, and needs be modulated, integrated, and controlled. Without such practice, children are inhibited to the extent that they remain unaware of their feelings and wants, timid and expectant in their interpersonal encounters, and inexperienced in making decisions.

When in such children self-induced dieting meets with success and affords them an occasion to feel competent through their own action, they seize this opportunity to direct their weight with unusual determination in the erroneous belief that thereby they can win control over themselves and their lives.

A Tentative Conceptual Model of Anorexia Nervosa

Anorexia nervosa cannot be fully explained on a psychological basis. Most likely it is the product of an interplay, at varying stations, of constitutional, biological, and psychological forces. I will discuss only the psychologic components, as they are accessible to direct observation via behavioral manifestations, through the accounts of patients, as reactions, and in interaction in the course of psychotherapeutic work. Psychologically, the patient's withdrawal to her body and its size can be viewed as a defensive reparative maneuver following an experience of inner upheaval leading to helplessness and a sense of worthlessness which the patient cannot dispel with available resources. This emotional impasse coincides with the requirement for the adolescent to rely and depend less on her parents and more on herself. Self-reliance and self-determination are interpreted concretely by these patients as severance of any ties and emotional dependence on others. The more patients emotionally disengage from human relationships, the more they become obsessed with their newly discovered form of self-approval and reassurance through the knowledge of having gained control over their body size. If meaningful relationships existed before but have become dormant, the investment in thinness will not be as exclusive, and it is easier for the patient to recover.

In anorexia nervosa, body size and consequently food function are the omnipresent intermediaries in an abnormally self-sufficient state. The sense of competence and approving self-regard still does not originate within the patient but in a self-initiated separately experienced part of herself, her thin body. In this way, food and physiological processes become perversely employed to regulate emotions. The gradual emotional reinvestment in body size after relinquishing relationships can be conceptualized as a failed restoration of the self in an ideal thin body (Kohut 1977). Food has lost its primary function of nourishment and is usurped for the regulation of feelings and intrapsychic tension states, with a thin body bearing testimony to superb self-control. This regulation occurs through cognitive mediation: the dominant, overvalued idea which can take on different forms (Benedek 1936). In anorexia nervosa, the simplest essential thought, "I must not be fat," is associated with and becomes elaborated into others, "I must run" or "I must avoid eating." These thoughts assail and preempt the patient's mind at any moment of emotional tension. The idea, for example, "I must ensure thinness at all cost" and its ensuing actions can with profound starvation be experienced as compelling, but without the additive effect of malnutrition, these ideas generally lack the alien coercive character of the obsessional thought.

Since the psychologic goals—a sense of identity, personal initiative, emotional equilibrium, and confidence in relationships—are the true motivation and cannot be attained even with exquisite thinness, patients never feel satisfied with themselves and continue to lose. But as we have shown (Casper et al. 1981), even at the stage of acute, severe anorexia nervosa, they stay aware of their emotional dilemma, and this prepares the way for treatment.

Principles of Treatment

1. ENGAGING THE PATIENT AS A COLLABORATOR

Since girls with anorexia nervosa strongly believe in their own solution, denying its dangers and misperceptions, few apply for treatment on their own. For those who do, the prognosis is better than for those who are pressured into treatment. The wish for treatment reflects the lessening of denial, initially the most formidable obstacle, and the recognition of having arrived at an impasse. The patient's lifelong distrust and skepticism and her more recent fear of losing control and becoming overweight impede cooperation. Assuming that, like any other pathological defense, the anorectic process has alleviated but not removed the patient's emotional distress, we best establish the alliance by addressing the patient's emotional isolation, her unhappiness, and propose to help her resume a normal life.

438

Our approach should differ from the methods used by the parents, who generally assume weight gain is all that is necessary to restore their daughter's wellness. We need to let the patient know of our concern for her future emotional and physical well-being, for which we regard normal weight as a natural prerequisite. In most cases, the patient can muster a glimpse of trust; yet the initial alliance is brittle, and it must be attended to and bolstered in every contact with the patient. We tend to fail with patients in whom denial is strong, who by frightening, inducing guilt, or splitting their parents and closest relatives have enticed their families into forsaking control. The situation is equally challenging when the emotional isolation on all sides has reached a point of no return, when parents or spouses care only about relieving their anger and frustration through ridding themselves of the patient. Fortunately, this occurs seldom. In the first case, we can assist the parents to regain control over their children by exploring their fear, guilt, and sometimes their shame at having failed. For the second patient, little can be done except to force-feed or hyperaliment (Pertschuk, Foster, Burby, and Mullen 1981) the patient in hope for change. The weight gained under duress will generally be lost once outside pressure ceases, although not always to the same degree.

2. RECOGNIZING AND CORRECTING THE PHYSICAL AND PSYCHOLOGICAL SEQUELAE OF STARVATION

Psychotherapy is inefficacious as long as the physical and psychologic effects of acute malnutrition and chronic starvation persist. Physical discomfort and the physical symptoms of starvation are as much as is humanly possible denied by the patient, who is interested in appearing well. The indifference toward physical symptoms can mislead physicians, who are attuned to hearing complaints, into ignoring them. This can have serious consequences. For example, if medication is used, the patient might be overmedicated with ill effects or she might not be restricted from strenuous physical exercise which can lead to injury. As another example, the physician who treats the invariably present sleep difficulties with sleeping medication instead of ensuring a sufficient nutritional intake will appear ill-advised. Depending on the severity of the weight loss and the duration and type of food restriction, the symptoms vary: from low blood pressure, a slow pulse, constipation, amenorrhea (Sydenham 1946), cold intolerance, sleeplessness, nocturia, and occasionally true anorexia to marked leucopenia, petechiae due to thrombocytopenia, increase in liver enzymes, arrhythmia due to hypokalemia, and inability to walk up stairs or lift themselves out of bed as a result of muscle wasting (Casper and Davis 1977). The endocrine changes are numerous (Brown, Garfinkel, Jeuniewic, Moldofsky, and Stancer 1977).

Experiments in normal volunteers or reports from prison camps under conditions of chronic starvation have furnished data on psychologic and behavioral effects (Keys et al. 1950). The starvation state engenders deprivation symptoms (such as thinking and dreaming about food), obsessive behavior (such as reading and conversing about food, picking up crumbs, and dwelling over meals), along with a narrowing of unrelated interests, indecisiveness, and restless overactivity which can be recognized in every patient with anorexia nervosa (Casper and Davis 1977). For malnourished anorectics, therefore, even if they sincerely try, it takes effort to consider seriously issues other than food or weight, and hence starved patients are unable at first to participate in conventional psychotherapy. Equally important is the dampening effect of starvation on emotions. Patients do not only seem indifferent, but they are truly detached; their masklike face is the physiological expression of a diminished capacity to experience emotions. In starvation, anxiety and anger lack the richness and flavor of the normal experience. Patients report often a resurgence of intense emotions when substantial weight gain has occurred. A sharpening of the visual and acoustic sense also observed in starvation has been reported by Bruch (1979). Therefore, the primary and principal goal of treatment as long as starvation persists is to devise ways to induce weight gain in order to remove the patient from the danger to her life and from the state of malnutrition.

3. ACKNOWLEDGING THAT ANOREXIA NERVOSA IS AN ADOLESCENT DISORDER

The patient's serious-mindedness and skill at verbal expression sometimes makes the physician forget the patient's young age and immaturity. It must be realized that the patient has been deprived of normal psychological growth, in a rare case even physical growth, for the duration of the illness. With regard to their physical appearance, it is not uncommon for patients to look as if they had stopped growing at the onset on the disease, for instance, to appear as if they were eleven years instead of looking their actual age. The longer lasting the illness, the more crucial developmental time patients will have lost. If treatment is effective, adolescent behavior with its turmoil and challenge is bound to emerge and is to be encouraged, even if patients should be in their twenties.

4. WEIGHT GAIN AND ITS PSYCHOSOMATIC ASPECTS

With the progression of the anorectic process, with increasing withdrawal from relationships and outside interests, the patient's body, its shape and sensations, becomes the arena for the patient's wishes and disappointments. A close link becomes established between emotions and physical, especially gastrointestinal, sensations. For example, the sensation of hunger does not simply give rise to a desire to eat, but may evoke, in fasting patients, a victorious feeling of being in control. In patients given to binge eating, hunger may stimulate tension, panic, and a fear of loss of control (Casper, Eckert, Halmi, Goldberg, and Davis 1980). Either the consumption of small amounts of food or emotional distress, for example, an unsettling family session, can make a patient instantly "feel fat." The mere thought of weight gain will create a feeling of heaviness or enlargement, whereas not only the actual occurrence of weight loss but also the mere assumption of weight loss can induce a feeling of lightness, freedom, and control. It is important to identify the defensive function and meaning of these connections. For example, for the fasting patient, "feeling full" after a meal might be experienced as defeat and surrender.

If we assume that a desirably thin body is the patient's concrete realization of herself, it follows that the patient's strongest emotions are invested in it and bound up in its defense. Hence, as long as weight is maintained or lost, we support this defense, and therefore no true psychological changes can occur. Conversely, promoting weight gain is the backbone of treatment and the only effective way to challenge the anorectic defense which will expose feelings and conflicts for work in psychotherapy. In a weight-gain program, emotions and behavior oscillate with weight changes. We must realize that weight gain is stressful for the patient, and once the patient has attained a safe weight we ought to proceed cautiously to set up a program which allows and encourages the patient to regulate her own progression. Our aim is to revive interests that are unrelated to food. Therefore, when we link weight gain to privileges, such as family visits or access to contact with friends and activities, we intentionally put the patient in a conflictual situation in which she cannot avoid reconsidering non-weight-related goals.

Although it follows from my remarks that body size and emotions in

441

anorexia nervosa are so closely interconnected that a change in one will produce a change in the other, this does not warrant the conclusion that the treatment sequence does not matter. If we assume that issues related to body size constitute the defensive overlay, attention to weight, eating habits, and exercise will take a certain precedence throughout treatment over the attention to emotional problems. This does not mean exclusive attention to weight gain since intensive psychotherapy occurs simultaneously; rather, it means that we must not cease our efforts to monitor, supervise, and structure the eating habits, food preferences, weight changes, and the tendency to conceal food, and we must be aware that the presence and severity of these symptoms signal the degree of emotional distress.

5. FAMILY THERAPY IS MANDATORY

True individuation cannot take place without the parents' emotional consent. Minuchin et al. (1975), who emphasize the intrafamilial and social roots of the illness, have outlined reasons for family therapy. They postulate the existence of a family organization that encourages somatization, involvement of the child in parental conflict, and a physiological vulnerability. These authors have proposed three factors in the structure and functioning of families with psychosomatically ill children: (1) the child has a specific organic dysfunction; (2) the family has the following transactional characteristics: enmeshment, over-protectiveness, rigidity, and lack of conflict resolution; furthermore (3) the sick child plays an important role in the family's pattern of conflict avoidance, which reinforces her or his symptoms.

Inasmuch as the parents have had a formative role in their child's development, they are indispensable to their child's treatment and continued development. If therapy is conducted within the family structure, the malfunctioning interaction patterns can be identified, explored, and corrected. If the patient's treatment and resocialization must be accomplished without the family's assistance, a highly skilled and mature staff is required to assume that function on the treatment unit and determine dysfunctional patterns in the patient's transactions to staff and other patients. In this situation it is more than likely that if the patient returns to the family following discharge, she will be held to her old ways which were instrumental in the evolution of the illness to begin with. The degree of family pathology will determine the prognosis: the better adjusted the family, the better is the prognosis for the child. The capacity for change in the family is another predictive sign; without change the prognosis will be guarded.

Treatment for the Anorexia Nervosa Patient

The psychiatrist's training, theoretical orientation, and style will determine his or her particular treatment approach to the anorectic patient. Of importance is a clear explicit arrangement in which individual modifications are negotiated through an ongoing dialogue with the patient. Unlike any other psychiatric illness, the treatment of anorexia nervosa calls for a great deal of activity in the form of intervention and guidance on the part of the psychiatrist.

In the following section I will describe some of our procedures in setting up treatment that other therapists might find useful for their practice.

THE INITIAL EVALUATION

The overall purpose of the evaluation is to gather the information needed for an expert recommendation to the patient and her family. This is best done by first encouraging the parents and the patient to express their concerns and questions, as this will minimize their anxiety and inspire confidence. If they expect to be questioned and seem more comfortable with it, we will guide them with questions. The evaluation essentially initiates treatment. Indirectly it is an invitation to the patient to retreat from the impasse in her physical and psychological development.

By and large, allowing for individual variations, the evaluation takes the following form:

1. Discussion of the patient's resistance to treatment and how the patient was persuaded to come in. The interaction around these and the following issues generates ample data for an evaluation of the parental relationship, the parents' expectation from the interview, and the mother's and father's relationship to the child. Assessing the parental relationship is important because if the parents cannot come to a relatively unambiguous decision about their child's need for treatment, all kinds of difficulties will arise once the parents are forced to seek help.

2. Assessment of the patient's physical condition, symptoms, and severity of weight loss expressed in percentage of normal weight. This involves actual weight and height measurements, including the pa-

tient's reaction to it, the strength of the denial, what would be considered a desirable weight, and the wish to gain, lose more, or stay the same.

3. Review of the patient's past and developmental history, her personality, friendships, interests, and talents, including a comparison with siblings and a search for precipitating factors or adjustment problems as well as the duration and course of the illness.

4. A separate interview with the patient. More than in any other psychiatric illness, this interview is crucial as it seeks to establish the patient's willingness to move from her antagonistic position into a cautious trial to explore an alternate way of leading her life. Every precaution must be taken not to support the patient's expectation that she be persuaded, coerced, pushed, or cheated into giving up her thinness. Interest and curiosity in the patient as a person, queries regarding her motivation and thinking about slenderness and her interpretation of fat accumulation as lack of self-discipline will help relax the patient's vigilance. Having reviewed the past, we examine the future: hopes, plans, and ambitions. At this point the patient cannot evade the realization of her predicament. Were the weight loss to continue, its result would be death; sustained thinness will perpetuate the emotional isolation.

The enhanced self-esteem and notion of superiority by virtue of having excelled in the art of slimming down is transitory in acute anorexia nervosa. Feelings of dissatisfaction and inadequacy remain, for which patients expect to be viewed critically and found wanting. In psychotherapy we must not cease our effort to convey to the patient that her tenacious attachment to her size is but one expression of a painful discontent with herself which needs to be comprehended in its own right, rather than confirm the patient's defensive notion that outside forces want to change her by altering her body weight against her will.

Usually I encourage the patient to tell me how she thinks she will get out of the deadlock. Most often the patient believes that with some help she will manage to gain weight on her own. In reality, this rarely works. Only under the most fortunate circumstances will weight gain alone correct her psychological maladaptation. A few patients decide to do it, usually with their parents' open or tacit consent, and a few gain enough to go on with their lives. Years later parents may call to tell that after initial improvement the patient relapsed or that despite a gain of weight the patient struggles with binge eating and is deeply unhappy with herself.

444

For those who have lost more than 25 percent of their normal body weight, the chances for restoring weight on their own at home are slim, even with concomitant outpatient psychotherapy. Chances are slightly better with family therapy. I usually advise patients about the odds, but if they insist on an outpatient approach, I will go along with them (provided they are not in physical danger) and set up a weight goal, for example, to gain one pound a week for a limited time, such as four weeks. We agree beforehand that hospitalization will become necessary if the patient's approach fails. For those who think one pound weekly excessive, we calculate the time required to return to normal weight at this rate; for example, a thirty-pound weight gain would require thirty weeks, a calculation which usually abates the patient's protests. Should the patient directly choose hospitalization, which rarely happens, I provide the patient with a detailed description of the program and encourage her to ask questions. I explain that I do not consider recovery to be complete without return to normal weight and that subsequent continued treatment may be required. I always negotiate a discharge weight in the low normal range, before hospitalization. Even if the ultimate plan is a referral elsewhere, I first discuss my recommendation with the patient alone, adjusting the level of sophistication to her age.

THE JOINT SESSION AND RECOMMENDATION

Based on the outcome of the interview with the patient, and taking my previous evaluation of the family into consideration, the strategy with the family will vary. As a rule, I first solicit their ideas about how to deal with the situation. If they profess ignorance or helplessness, I endeavor to review their past attempts and why and how they failed. Then I ask the patient to share her thoughts with her parents. If she declines, I inform the parents in a general way of our discussion concerning treatment, inviting the patient to correct me. Most parents are infinitely relieved once they discover the slightest sign of cooperation on their child's part. Parents, who dislike the idea of hospitalization (which is often related to their feeling guilty about having failed as parents, aside from financial considerations), welcome the child's decision to try it on her own and are eager to discuss the details. Even in this situation, I assume that they have come to hear an expert opinion and review my recommendation with them.

Most commonly the parents admit that their patience and tolerance are exhausted and accept the recommendation for hospitalization, with the patient being opposed to it. What then ensues is a negotiating process during which it is important for the psychiatrist to help the patient accept hospitalization as a faster and more effective alternative than home treatment and at the same time to support the parents in their decision. Under these circumstances, the recommendation for regular family sessions is usually well received. Unless an emergency exists—for example, when the patient has refused fluids, which prevents much of the foregoing discussion, only to have it take place at some later date—I do not advise instant hospitalization but prefer to set a date at the beginning of the following week to have the patient and the parents prepare for hospitalization and reconsider the decision. Hospital admission on a Monday gives the staff a chance to acquaint themselves with and to monitor the patient closely for a full week. This is usually sufficient for stabilizing the patient nutritionally before the next weekend.

TREATMENT IN THE STARVATION PHASE

The separate description of the physical and psychological treatment does not imply that they are to be kept apart. In reality they cannot be separated. For example, any weight gain elicits a strong emotional response from the patient. As the patient's condition changes, one or the other will be in the foreground. With a severely malnourished, emaciated patient the greatest effort will go into nourishing the patient until she is physically stable. The program we devise is a generous variation of Sir William Gull's regime (1964):

> I would advise warm clothing, and some form of nourishing food every two hours, as milk, cream, soup, eggs, fish or chicken. I would conjoin a dessertspoonful of brandy every two or three hours. Whilst the present state of weakness continues, fatigue must be limited, and if the exhaustion increases beyond its present degree the patient should for a time be kept in a warm bed.

Restoration of normal body weight is achieved in a two-step approach. The first involves correction of the malnutrition and the acute starvation state until most physical signs of starvation including sleep difficulties, restlessness, and morbid dwelling on food have subsided. This means refeeding to a weight loss not exceeding 20 percent of normal weight. The second urges the patient to regain her normal age-appropriate weight.

446

The first phase is considered primarily medical treatment and the patient is advised of this. In this situation the patient's character structure, her compliance, and her wish to please and be persuaded comes to our aid. In almost every case, provided enough time is spent with the patient, patience and kind attention combined with firmness will entreat the patient to eat. If this fails, we have no choice but to ignore the patient's wishes and resort either to intravenous hyperalimentation or gastric tube feeding. This approach is important because enfeebled patients may have truly lost their appetite, which is generally restored after a few days on a balanced diet.

The first week of hospitalization is devoted primarily to convincing the patient to resume eating. At the same time, a thorough physical and psychological evaluation take place. The physical evaluation includes consultation with an internist; blood (including platelet count), urine, and electrolyte determinations; plasma cortisol, liver, and urinary function tests; thyroid status; an electrocardiogram; electroencephalogram; skull X-ray and chest X-ray. If the laboratory is equipped for radioimmunoassays of pituitary hormones, then growth hormone (GH), luteinizing hormone (LH), follicle stimulating hormone (FSH), thyrotropin (TSH), prolactin (PRL), and adrenocortico-stimulating hormone (ACTH) ought to be determined. The psychological evaluation involves a thorough history and family evaluation.

The diet is (Halmi and Larson 1977) a well-balanced liquid nutrient containing vitamins and trace metals (Meritene, Sustagen, or Ensure), offered in six divided meals. Its amount is determined by the age, height, and condition of the patient. For the first three days, approximately 1,450–1,800 calories per day, that is, 250–300 calories per meal (about one cup of liquid nutrient), provide sufficient calories and fluid. The patient is allowed between thirty or forty-five minutes to finish a meal. No extra fluids are permitted, and a strict record of fluid and caloric intake and output (urine collections) is kept. The patient is weighed every morning after voiding her bladder in the same gown or clothes, whereupon the weight is recorded and plotted on a weight chart. Every detail of the program is explained to the patient. If the patient refuses to drink the nutrient, the psychiatrist is called, the reasons for her refusal are explored, and she is told that her precarious physical condition does not allow her to starve herself. The expectation that she drink the prescribed amount is repeated. Justification for ignoring the patient's wishes is the existence of a potentially harmful starvation state. The patient's emotional reaction to eating is discussed and attended to carefully.

With firmness, warm praise, and constant supervision, most patients eat on their own by the third day (Galdston 1974). Sitting with the patient and using gentle persuasion requires, during this first week, hours of the nurses' and the psychiatrist's time, aside from talking with the patient for the purpose of conducting the psychological evaluation. It is important to realize that in order to gain weight, calories in excess of the normal amount have to be consumed; most outpatient treatment fails because too few calories are offered.

At the end of the first week, a short-term and a long-term treatment outline is developed and discussed with the patient and her family before being finalized. There are great advantages to a well-designed treatment program: it allows consistency and eases communication; it solicits the patient's cooperation and encourages planning into the future; it counteracts the patient's ubiquitous tendency to subterfuge and offers predictable sanctions, if it is violated.

The short-term treatment prospect is designed to ensure a stable physical condition, achieved when between 2,000 and 3,000 calories are consumed and the weight loss does not exceed 20 percent. Unless every management aspect is clearly spelled out, an undue amount of effort and staff time continues to be spent in anxious concern over the patient's physical well-being, which then prevents everyone from attending to the psychological problems.

Patients with the habit of regurgitating or vomiting after meals remain in the day area under direct supervision for an extra forty-five minutes subsequent to their meals. This way, most food stuff is absorbed. Between mealtimes a deliberate attempt is made to engage patients in discussions and activities unrelated to eating, counteracting the patients' tendency to have every activity revolve around food, weight, or eating.

RESTITUTION OF NORMAL AGE-APPROPRIATE BODY WEIGHT AND NORMALIZATION OF THE BODY IMAGE

Once the patient eats regular meals containing a minimum of 1,800–2,100 calories day and there is no danger that minor weight fluctuations will jeopardize her health, as a rule at a weight about 80 percent of her normal weight, the patient is given more leeway to gain according to her own pace. A comprehensive care plan reviewed in a weekly team meeting consists of a continuing detailed weight-gain regime, school for the younger patients, psychotherapy, and family treatment coordinated with the staff's corrective approach to the patient's interactions or lack of contact with other people on the treatment unit.

The weight-gain program imaginatively identifies the patient's preferences and uses them as incentives for slowly increasing weight goals. With several patients on the same ward, a uniform approach is easier since patients will jealously watch minor inequities among each other, but it is not necessarily better. What might be desired by one patient, for example, family visits, may be a deterrent to another. Initially, the prospect of discharge is a strong incentive, but it loses its glamour as the family and the patient change. Eventually, when discharge is imminent, the reactions are much more realistic, with apprehension overshadowing the return to normal and everyday life without the protection, structure, and reassurance of the hospital. For patients many activities can be wants, once they are disallowed: access to telephone calls, mail delivery, visits by family or friends, passes to leave the unit, trips, athletic activities, tennis, jogging, walks, and swimming. Any type of physical activity (exercises, dancing, walking, playing tennis) heightens the patient's sense of mastery and reduces her helplessness. Provided the patient is physically well, gaining weight, and not exhausting herself, physical activity is encouraged. The well-defined structure in the treatment program replaces and thus disfranchises the patient from her self-imposed rules and regulations; she struggles with the staff instead of only within herself, which makes her behavior accessible to observation, analysis, and corrective measures. Punitive measures or so-called negative reinforcements are not employed. This does not preclude that patients will interpret and experience withdrawal of privileges or restrictions as punitive or that any schedule for regular balanced meals is seen as coercive.

The distorted sense of bodily proportions, for instance, overestimation of body size, extends to meal size. The patient can, however, modify her assessment according to the caloric content of the food, for example, a drop of gravy counts more than a celery stick. Patients generally complain about the size of each meal, a reason for offering frequent small meals. Agras, Barlow, Chapin, Abel, and Leitenberg (1974) observed that meal size related positively to the amount consumed by the patient, and this led some centers to offer huge meals. Such a policy raises the danger of teaching patients to overeat. For this reason, we offer meals containing slightly above normal caloric requirements and encourage a slow but steady weight gain. Many patients, after initial protests, prefer to drink the liquid nutrient to avoid contact with food, especially those who are strongly obsessive or crave sweets. Before discharge, all patients are encouraged to master regular food at mealtime. At all times, the patient's eating habits ought to be closely followed. Unsupervised patients will determine when to eat and tend to postpone meals; they tend to skip breakfast, sometimes lunch, and end up eating the bulk of their meals at night, alone. We do not know whether a physiological unbalance contributes to the selection of this night eating pattern. Supervision of the eating pattern and weight-gain plan requires an indefatigable staff. Patients will resort to every imaginable maneuver, such as hiding, cheating, lying, manipulating, and denying in order to escape weight gain. Bathroom or kitchen privileges may need to be revoked to oversee the patients' where-abouts. When discovered, patients invariably are ashamed and guilty. This reaction provides a natural starting point for psychotherapy.

PSYCHOTHERAPY

Traditional psychotherapy has little impact on the patient with anorexia nervosa. Bruch (1979) has repeatedly emphasized that insight-oriented interpretations suggesting to patients how and what they feel not only do not suffice but may reinforce the notion of in-adequacy. The type of psychotherapy required in anorexia comes closest to that employed in adolescents. Psychotherapy with bulimic patients demands further modifications, in that more active assistance is needed to provide internal control and structure. This special form of treatment will not be considered here.

We have to ask ourselves what we want to achieve in psychotherapy and then contemplate how and whether we can achieve it. The pa-tient's self-concept and her relationships with people are the prime targets for psychotherapy; through her pathology the patient has found a temporary solution to both. Being exquisitely thin is a defense against being nobody. The thinness has removed patients to an exalted special position in which they reign over others in the belief that others admire and envy them. Mutual relations with her parents and others have been replaced by a self-sufficient relationship to an idealized thin body, a maneuver that has improved the patient's self-concept and self-image. When this structure is interfered with as it occurs in treatment, the patient is deprived of the approving or satisfying agency within herself, as well as of the goal and purpose she has set for herself in an attempt at self-determination. Psychological treatment in connection with weight gain will lead to the disintegration of this structure and expose a deficient and critical self-concept, despair, and sometimes suicidal thoughts. Fortunately, this process occurs over a period of time; it must be carefully monitored and assuaged by the treating psychiatrist. A certain understanding of these dynamics can be alluded to in psychotherapy. They ought not to be imparted to the patient through interpretations until the patient is in fact undergoing the painful experience of giving up what she considers her most valued possession, her thinness, and is close to the realization that the thin body and all activities ensuring it provided her with a sense of herself which was not there before the illness. The patient's sensitivity and anxiety about her body size is the most enduring sign of the illness; its fluctuation therefore can be used as a marker for treatment progress.

The description of the gradual movement and progression in psychotherapy exceeds the purpose of this chapter. Here I intended to convey some practical information about how to create certain conditions, such as a predictable, consistent, protective environment, that then would enable the patient with anorexia nervosa to participate fully in the psychological treatments offered.

Conclusions

As long as we cannot correct the presumptive and unidentified biological contributions to anorexia nervosa, treatment consists of nourishing the patient in a closely supervised program with the aim of restoring normal body weight and at the same time assisting the patient in individual psychotherapy and family therapy to acknowledge and correct the psychological deficits that have led to the pursuit of thinness. The most important treatment issue is improvement of the patient's self-concept through expressing and integrating previously unacceptable wishes and feelings in renewed, meaningful, interpersonal relationships with the psychiatrist and within and outside the family.

REFERENCES

Agras, W. S.; Barlow, D. H.; Chapin, H. N.; Abel, G. G.; and Leitenberg, H. 1974. Behavior modification of anorexia nervosa. *Archives of General Psychiatry* 30:279–286.

Benedek, T. 1936. Dominant ideas and their relation to morbid cravings. *International Journal of Psycho-Analysis* 17:1–17.

Brown, G. M.; Garfinkel, P. E.; Jeuniewic, N.; Moldofsky, H.; and Stancer, H. 1977. Endocrine profiles in anorexia nervosa. In R. A. Vigersky, ed. *Anorexia Nervosa*. New York: Raven.

Bruch, H. 1974. *Eating Disorders: Obesity, Anorexia Nervosa and the Person Within*. London: Routledge & Kegan Paul.

Bruch, H. 1979. Island in the river: the anorexic adolescent in treatment. *Adolescent Psychiatry* 7:26–40.

Bruch, H. 1980. Preconditions for the development of anorexia nervosa. *American Journal of Psychoanalysis* 40:169–172.

Bruch, H. 1981. Developmental considerations of anorexia nervosa and obesity. *Canadian Journal of Psychiatry* 26:212–216.

Cantwell, D. P.: Sturzenberger, S.; Burroughs, J.; Salkin, B.; and Green, J. K. 1977. Anorexia nervosa: an affective disorder? *Archives of General Psychiatry* 34:1087–1093.

Casper, R. C., and Davis, J. M. 1977. On the course of anorexia nervosa. *American Journal of Psychiatry* 134:174–178.

Casper, R. C.; Eckert, E. D.; Halmi, K. A.; Goldberg, S. C.; and Davis, J. M. 1980. Bulimia, its incidence and clinical importance in patients with anorexia nervosa. *Archives of General Psychiatry* 37:1030–1035.

Casper, R. C.; Offer, D.; and Ostrov, E. 1981. The self-image of adolescents with acute anorexia nervosa. *Journal of Pediatrics* 98:656–661.

Crisp, A. H. 1980. *Anorexia Nervosa: Let Me Be*. New York: Grune & Stratton.

Dally, P. 1969. *Anorexia Nervosa*. New York: Heineman.

Dally, P.; Gomez, J.; and Isaacs, A. J. 1979. *Anorexia Nervosa*. London: Heinemann.

Falstein, E. I.; Feinstein, S. C.; and Judas, I. 1956. Anorexia nervosa in the male child. *American Journal of Orthopsychiatry* 26:751–772.

Galdston, R. 1974. Mind over matter: observations of 50 patients hospitalized with anorexia nervosa. *Journal of the American Academy of Child Psychiatry* 13:246–263.

Greenblatt, R. B.; Barfield, W. E.; and Clark, S. L. 1951. The use of ACTH and cortisone in the treatment of anorexia nervosa. *Journal of the Medical Association of Georgia* 40:299–301.

Groen, Y. Y., and Feldman-Toledano, Z. 1966. Educative treatment of patients and parents in anorexia nervosa. *British Journal of Psychiatry* 12:671–681.

Gull, W. W. 1964. The address on medicine (1868). In R. Kaufman and M. Heiman, eds. *Evolution in Psychosomatic Concepts*. New York: International Universities Press.

Halmi, K. A., and Larson, L. 1977. Behavior therapy in anorexia nervosa. *Adolescent Psychiatry* 5:323–351.

Halmi, K. A.; Powers, P.; and Cunningham, S. 1975. Treatment of anorexia nervosa with behavior modification. *Archives of General Psychiatry* 32:93–96.

Keys, A.; Brozek, J.; Henschel, A.; Mickelsen, O.; and Taylor, H. L. 1950. *The Biology of Human Starvation*. Minneapolis: University of Minnesota Press.

Kohut, H. 1977. *The Restoration of the Self*. New York: International Universities Press.

Minuchin, S.; Baker, L.; Rosman, B. L.; Liebman, R.; Milman, L.; and Todd, T. C. 1975. A conceptual model of psychosomatic illness in children. *Archives of General Psychiatry* 32:1031–1035.

Moldofsky, H., and Garfinkel, P. E. 1974. Problems of treatment of anorexia nervosa. *Journal of the Canadian Psychiatric Association* 19:169–174.

Needleman, H. L., and Waber, D. 1976. Amitriptyline therapy in patients with anorexia nervosa. *Lancet* 2:580.

Pertschuk, M. Y.; Foster, J.; Burby, G.; and Mullen, Y. L. 1981. The treatment of anorexia nervosa with total parenteral nutrition. *Biological Psychiatry* 16:539–550.

Plantey, I. 1977. Pimozide in the treatment of anorexia nervosa. *Lancet* 1:1105.

Rahman, L.; Richardson, H. B.; and Ripley, H. S. 1939. Anorexia nervosa with psychiatric observation. *Psychosomatic Medicine* 1:335–365.

Rollins, N., and Blackwell, A. 1968. The treatment of anorexia nervosa in children and adolescents: stage I. *Journal of Child Psychology and Psychiatry* 9:81–91.

Russell, G. F. M. 1977. General management of anorexia nervosa and difficulties in assessing the efficacy of treatment. In R. A. Vigersky, ed. *Anorexia Nervosa*. New York: Raven.

Schiele, B. C., and Brozek, J. 1948. "Experimental neurosis" resulting from semistarvation in man. *Psychosomatic Medicine* 10:33–50.

Selvini-Palazzoli, M. 1978. *Self-Starvation*. New York: Aronson.

Stonehill, E., and Crisp, A. H. 1977. Psychoneurotic characteristics of patients with anorexia nervosa before and after treatment and at follow-up 4–7 years later. *Journal of Psychosomatic Research* 21:187–193.

Swann VanBuskirk, S. 1977. A two-phase perspective on the treatment of anorexia nervosa. *Psychological Bulletin* 84:529–538.

Sydenham, A. 1946. Amenorrhea at Stanley Camp, Hong Kong, during internment. *British Journal of Medicine* 159:249–256.

31 PSYCHOTHERAPEUTIC APPROACHES WITH DEPRESSED, ACTING-OUT ADOLESCENTS: INTERPRETIVE TACTICS AND THEIR RATIONALE

PAUL G. ROSSMAN

A consideration of treatment issues with depressed adolescents raises two broad concerns: the concept of depression in adolescence, related etiological factors, and the clinical manifestations of depression in this age group; and particular therapeutic tactics and approaches which appear to be helpful in establishing treatment relationships with this patient population. This chapter considers the initial treatment approach with depressed adolescents who are amenable to outpatient treatment, with an emphasis on issues arising in individual psychotherapy. A discussion of initial psychotherapeutic strategies requires a brief review of the concept of depression in adolescence and the means by which adolescents cope with depressive symptomatology.

The etiology of adolescent depression may reflect acute environmental stress such as family disruptions through death, divorce, or separation; developmental tasks which cannot be mastered; the broad psychosocial demands when entering or leaving high school to begin work or enter college; and chronic environmental stress such as ambivalent or ungratifying relationships with family members, or an inability to establish satisfying relationships with peers. The adolescent with a genetic vulnerability to depressive illness is at particular risk in the face of such vicissitudes (Cadoret and Tanna 1979; Conners, Himmelhock, Goyette, Ulrich, and Neil 1979; Thomas and Chess 1977; Welner, Welner, and Fishman 1979).

Depressive symptomatology in adolescents may be manifested by sadness, guilt, loss of interest in customary areas of pleasure or activity, or sleep and eating disturbances. Carlson and Cantwell (1979) suggest that depressive symptomatology in adolescents may reflect a primary depressive syndrome, or the symptoms may be linked with other psychiatric disorders (identity, adjustment, and behavioral disorders). Often, nonspecific depressive symptoms (low self-esteem, mood disturbance) may reflect the adolescent's unhappiness with specific life circumstances, called "situational dysphorias" by Gittelman-Klein (1977). When interviewed, the teenager may appear unhappy, anxious, emotionally needy, withdrawn, or preoccupied with bodily concerns. However, it is common for the teenager to cope with underlying feelings of unhappiness through mechanisms of denial, projection, and some form of acting out or passive-aggressive behavior.

The concept of "masked depression" or "depressive equivalents" has been utilized to describe the propensity of adolescents to employ action-oriented defenses—insisting that the surrounding environment is to blame for their predicaments (Malmquist 1971). Family members, school personnel, or the community itself will often be the object of the adolescent's provocative behavior. The use of acting-out or disruptive behaviors enables the adolescent to translate depressive thoughts or feelings into action equivalents. The emotional pain attendant upon conscious awareness of such thoughts and feelings is thereby blunted. The teenager thus seeks actively to preserve a sense of integrity, to avoid the experience of helplessness, and to ward off painful, persecutory feelings.

Unhappy adolescents often cope with psychic pain through the increased expression of anger and irritability, suicidal gestures, power struggles with family members, sabotage of school or vocational performance, delinquent behavior with the peer group, increased use of drugs, and running away (Feinstein 1973). Burdened with inner pain, the disturbed adolescent often feels helpless and may experience the underlying dysphoria as tormenting or persecutory (D. Miller, personal communication, 1979). Through disruptive, acting-out behavior the inner feelings of persecution are externalized, and the teenager often succeeds in eliciting persecutory or angry responses from the environment.

Unlike adults, adolescents are rarely self-referred for help, and may not—through the use of denial and projection—initially complain of typical depressive symptoms. Similarly, some vegetative signs of depression (frequently seen in adults) may not be apparent at first in teenagers who otherwise seem to be depressed. When interviewed, the adolescent may deny or attribute to others even those depressive symptoms which are rather nonspecific. Thus, when evaluating adolescents who initially present with irritable and provocative behavior as a major symptomatic disturbance, the clinician should consider the possibility of underlying depressive problems in the area of academic and social functioning, self-esteem, and mood regulation.

Engagement in Individual Psychotherapy

This chapter considers adolescents who present with depressive symptoms as an overt or underlying problem and who utilize acting-out behaviors to cope with depressive cognitions and affect. This outpatient psychotherapeutic approach is indicated for teenagers whose capacity to make relationships is not markedly impaired and who possess some ability to experience and tolerate ambivalent feelings toward significant people.

The immediate psychotherapeutic goal is to engage the adolescent in a treatment relationship which may contain the teenager's burdensome feelings of dysphoria, felt torment from others, and helplessness. The teenager needs to relinquish the gratification obtained through disruptive behavior and find socially acceptable means to express underlying feelings and impulses. Compensatory satisfactions must be offered, and the therapist needs to establish rapidly a treatment setting perceived as gratifying, supportive, and helpful. Unless the teenager perceives the treatment setting to be sufficiently gratifying, the expression of disruptive behaviors continues, the underlying depressive conflicts endure, and the viability of outpatient therapy is jeopardized.

Initial Treatment Strategies and Interpretive Tactics

It may be said that all adolescent patients initially distrust the therapist, but the particular form of distrust must be clarified early in treatment or therapy will not likely succeed. Without attention to the initial treatment issue of underlying suspiciousness and mistrust, many of the therapist's interventions will simply fall on deaf ears as the adolescent persistently believes that the therapist works for somebody else.

Particularly with early and mid-stage adolescents, who may come to interviews only because of parental insistence, the issue of who benefits from treatment must be addressed immediately. Often it is helpful to acknowledge that the adolescent is quite justified in feeling some type of distrust and suspiciousness toward the therapist. In fact, one can agree with the teenager that only a foolish person would immediately trust a stranger or feel comfortable about sitting down to talk. Supporting the teenager's "paranoia," so to speak, relabeling the attitude as understandable rather than unacceptable, lessens the patient's need to justify maintaining distance.

Additionally, it is important to interpret or clarify the adolescent's fantasy about treatment, as seen as the therapist comes to some understanding about this issue. For example, if an adolescent boy is referred because of aggressive behavior, he may believe that the purpose of the therapy is a type of psychological castration. The function of the therapist is to take his anger away so that the teenager becomes more acceptable to his family, community, or school.

Nevertheless, it is pointless to reassure the teenager that the therapist is interested in working with and for the patient; indeed, such comments may be heard as seductive. As an initial approach, it is helpful for the therapist to share his apparent dilemma with the teenager. The therapist may comment to the adolescent, "If I question your willingness to behave in such nasty ways, you may believe that the purpose of sessions is to make you more presentable for your family; if I say nothing, you might conclude that any change in your life is a hopeless matter." The therapist can then insist that the adolescent not make rash judgments about the trustworthiness of the therapist or the value of therapy. The teenager should be encouraged to accumulate personal observations regarding the treatment, consider whether such distrust is justified, and then make up his own mind, in his own way, and in his own time.

The Benefits of Treatment and the Issue of Disappointment

Depressed adolescents often have rather harsh consciences and are, resultantly, burdened by intolerable feelings of guilt. The teenager may project this guilty conscience onto others and then behave provocatively—to incur a punishment perceived as deserved. Alternatively, if the adolescent is allowed to externalize his conscience onto the therapist, the teenager will likely feel increasingly persecuted, criticized, and tormented—with the result that he flees treatment.

Because many of the therapist's initial comments or inquiries will be experienced as critical, it is helpful for the therapist to recognize the importance of explaining the purpose of sessions to the teenager from the outset of treatment. After all, the idea that the teenager comes in and talks to a stranger about matters which may be more or less personal is, from the adolescent's point of view, rather peculiar.

To foster motivation for treatment, the therapist needs to convey that the teenager can be helped to understand more about himself and about family members, to have more gratifying relationships with others, and to achieve a sense of self-respect and competence. As many unhappy adolescents feel a sense of underlying powerlessness, the therapist can forcibly convey that a principal benefit of treatment is that the teenager will come to feel more powerful, a power reflected both in increased self-understanding and in a genuine sense of choice about his life—rather than the compulsive power to simply hurt himself or injure others.

Psychotherapeutic treatment takes time, however, and most teenagers do not like to wait. Additionally, many depressed adolescents desperately wish to be freed of unpleasant feelings and often expect the therapist magically to alleviate symptoms. It is helpful, therefore, to predict that the adolescent will often feel disappointed during the interviews, feeling that the therapist does not act fast enough or could do more for the teenager if he were so inclined. The teenager's subsequent temptation to behave disruptively, in the face of disappointment with the therapist, should also be predicted. The intervention is designed both to provide structure to the treatment setting and to lessen the gratification obtained by the teenager through disruptive behavior, since many angry and oppositional adolescents are not interested in behaving in a predictable manner.

The Importance of Taking a Stand

Many depressed adolescents come from families in which one of the parents is chronically depressed. The adolescent may identify with the parental style—identifying with the aggressor, so to speak—as a way of obtaining love, fulfilling parental needs and expectations, or seeking revenge. In such families, the emotionally burdened parent(s) often behaves in a rather inconsistent manner, vacillating around important issues in the teenager's life. And yet, it is important for the teenager to have the experience of pushing against nonretaliatory interpersonal limits as an ingredient of the adolescent separation-individuation ex-

459

perience. As many depressed teenagers will present with some type of aggressive or self-destructive behavior, sooner or later the therapist will have to take a stand regarding the expression of these behaviors (Rachman 1975). Additionally, the therapist can probably assume that whenever the teenager talks about self-destructive action, it is because he wishes to be stopped.

As an initial tactic, the therapist may indicate that many symptoms of apparent failure are in fact "symptoms of success." For example, academic failure often succeeds in punishing or tormenting parents. The therapist can also convey his appreciation that much of this destructive behavior does offer the teenager a sense of power and is, so to speak, an effective way of getting important people over a barrel. However, the therapist must repeatedly question the teenager about the genuine gain accrued from this kind of power. If the therapist is indecisive, he runs the risk of simply recreating the family situation in treatment, unfortunately with the same outcome. As a way of fostering motivation for change, it may be helpful for the therapist to be openly contemptuous about the gain derived from destructive behavior, conveying that the teenager is really driven to do as he does rather than having the real power of reasonably free choice.

The therapist should offer a rationale for his opposition to acting-out behavior—that is, such behavior can only leave the teenager feeling worse about himself, and exploiting or tormenting others ultimately leaves the adolescent stuck in revenge. It is not crucial for the teenager to behave less destructively as soon as the therapist takes a stand; it is not up to the therapist to permit or actually control the patient's behavior, except where issues of danger to life arise. What is important is for the therapist to display conviction about what kind of behavior leads to self-respect and then deal with the adolescent's response to the therapist's stand.

Disturbed adolescents seem to view their interpersonal world through the filter of their own impulses and conflicts. When the therapist deliberately assumes a powerful and authoritative stance, approximating the adolescent's own omnipotence (expressed through disruptive behaviors), the therapist may then become more intelligible to the teenager. Thus, it is often helpful for the teenager to perceive the therapist as competent, powerful, and at times blunt and direct in the expression of convictions regarding impulsive or self-destructive behavior. If the therapist does not take a firm stand when the adolescent consistently behaves in self-destructive ways or blandly rationalizes his destructive behavior toward others, the adolescent will justifiably conclude that the therapist is a colluding partner in the acting out, or worse, that the therapist expects that the patient can do no better than to hurt himself or others.

The Importance of Negative Transference

Most depressed adolescents are not only sad but angry. The anger may be defensive or retaliatory. It may be related to accurate or fantasied perceptions of the parents or significant adults as distant and uncaring. To arrive at underlying problems of self-esteem, sadness, or helplessness, the therapist intervenes to interrupt the expression of acting-out behaviors and indicates a willingness to deal firmly with the expression of the adolescent's anger and bitterness.

The therapist should understand that the adolescent needs an experience in which anger, bitterness, or irritability provokes neither capitulation (the therapist avoids the expression of firm convictions regarding the consequences of the teenager's behavior) nor the experience of retaliation (the therapist becomes defensively angry because he cannot "control" the teenager's actions). Many disturbed adolescents appear to be on a desperate search for an adult perceived as sufficiently powerful to cope with the teenager's anger (Rossman and Knesper 1976). Therapy should provide a setting in which these intense feelings of ambivalence may be contained.

Within the treatment setting, the teenager's anger is often multiply determined. For example, when the therapist is perceived as omnipotent, the adolescent may angrily blame him for predicaments in the teenager's life. On other occasions, the anger arises as a reaction to the teenager's perception of the therapist as critical or else as a source of disappointment when magical expectations have not been fulfilled. The adolescent may then seek to rationalize and justify his anger, to cope with expected retaliation from the therapist. Many depressed adolescents harbor underlying fantasies that irritability and anger destroy relationships and drive others away. Anticipating such an outcome, the adolescent must frequently test the capacity of the treatment setting to endure when angry impulses or feelings are expressed.

As an initial approach, it is important to accept the adolescent's perception of the treatment setting as fragile while conveying that the teenager clearly wishes to be angry with the therapist. The therapist may then indicate that the adolescent has been angry for some time and that any adult who wishes to be helpful to the teenager would certainly have to deal with these feelings. The therapist may comment, "It is certainly not pleasant to be the object of your bitterness and anger. However, at least it is an honest feeling and emotion, and if nothing else, therapy offers a safe place to work on this problem." In this manner, the therapist conveys a sense of comfort with the expression of the adolescent's irritability during the sessions. Finally, the therapist should indicate that the goal of treatment is not necessarily to help the teenager to be less angry, but to aid the adolescent to find less destructive means of expressing these feelings and impulses.

Acceptance and Reassurance

Many disturbed adolescents feel unloved and unlovable and then fear that the therapist, as if he were omniscient, will perceive or discern their underlying feelings of unworthiness. If an adolescent is behaving in ways that are either destructive or self-destructive, the therapist needs to find a way to separate the behavior from the personality of the teenager. Therapeutic acceptance does not mean acceptance of the teenager as he is—often he may be behaving in ways that are distinctly unpleasant. Rather, the therapist must convey implicitly or explicitly a conviction that the patient himself is worthwhile.

As an initial interpretive approach, the therapist conveys that the teenager surely had understandable reasons which motivated past behavior, even if the consequences of the behavior were problematic or disastrous. The treatment issue then becomes whether these reasons are still good enough for the teenager to act upon them. This does not imply that the therapist should ask the teenager, "Why do you do as you do?" Often adolescents perceive such questions as tormenting. Nor does it imply telling the teenager why he behaves as he does. A more helpful approach is to offer comments like, "I can understand how you would behave, given your feeling that . . . ."

The therapist's task is to formulate the factors which motivate the patient's behavior, based upon assessment of stress areas in the teenager's life. This treatment approach implies a search for the understandable reasons which underlie apparently incongruous or irrational behaviors, with a corollary focus on wishes or impulses felt as unacceptable. In particular, with disturbed adolescents, this maxim suggests that the therapist always accepts the teenager's impulses as sensible and logical given the way the teenager looks at the world. Thus, impulses are never bad in themselves; it is only the resultant behavior that may have serious consequences. In effect, the therapist firmly states that he would like to help the teenager to misbehave in ways that will hurt the teenager less and, it is hoped, hurt others less. As indicated, the adolescent will often externalize his punitive conscience onto the therapist, and the latter's initial interpretive tactics should reflect a deliberate effort to avoid this (superego) position.

As the therapist seeks to understand the teenager, he has to get across a feeling of excitement and interest in establishing a treatment relationship. This is a crucial ingredient in the psychotherapy of depressed adolescents. The teenager will need to feel that to be taken seriously by the therapist is at least as exciting or rewarding as the gratification of acting-out behaviors and preferable to the safety of remaining isolated and distrustful toward adults. After all, the basic gratification of psychotherapy is that the teenager feels valued, understood, and taken seriously.

The therapist cannot offer reassurances that the patient is alright or basically decent. The teenager does not feel at all this way, and such empty support basically conveys the therapist's reluctance to learn how bad the teenager really feels. The basic reassurance which can be offered is that the teenager does not do things for stupid or dumb reasons, but only for reasons which make excellent sense to the adolescent. Thus, whenever the teenager says he does things because of stupidity or dumbness, the therapist must immediately challenge and confront, insisting that "smart adolescents do not do things for dumb reasons." Similarly, when the adolescent does behave in ways that are indeed foolish, the therapist can then ask, "How come a smart person like you does such dumb things?" Thus, it is possible to confront the teenager about the implications of his behavior without tearing down his fragile sense of self-esteem.

The Therapist as an Ego Ideal

Much of the treatment with depressed adolescents, particularly early adolescents, may not primarily utilize verbal communication, conscious understanding, or insight. Often a crucial therapeutic ingredient is the identification a patient makes with the therapist or aspects of the therapist's personality, style, and way of handling problems. Because many depressed adolescents enter treatment burdened with feelings that they must live up to unattainable standards in order to feel lovable and worthwhile, it is helpful for the therapist to offer a model of flexibility and a tolerance for mistakes—with emphasis on what is positive and valuable in the teenager rather than what is missing or needs to be accomplished. The therapist should not retreat from expressing, at an appropriate time, personal values and standards in regard to relationships with others, the importance of self-respect, and the need for reasonable achievement in academic work. Such communications must always be coupled with a therapeutic stance that the adolescent will take away from treatment only what really makes sense to him.

These identifications with therapy take place only when the adolescent perceives the treatment relationship as reasonably gratifying and helpful—the importance of being taken seriously. Additionally, depressed teenagers will often use the treatment relationship to gratify their hunger for interpersonal relationships. However, as a way of coping with underlying feelings of hopelessness, depressed adolescents often view themselves as powerful and omnipotent, and, early in treatment, such feelings are frequently projected onto the therapist.

Thus, depressed adolescents may establish narcissistic transference relationships with the therapist (Kohut 1968). The adolescent then perceives the therapist either as an extension of himself or else as a powerful parental figure whose interest somehow lends meaning to the teenager's life. The therapist should feel comfortable in accepting and tolerating this type of relationship, particularly where the gratification of the treatment relationship is helpful in reducing the sense of isolation and estrangement that many depressed adolescents experience. However, the therapist must remember that the teenager will probably experience intense disappointment as therapy progresses, especially when the adolescent realizes that he cannot omnipotently control the response of the therapist. The treatment focus will then shift to the adolescent's resultant feelings of helplessness and reactive anger.

Humor

As noted, a crucial therapeutic stance is for the therapist to convey that the adolescent's feelings, motives, and perceptions are taken seriously in sessions. This stance does not imply, however, that the therapist should interact with the teenager in a ponderous or heavy-handed manner. Particularly with depressed adolescents, it is important to help the teenager gain some distance from grimly perceived problems and conflicts with others—particularly as a way of fostering the teenager's interest in self-observation.

Early in treatment, the therapist will need to challenge some of the adolescent's basic assumptions, that is, parents or siblings are to blame for life predicaments, running away solves problems, the future remains eternally bleak, and so forth. Use of humor or gentle sarcasm may foster a perception of the therapist as playfully omnipotent or provocative. As noted, a deliberate "mirroring" of the adolescent's omnipotence often allows the therapist to become more intelligible to the patient. The therapist's willingness to interact playfully and creatively with the adolescent implicitly encourages the teenager to do likewise.

For example, many depressed adolescent girls will complain about their mothers, frequently criticizing their parental shortcomings. However, this vigorous criticism may conceal underlying feelings of loyalty to the family. The therapist needs to acknowledge the adolescent's feelings and perceptions while not siding with the teenager against the parent. While there may be a reality basis for some of the complaints, if the therapist simply listens to the verbal diatribe, the teenager may assume that the therapist views the mother as bad and useless. The teenager may then abandon treatment—to preserve the hidden loyalty tie.

As an initial strategy, the therapist may playfully challenge the adolescent's perception and comment in a somewhat offhanded manner, "From what you have told me, it is obvious that your mother is a most foolish person; of course it would be impossible for any teenager to live with her." And again, in a playful manner, "I suppose that the only problem is whether her foolish brain genes have been transmitted to you and your sibs."

The use of playfulness as an initial treatment approach may provide a nonthreatening challenge to the adolescent's beliefs and implicitly conveys the therapist's interest and concern for the burdened teenager. Humorous support may also allow the adolescent to bear feelings and perceptions previously experienced as unbearable.

The Issue of Autonomy

An initial treatment issue for depressed adolescents is the fear of being molded or controlled by adults. It is important that the therapist recognize that many depressed teenagers need the experience of angrily saying no as a way of preserving a fragile sense of personal autonomy. Sometimes the adolescent may agree with what the therapist has said or with the position the therapist has taken, but nevertheless needs to disagree angrily until the anxiety about being controlled by others has lessened.

The fear of external control is part and parcel of the adolescent's disturbance, as he experiences himself as incompetent or unlovable while hungering for dependency or caretaking relationships with powerful adults. Adolescents who are not overwhelmed with their depression may, of course, vigorously deny this unconscious wish and fear and loudly proclaim their independence. The allergy to perceived external control is proportional to the adolescent's anxiety about his capacity to manage his life successfully.

Nevertheless, the therapist has to establish an authoritative (as opposed to authoritarian) position in the session—otherwise therapy may have no direction. The adolescent then justifiably wonders why he comes to see someone who has no convictions about what therapy is or should be about. It is sometimes helpful to make a distinction between the adolescent, who is in charge of his own life and will always know more about himself than the therapist will ever learn, and the therapist, who knows more about therapy and what is needed in the treatment for the teenager to benefit.

Thus, the therapist should never make comments that the teenager can only accept with a loss of face. Sometimes it is useful to make general comments like, "Many teenagers in your position would behave or feel . . . " as a way of leaving space for the teenager to decide whether the comment should apply to him (Miller 1974). Similarly, it is helpful if the therapist makes direct comments while indicating that he is simply communicating personal opinions and encouraging the teenager to think matters over and decide whether the comments make sense to him.

A final interpretive approach. To support the adolescent's fragile sense of autonomy, the therapist must systematically intervene when the teenager seeks to blame others for his own predicaments, especially when such blame is placed upon the parents. As long as the therapist implicitly agrees with the teenager that "other people make me do as I do, " he cannot also be supportive of the teenager's sense of autonomy and capacity to choose among behavioral options. Although it may be true that parents cause disturbance in their children, the responsibility for the form of the disturbance must rest with the teenager himself.

466

Conclusions

Many treatment issues in individual psychotherapy with depressed teenagers focus on the therapist's initial interpretive approaches. The aim is to offer the adolescent a gratifying but unexpected encounter with a significant adult. This treatment approach recognizes the teenager's need to perceive the therapist as competent, powerful, interested, interesting, and concerned—so that the expression of disruptive behaviors may be contained.

The self-esteem of the depressed adolescent is built up, not through simple reassurance, but through the therapist's conviction that there is a wisdom behind the adolescent's behavior, motivated by good reasons—even where the therapist directly opposes the expression of the adolescent's symptomatic actions. In addition, the therapist must be sensitive to aspects of adolescent growth process: the teenager's need to make socially acceptable identifications with extrafamilial adults who freely express their convictions, take the teenager seriously, tolerate the adolescent's anger and bitterness, and yet remain sensitive to the teenager's need for autonomy and self-assertion. It may be argued that the successful ingredients of psychotherapy with depressed adolescents center not so much on the content of the treatment process as on the degree of perceived gratification in the therapist-patient interaction, and the type of adult model which the therapist offers to the adolescent.

REFERENCES

Cadoret, R., and Tanna, V. 1975. Genetics of affective disorders. In G. Usdin, ed. *Depression*. New York: Brunner/Mazel.

Carlson, G., and Cantwell, D. 1979. A survey of depressive symptoms in a child and adolescent population. *Journal of the American Academy of Child Psychiatry* 18:587–600.

Conners, C. K.; Himmelhock, J.; Goyette, C. H.; Ulrich, R.; and Neil, J. F. 1979. Children of parents with affective illness. *Journal of the American Academy of Child Psychiatry* 18:600–608.

Feinstein, S. 1973. Adolescent depression. In E. J. Anthony and T. Benedek, eds. *Depression and Human Existence*. Boston: Little, Brown.

Gittleman-Klein, R. 1977. Definitional and methodological issues concerning depressive illness in children. In J. G. Schulterbrandt and A. Raskin, eds. *Depression in Childhood*. New York: Raven.

Kohut, H. 1968. The psychoanalytic treatment of narcissistic personality disorders. *Psychoanalytic Study of the Child* 23:86–113.

Malmquist, C. P. 1971. Depression in childhood and adolescence. *New England Journal of Medicine* 284:887–894.

Miller, D. 1974. *The Psychology of Adolescence*. New York: Aronson.

Rachman, A. 1975. *Identity Group Psychotherapy with Adolescents*. Springfield, Ill.: Thomas.

Rossman, P. G., and Knesper, D. J. 1976. The early phase of hospital treatment for disruptive adolescents. *Journal of the American Academy of Child Psychiatry* 15:693–708.

Thomas, A., and Chess, S. 1977. *Temperament and Development*. New York: Brunner/Mazel.

Vaillant, G. E. 1972. Theoretical hierarchy of adaptive ego mechanisms. *Archives of General Psychiatry* 33:535–545.

Welner, A.; Welner, Z.; and Fishman, R. 1979. Psychiatric adolescent inpatients. *Archives of General Psychiatry* 36:698–701.

32 THE DILEMMA OF DISPOSITION: PSYCHIATRIC DECISION MAKING AND THE COLLEGE-BOUND HIGH SCHOOL SENIOR

EUGENE H. KAPLAN

Each year adolescent psychiatrists receive a flurry of referrals as the deadlines for college applications and departures approach. High school seniors and their parents, who had hoped problems of separation, sexual identity, peer relationships, eating and sleeping disturbances, and a host of other complaints would be outgrown, begin to worry about whether they will interfere with successful functioning in college.

The psychiatrist is faced with several challenges. He must decide whether and when treatment is indicated, predict what the effect of removal from the old family surround will be, and try to project the influence of the new university setting on the present psychopathology and continuing development of the adolescent. This tests our mastery of the developmental vicissitudes of adolescence (Kaplan 1980).

Should the student remain at home and attend a local college? As an institutionalized transition, the move from home to the university is very valuable developmentally—for those who can utilize it. While the schools no longer act *in loco parentis,* they still assume many parental functions, providing for housing, health care, and recreation. In this facilitating and enriching setting, the young person can work on the late adolescent tasks of inner consolidation and external adaptation (Arnstein 1980).

Are suitable therapists available at the school away from home? In my experience, acute emergencies, crisis intervention, and brief therapy for adjustment reactions are dealt with adequately by many university health services, whereas longer treatment with a skilled and seasoned therapist is not uniformly available. Therefore, adolescents who begin analysis or long-term psychotherapy earlier in high school should be informed at the outset of the postgraduation alternatives: termination, remaining at home and continuing therapy, interruption with appointments during college recesses, or transfer to another analyst. Where the last is necessary, the choice of schools may have to be limited to the large metropolitan areas where psychoanalysis is available. When the adolescent begins therapy during his senior year, it is often too late to make such a disposition.

Consolidation of Sexual Identity in Late Adolescence

The consolidation of sexual identity and formation of an adult sexual pattern, requiring the resolution and integration of sexual and aggressive conflicts, is a salient developmental task facing the high school senior. This issue is often a strong motivation for seeking psychotherapeutic intervention, with the advantage that sexual preferences are much more amenable to change during late adolescence than in early adulthood.

CASE ILLUSTRATION: GARY

Gary, age seventeen, asked to see a psychiatrist in the fall of his senior year in high school. Slim, lithe, modishly dressed, he was quite nervous in articulating his reasons for coming, presenting them in order of increasing painfulness.

Gary considered himself fortunate to have an intact, close-knit family. His father was "good"—compassionate, forbearing, fair, amenable to reason—and Gary despaired of ever living up to such an ideal. The youngest of three sibs, he saw his brother (seven years older) as very much like and very close to father, while his sister (five years older) had a counterpart identification and closeness with mother. It made him feel left out. Father and brother were both "jocks," and his lack of athletic ability accentuated his difference from them. Sister had just married, and brother was just about to. His mother's depression bothered him—for the past year she had been crying frequently without reason, putting on weight, and withdrawing from social contacts; she was in therapy.

Gary was an outstanding student, much better than his brother, active in school affairs, and was aiming for an Ivy League college. He had worked two days a week for the past year, spending his wages on fashionable clothes. While he had a circle of good friends of long standing, Gary was aware of a tendency to alienate both peers and teachers.

Finally, the youth revealed his reason for coming—homosexual erotic fantasies and attraction. These coexisted with a series of real girl friends, about whom he felt quite romantic, and with whom he had repeated mutual oral-genital intimacies for over two years. Several months previously, however, Gary had lost his erection on attempting vaginal penetration.

While he objected to my seeing his parents, Gary unconsciously revealed his difficulty to them, between his first and second appointments, by leaving a homosexual magazine out in his room. His motivation, self-reliance, intelligence, articulateness, and introspective capacities led me to dispense with parental interviews and psychological testing. My preliminary assessment excluded psychosis, the borderline conditions, and early pervasive developmental deviations and arrests.

His powers of self-observation and self-criticism, together with developed conscience, allowed for object relations with awareness and consideration of the other as separate and different. While Gary had some trepidation about the university as initiating the ultimate departure from home, there was no significant separation problem. Essentially, he had achieved the developmental tasks through latency up to mid-adolescence, with progressive weakening of the infantile attachment to the parents, increasing cathexis of peer group, heterosexual object choice (albeit conflicted), with advances in ego and superego development promoting autonomous functioning.

Assessing his presenting complaint, I noted the absence of a latency history of conscious homoerotic wishes or preference for playing with girls, so commonly reported by male homosexuals. Moreover, his enthusiastic cunnilinctus was clearly different from the obligatory homosexual's horrified avoidance of the female genital. At the same time, Gary's arousal from the girl's excited response to his oral stimulation indicated his identification with her. When she fellated him, Gary imagined himself fellating a muscular athlete. This was his masturbatory fantasy for the past three or four years, varied occasionally by images of actively penetrating one of those athletic types anally.

Gary ardently desired heterosexual relationships with full sexual intimacy, marriage, and children, so these homosexual masturbatory fantasies were painfully ego-alien: "They . . . they kill me . . . I'd rather be neuter."

I told Gary that there were reasons for his conscious homosexual feelings and fantasies which should be clarified and understood in an uncovering psychotherapy. It was most unlikely that the underlying conflicts could be resolved before he left for college, so if he began with me, he would have to transfer to another therapist there. Gary refused to wait, so I saw him for nine months, from November through July. Problems of scheduling and distance limited frequency to twice weekly, and he was seen for a total of fifty-seven sessions.

Almost immediately, it was possible to link the homosexual fantasies with his idealization of muscular athletes, like father and brother, together with his conflicted avoidance of competition. Eschewing their sports, he could compete scholastically because it was not their bailiwick. Following this correlation, he enjoyed being fellated by his girl friend to ejaculation without a homosexual fantasy, but then dreamt of attempting anal penetration of a muscular youth with the same thoughts and feelings which accompanied his failed attempt at vaginal penetration.

Soon after, he became aware of his resentment at both parents for their rejection of him as an "unwanted accident." His mother had an abortion after his birth; father never had time for him when he was little, working long hours or playing golf with his brother. As Gary became more critical of his hitherto idealized father, we considered his procrastination and provocation as passive masochistic reactions to the father's preference for his brother.

Two-and-a-half months after we began, Gary's father called me for an appointment, which the patient firmly vetoed. However, he spoke to his father at length, but in generalities, and when the father acceded to the veto, felt much closer to him.

The defensive function of the homosexual fantasies was demonstrated by their containment in the compulsive daily ritual of masturbation or during heterosexual intimacy. Masturbation was initiated without arousal, as an affectively isolated decision, followed by the evocation of the homosexual fantasy to stir excitement. Talking about it was extremely difficult, but Gary was encouraged by increasingly frequent spontaneous desires for, and dreams of, vaginal penetration.

Five-and-a-half months into the treatment, Gary reported a nightmare: he had just had intercourse and both he and the girl were pregnant; from his hospital room he could see his parents having dinner in a restaurant across the street, they could see him, too; he felt pains, squatted on a stool, and the baby came out, hitting the floor with a "splat"; he asks his mother and his girl friend to confirm that the baby is dead; mother says they knew before, but did not want to upset him.

While the manifest content suggested many possibilities, including primal scene, denial of the anatomical difference between the sexes, identification with the woman's envied procreative powers couched in a regressive equation of baby with feces, perhaps alluding to mother's abortion, I did not go much beyond his associations: he awoke from the nightmare and since he was unprepared for English and Spanish, stayed home; the English teacher was an avowed homosexual, "Oscar Wilde with three concubines . . ."; and Gary was failing despite his high grades because he had turned in only three of five required papers. I pointed out his motive for provoking, to recreate the original situation of father preferring brother over him. The Spanish teacher, who was tolerant of his procrastination, was very pregnant. Her big belly seemed so vulnerable, the baby so exposed to damage. Gary then recalled his fear of fights ever since losing one at age seven, linking the vulnerability of the unborn child to his aggressive-sadistic impulses and implicating his homosexual fantasies as a defense against the fears of injuring the girl in coitus arising from these impulses.

After this dream, Gary's focus shifted from father's preference for brother to the demoralizing effect of mother's depression. Her helpless self-blame in reaction to Gary's urgings for involvement and activity left him frustrated and guilty for attacking his already damaged mother. A month later, after seven months of treatment, his antagonism toward the homosexual English teacher abated. Gary attempted vaginal penetration several times, stopping short at his girl friend's complaints of pain.

In the eighth month of treatment, a homosexual masturbation fantasy following one such abortive vaginal penetration led to significant genetic material. He confessed that the idea of homosexual submission was exciting, connected with two recurrent dreams from approximately age seven. In the first, young men poke him, naked and chained, with sticks. In the second, a nightmare after his first sleep-away camp summer, a bear clasps him "the way a father carries a child" (chest-to-chest, the child's limbs encircling). The humiliating loss of the fight at seven was compounded by an apology forced from his conqueror through the intervention of their mothers. Gary confessed that he felt drawn to the company of girls at that point. These dreams were the forerunners of his homosexual fantasies. At the onset (around fourteen), the theme was submissively fellating a motorcycle gang.

Gary came to understand that his strong conscious stirrings for vaginal penetration had the unconscious meaning of a damaging sadistic attack, forcing the submission of a vulnerable, already damaged partner, and that he defended against this unconscious sadism by a masochistic identification with her. Gary soon reported that his masturbatory fantasies had become exclusively heterosexual and, shortly before termination, that he had experienced complete and gratifying coitus.

The patient saw no need for a referral to a therapist in his college town. He left, very pleased with the outcome, and with the option of an appointment during vacation breaks. I did not see the patient until a year later, and he had a confession to make.

The year before, Gary had been too ashamed to reveal the two homosexual episodes with a fellow student which had prompted his initial request for treatment. It had happened twice more at college, with another student, and he had begun to frequent gay bars since his return home the month before. Each time, the patient felt terribly afraid before, then wracked with shame and guilt for days afterward. Only the last of the five men really attracted him, but this man's offer of a continued relationship made Gary recoil in disgust and call for an appointment.

Gary still had the same girl friend. It was great to be adored, but he deprecated her beauty and intelligence and was afraid to approach other girls. They had intercourse frequently; he had no erectile difficulty and she had orgasm regularly, but he did not.

The patient could ejaculate only by masturbating with a homosexual fantasy after coitus.

Gary would not be categorized satisfactorily by DSM III. While his overt homosexual arousal, strong internalized negative feelings about homosexuality, and persistent desire to change sexual orientation match the criteria for ego-dystonic homosexuality, his capacity for strong, sustained, heterosexual arousal and relationships does not.

Rather, Gary's predicament could be understood developmentally, utilizing Freud's (1914) conceptualization of the genesis of the ego ideal in the negative oedipus complex. Ritvo (1971) elaborated this in connection with the late adolescent's approaches to the new object and to reality choices, crucially bound up with self-esteem. At this time, conscious homosexual fantasies and episodes of homosexual activity may occur, simultaneously or in alternation with moves toward the heterosexual object. This developmental view was the basis for my guarded optimism at the beginning of the treatment.

Let us review the diagnostic evaluation and disposition in the light of Gary's revelatory follow-up. There had been no indication to keep him home nor any problem leaving. His excellent academic performance had continued at college and he had made friends, though inhibited from approaching girls for sexual intimacy. In view of his mounting contempt and impatience with his depressed mother, whom he blamed for making him like her, the separation was helpful. As a result of the therapeutic focus on Gary's provocativeness, his relationship with father had improved appreciably. Gary's confession served to support the initial dynamic developmental formulation and prognostic optimism.

Ritvo points out the multiple, shifting meanings of the homosexual fantasies and behavior in the same adolescent (1) as a defense against fears of engulfment by the castrated/castrating phallic woman because of intense passive strivings arising from revived preoedipal object ties and pregenital wishes; (2) as an identification with the woman in the passive-feminine defense against oedipal strivings stirred up by the move toward the new heterosexual object; and (3) when the main threat is narcissistic, in adolescents who cling compensatorily to a grandiose self-image. In a desperate bid to maintain self-esteem, a regressive reinstinctualization may occur, with repersonification of the ego ideal in the homosexual object, expressed in the wish to love and be loved by the kind of person he would like to be. There were hints of all these multiple meanings in Gary's case as he spoke of his identification with his depreciated mother who had made him the same way and viewed his girl friend in the same light.

Infantile Object Ties, Current Reality, and Emancipation from the Family

Recommendations that an adolescent remain at home or go away to college may be flawed by the failure to distinguish between intrapsychic and external reality. Blos's (1967) conceptualization of adolescence as a second individuation process refers to an intrapsychic transformation involving disengagement from the infantile objects or, more precisely, their representations. He characterizes the actions of some adolescents who break with their families and their past as an extreme defense against the regressive pulls of the inner infantile tie, substituting geographical or ideological distance for intrapsychic separation.

Schafer (1968) makes this distinction between internal and external with great clarity. In his struggle for detachment, the adolescent consciously regards the locus of his problems as his actual contemporary parents. Unconsciously, however, his inordinate fear of parental influence is based on a defensive regression from revived incestuous oedipal tendencies, persisting wishes for closeness or merger with his parents, and a tendency to endow them with infantile grandiosity. Schafer concluded that this unconscious situation makes it impossible for the adolescent to resolve his developmental problems by avoiding or overwhelming his actual parents of the present. Rather, a transformation of his archaic inner world is required. Such psychic restructuring is more likely to occur when the actual parents of today continue providing a stable phase-adequate holding environment so that the adolescent's development advances through succeeding phases.

On the other hand, we may be able to determine that the actual contemporary family environment is pathological and interfering significantly with the adolescent's further development. When parents are seductive, clinging, and grandiose in actuality, or oppose the adolescent's striving for autonomy in other ways, his task of inner transformation may be hopelessly blocked. Winnicott (1972) holds that many of the adolescent difficulties for which professional help is sought derive from environmental failure. Without extraparental adult support, disturbed middle and late adolescents find it difficult to surmount regressive dependency needs and free themselves from the childish component of the tie to the original objects (Miller 1973).

Unfortunately, the deterioration of social networks has reduced the availability of suitable adults for individual adolescents. Statistics of social pathology indicate that in a fifteen-year period, the homicide rate for white males, age fifteen to nineteen, has more than doubled, as has the suicide rate, the rate of illegitimacy for young white females, and the reported cases of gonorrhea in this age group. Adelson (1981), citing these figures, suggests a correlation with the decline in family stability, increase in divorce rate, and percentage of one-family households. The case examples I will cite are from intact families with marked psychopathology, where departure for college was one form of face-saving escape.

CASE ILLUSTRATION: SANDRA

Sandra entered psychotherapy at her own request when she was seventeen and a high school junior, complaining of extreme emotional lability and multiple somatic symptoms which were causing excessive absences from school. She was the middle child in her family and the only girl. Her older brother was a high school dropout and substance abuser; her younger brother had learning disabilities and predelinquent behavior. Both parents were depressed, with drinking problems. The mother, whose family history was loaded heavily with affective disorder, became more blatantly alcoholic in the course of Sandra's treatment.

Sandra had never manifested any separation difficulties, but it took seventeen months of twice weekly psychotherapy (130 sessions) focused on her guilt-ridden, masochistic acting out and somatization before the patient was able to move out. During this time I had to intervene forcefully with the parents about treatment for themselves and permitting their daughter to share an apartment with a girl friend.

The impact was immediate. Sandra felt calmer, more substantial, and better able to cope once away from the parental depression and drunkenness and sibling intrusiveness and abuse. Several weeks later, she decided to stop treatment. Sandra went away to college five months later and made the dean's list her first semester. Finding it easier to talk with a woman counselor, she asked me

477

for a referral to a female psychiatrist at the end of her freshman year.

Sandra sought me out two years later to express her gratitude and gave me a brief follow-up. After two years away at college, she had dropped out to work for a year. Now she was at a local school with her own apartment, self-supporting, with encouraging prospects in a creative-performing career. Sandra was still in treatment with the woman psychiatrist and had a continuing, but more detached, relationship with her family.

CASE ILLUSTRATION: MEG

Meg, almost eighteen, was referred for psychoanalysis after consultation with her mother's psychiatrist in the spring of her senior year in high school. Her mother, misconstruing Meg's worsening somnolence as evidence of drug abuse, had initiated the consultation.

The patient readily admitted feeling depressed for several years, with progressively mounting anxiety in the preceding six months, but denied any substance abuse. A gauche awkwardness suggested a strong bisexual conflict, and she soon revealed an intense, long-standing, sadomasochistic fantasy life. Since approximately age nine, she had lulled herself to sleep with elaborate fantasies of a boy abused and beaten by grownups, as a distraction from the loud protracted arguments in the adjacent parental bedroom.

I was impressed both by Meg's need for analysis and her analyzability. Bright, talented, psychologically minded, and free of any thought disorder, she was eager for therapeutic contact. The ideal prescription would have been analysis at college, away from the destructive family influences. Her obese, phobic mother sought repeatedly to involve Meg in the endless parental quarrels, and I construed the girl's sleepiness as a manifestation of depression and a retreat from the marital conflicts.

However, analysis was feasible only if the patient remained at home. Meg was prepared, albeit with deep disappointment, to give up her out-of-town college. Instead, I recommended that analysis be deferred and that she go away as originally planned, with the expectation that removal from the highly conflicted family setting would provide some relief and allow for further development, despite her internalized neurotic conflicts. The corollary to this recommendation was that the destructive family influence would make analysis extremely difficult. I suspected further that her mother sought unconsciously to keep Meg at home since her departure would empty the nest.

I saw the patient for thirty-eight sessions before she left for college and during visits home. In June, Meg reported the completion of an extremely successful freshman year. The depressive and defensive emotional numbness, fatigue, immobilization, and insomnia had yielded to a preponderantly mild hypomanic state, punctuated by brief depressive episodes. She achieved a good academic average while immersed in extracurricular activities. For the first time in her life she was popular. Meg's boyfriend for the year was very considerate, even indulgent, but she found him lacking in forcefulness and passion and became restless in the relationship. At home, her parents were getting along as poorly as ever. I concluded that she had made significant developmental advances following separation from her pathological home situation and left future appointments up to Meg.

In her sophomore year, the patient came in once at Thanksgiving and several times during the Christmas recess. At home the previous summer, she had become enamored of a carhiker, with whom she had had her first intercourse. Back at college, Meg quickly established a liaison with an impulsive, alcoholic professor while his wife was hospitalized. Meg realized that she was still in the grip of sadomasochistic fantasies which she now was living out in her actual relationships.

Meg was upset that these fantasies were sexually exciting. Seeing the link between the fantasy and her reality choices, she broke off with the professor. Soon after, she masturbated for the first time, with the fantasy of an airline stewardess submitting with sexual abandon to the desires of a stranded male passenger. Confronted with masochistic submission as a requirement for sexual excitement led to the insightful clarification of her relationship to the "nice boyfriend." She lost interest precisely because his love for her gave her the upper hand. At that point, she had hurt him by expressing her wish to date other men.

With these insights, Meg sought and won parental support for intensive treatment. Convinced that her year away had promoted her development significantly, she rejected transfer to a local college, beginning psychoanalytically oriented psychotherapy in March of her sophomore year.

As treatment continued through the summer between her sophomore and junior years, her academic performance rebounded and promiscuity yielded to a healthier heterosexual relationship. When her interest waned because the young man lacked aggressiveness, Meg saw the parallel with her parents' relationship and her identification with mother, the destroyer of men. She interrupted treatment with Dr. B at the junior year Christmas recess, resuming later for the first senior semester because of recurrent promiscuity.

After studying abroad for the final semester, Meg consulted me. For the next two years, she pursued graduate studies at a school remote from well-trained therapists. During this time I conducted what might be termed episodic or intermittent analysis during breaks. The patient was treated on the couch for a total of 123 sessions in twenty-seven months.

Back home the following summer, Meg simultaneously conducted affairs with two older married bosses while sexually involved with a student her own age. The bosses were brothers, and she swore each to secrecy from the other. The patient was excited by the danger of exposure of her deceit and by receiving money from them after each rendezvous.

Abroad, Meg had a similar experience. She engaged in a sexual threesome with two older men while her young lover was away. I pointed out that all the older men were characterized as gentle (read passive), which was like her father. Moreover, those two pairs of older men represented her two therapists. Meg had kept the details of her sexual activity and her continuing investment in me secret from Dr. B, while she kept her presence at home that summer secret from me.

This intervention enabled the patient to remember her early erotic closeness to father. Around age three, both parents amusedly encouraged her game of pulling the tiestring to drop father's pajamas. Sometime before age four, he turned stern and angry when she sought to play this game in mother's absence. A strong positive oedipal attachment persisted nevertheless, and Meg would run excitedly every evening to greet his return home. As mother became increasingly depressed and quarrelsome, her evening greeting became a conspiratorial warning to father about the state of mother's moodiness.

Their secret oedipal alliance ended abruptly at age seven when mother overheard the two of them and exploded with rage. Father immediately broke off all contact with his daughter except in the mother's presence. The fantasies appeared then, as a substitute for the loss of this special relationship, while her personality change represented an identification with the submissive compliance of the abandoning object.

A more detailed account of the analysis would document contributions to her bisexual conflict, as well as to the masochistic acting out in the sexual and professional spheres. Mother, a depressed, obese, unattractive housewife, viewed all attractive women as whores and constantly accused father of infidelity; father not only rejected Meg's femininity but actively encouraged her tomboyishness. On completion of graduate school, Meg resumed treatment, working very productively. She was pleased at her newfound equanimity in the face of the parental arguments and at a new capacity for maintaining independent relationships with both parents.

Meg reported two significant initiatives in quick succession. She had taken an apartment in the city, and mother's tearful objections now angered her; formerly she would have backed down guiltily. Then she actively had obtained a highly promising position in her field, which, she claimed, forced her to discontinue treatment immediately. Her awareness of residual oedipal conflicts led Meg to anticipate continuing difficulties in heterosexual relationships. However, she described self-analysis in my absence and felt emancipated.

Although Meg was twenty-four by this time, her decision to stop therapy had a markedly adolescent flavor since it followed immediately on her full emancipation. She had become self-supporting and had moved into her own apartment. Remaining in treatment would have required a continuing parental subsidy.

In addition to this phase-appropriate reworking of separation-individuation, I speculated on the multifaceted transference significance of the termination. The analysis of her resistances stemming from the revival of oedipal wishes in the transference had resulted in considerable lifting of repression with retrieval of important childhood memories and decreased inhibitions. To the degree that her consequent improvement connoted success, Meg reacted guiltily, turning away masochistically from what she regarded as too good for her. In addition, becoming the abandoner rather than the abandoned was an unconscious motive which may have been aggravated by the episodic nature of the treatment reviving the repeated rejections by father in childhood.

Adatto (1980) points out that the threat of regression, experienced in relationship to the analyst, interferes with the development of a full transference neurosis and is reflected in an inability to fully explore the infantile neurosis and its later versions. Analysis in adolescence is particularly subject to interruption or premature termination. Adatto observes that many late adolescents interrupt psychoanalysis once satisfying love relationships are made. Friend (1980) notes that the analyst may regret having accomplished only a "piece of analytic work," but is reluctant to analyze an adolescent's wish to leave home and treatment to attend college or seek work as a resistance rather than an adaptive step.

Some follow-up was provided by Meg's older sister three-and-a-half years later, when she consulted me at Meg's suggestion. At that time, Meg was reported to be coping, self-sufficient, living alone, and without a boyfriend. There was no indication of the old masochistic promiscuity or of frequent contact with her parents. Although happy with her work, she did not seem to be fulfilling her earlier promise, and the lack of an enduring heterosexual relationship was strongly suggestive of the continuing influence of her masochistic tendencies.

Conclusions

In addition to decisions about diagnosis and the nature and timing of treatment when indicated, the high school senior's college plans also compel our predictive judgments about the effects of removal from the family setting and the influence of the new college environment on his or her present psychopathology and continuing development.

The choice of school may be influenced by the availability of therapists if treatment is indicated after departure from high school. Recommendations that an adolescent remain at home or go away to college should be based on the therapist's informed grasp of the distinction and complex interaction between intrapsychic and external reality. The case examples illustrate how the impending deadline of departure may motivate the adolescent to seek therapy, the therapeutic effect of removal from destructive family influences, the efficacy of intermittent or episodic psychoanalysis, the uncertainty and difficulty of such decisions, and the importance of follow-up.

NOTE

Presented in an earlier version to the American Society for Adolescent Psychiatry, New Orleans, Louisiana, May 10, 1981.

REFERENCES

Adatto, C. 1980. Late adolescence to early adulthood. In S. Greenspan and G. Pollock, eds. *The Course of Life: Psychoanalytic Contributions toward Understanding Personality Development.* Vol. 2. *Latency, Adolescence and Youth.* Washington, D.C.: Government Printing Office.

Adelson, J. 1981. What happened to the schools. *Commentary* 71:36–41.

Arnstein, R. 1980. The student, the family, the university and transition to adulthood. *Adolescent Psychiatry* 8:160–172.

Blos, P. 1967. The second individuation process of adolescence. *Psychoanalytic Study of the Child* 22:162–186.

Freud, S. 1905. Three essays on the theory of sexuality. *Standard Edition* 7:135–243. London: Hogarth, 1953.

Friend, M. 1981. Indications and contraindications for the psychoanalysis of the adolescent. In S. Orgel and B. Fine, eds. *Clinical Psychoanalysis.* New York: Aronson.

Kaplan, E. 1980. Adolescents, age fifteen to eighteen: a psychoanalytic developmental view. In S. Greenspan and G. Pollock, eds. *The Course of Life: Psychoanalytic Contributions toward Understanding Personality Development.* Vol. 2. *Latency, Adolescence and Youth.* Washington, D.C.: Government Printing Office.

Miller, D. 1975. The drug-dependent adolescent. *Adolescent Psychiatry* 2:70–97.

Ritvo, S. 1971. Late adolescence. *Psychoanalytic Study of the Child* 26:241–263.

Schafer, R. 1968. *Aspects of Internalization.* New York: International Universities Press.

Wallerstein, R. 1975. *Psychotherapy and Psychoanalysis: Theory, Practice and Research.* New York: International Universities Press.

Winnicott, D. 1972. Adolescence: struggling through the doldrums. *Adolescent Psychiatry* 1:40–50.

33   THE PROGNOSTIC SIGNIFICANCE OF ADOLESCENT INTERPERSONAL RELATIONSHIPS DURING PSYCHIATRIC HOSPITALIZATION

WILLIAM S. LOGAN, F. DAVID BARNHART, AND JOHN T. GOSSETT

The importance of interpersonal relationships in adolescent and child development has long been recognized (Blos 1962). The relationship skills of hospitalized adolescents are frequently disturbed, and a primary focus of adolescent unit milieu is the recognition and treatment of dysfunctional relationship patterns.

Validating this treatment approach, past evidence suggests that the quality of peer relationships may have prognostic significance. In a comprehensive review of the predictability of adult mental health from childhood behavior, peer adjustment added substantially to predictions based on intelligence and antisocial behavior, the two strongest predictors of adult functioning (Kohlberg, LaCrosse, and Ricks 1972). Other studies have identified good preadolescent and adolescent peer relationships to be predictive of later healthy adult functioning, both in follow-up studies of children and in preadmission histories of hospitalized adolescents (Carter 1947; Hartmann, Glasser, Greenblatt, Solomon, and Levinson 1968; Havighurst, Bowman, Liddle, Matthews, and Pierce 1962; Pollack, Levenstein, and Klein 1968; Van Alstyne and Hattwick 1939).

In addition, correlations between poor peer relations and future antisocial behavior, neurosis, and schizoid personality have been established (Robins 1966; Roff 1961).

Masterson and Costello (1980), in a recent follow-up study of hos-

484

pitalized borderline adolescents, found preadmission social functioning and admission peer object relations to be predictive of outcome.

While several studies have identified various preadmission, hospital course, and postdischarge variables that affect the prognosis of hospitalized adolescents, few systematic attempts have been made to assess the interpersonal relationships of adolescents during their hospitalization or to correlate these ongoing relationship skills with long-term treatment outcome (Gossett, Barnhart, Lewis, and Phillips 1977, 1980; Gossett, Lewis, Lewis, and Phillips 1973; Gossett, Meeks, Barnhart, and Phillips 1976; Lewis, Beavers, Gossett, and Phillips 1976; Masterson and Costello 1980).

In a large follow-up study of hospitalized adolescents, Garber (1972) identified the adolescents' involvement with the peer group as a significant outcome predictor but did not specify the technique used to measure these relationships.

This report focuses on the development of a practical technique for measuring adolescents' perceptions of closeness to peers and to members of the treatment team during psychiatric hospitalization and on the relationships of these assessments to future functioning. It was hoped that assessment of these skills would yield not only significant prognostic data but also important clinical information for treatment-planning purposes.

Methodology

Patients for this study were selected from a group of 120 consecutive admissions to the Timberlawn Adolescent Service occurring between September 1968 and November 1972. Of this group, thirty-two adolescents (sixteen boys and sixteen girls) met the selection criterion (see In-Hospital Procedures below). The ages at admission ranged from thirteen to seventeen, with a median of fifteen and one-half years. The median IQ was 116. The majority of the group derived from middle- or upper-middle-class families. In diagnoses, the group represented a variety of personality disorders ($N = 21$), a smaller group exhibited psychotic symptomatology ($N = 8$), and three had profound neurotic disorders. In retrospect, many of the patients would fit DSM III criteria for Borderline Personality Disorders.

Common symptoms included drug and alcohol abuse, delinquent acts, promiscuity, severe academic underachievement, runaways, and chronic conflict with authorities. Over one-half had prior outpatient and inpatient treatment, while all except three of the remainder had prior outpatient treatment without previous hospitalization. The youngsters in this study were hospitalized at Timberlawn for periods of time ranging from seven to thirty-nine months, with a median length of stay of nineteen months. Demographically, the group of thirty-two adolescents did not differ significantly from the larger group of 120 patients described elsewhere (Gossett et al. 1980).

IN-HOSPITAL PROCEDURES

During hospitalization, the patients were surveyed at approximately three-month intervals regarding their perceptions of closeness to the other adolescents in the hospital and to the unit staff. The surveys were conducted for a two-and-one-half-year period from January 1972 through May 1974. Each adolescent was asked to select the three peers on the Adolescent Service to whom he or she felt closest and to select the three staff members to whom they felt closest. In addition, staff of the Adolescent Service (administrative psychiatrists, individual therapists, schoolteachers, nurses, and aides) were asked to list members of the adolescent group in rank order in terms of how close the individual staff member felt to each patient.

In order to obtain measures of consistency of interpersonal relationships, the criterion for selecting the sample from the group of 120 patients was participation in three consecutive closeness surveys. While this procedure resulted in a considerable reduction in sample size, it allowed a focus on relatively long-term relationships, which was felt to be consistent with the program's emphasis on intermediate to long-term reconstructive treatment with a highly resistant patient population.

POSTDISCHARGE FOLLOW-UP

Follow-up assessment consisted of a ninety-minute interview with the former patient and a separate ninety-minute interview with his or her parents. The interviews were conducted from June 1975 through September 1978. The median elapsed time between hospital discharge and follow-up assessment was five years, with a range from two years, eleven months, to seven years, eight months.

The follow-up interviews began with an open-ended request for the former patient (or parent) to review the period of time since discharge. Subsequently, the interviewer asked more focused questions pertaining to the former patient's current peer relationships, relationships with parents and other family members, educational and vocational history, alcohol and drug usage, contacts with legal authorities, and additional psychiatric treatment. Additional details of the interviewing procedures have been described elsewhere (Gossett et al. 1980).

The follow-up material was summarized in writing, together with the interviewer's comments concerning the subject's current mental status. These deidentified summaries were evaluated independently by three raters (not members of the Adolescent Service staff) who assessed the former patient's level of functioning, focusing specifically on occupational adjustment, family relationships, and peer relationships. Their numerical ratings were based on the following scales.

FOLLOW-UP LEVEL OF FUNCTIONING SCALES

I. PEER AND SOCIAL FUNCTIONING

1. *Good:* At least one intense, mutually gratifying relationship with a peer of either sex. Relationships with other peers of both sexes are not grossly restricted.

2. *Fair:* Clear evidence of marked restriction in some aspect of relationships with peers. Such restriction may be either that relations are superficial or that despite having one intense relationship, there is some marked restriction, as, for example, definitely impaired relationships with persons of the opposite sex.

3. *Poor:* No friends at all or only superficial acquaintances.

II. RELATIONSHIP WITH PARENTS

1. *Good:* A stable relationship, showing age-appropriate independence, and demonstrating mutual respect and affection.

2. *Fair:* Relationship clearly impaired. (No attempt is made to assess how much of this might be attributable to the patient rather than the parents.)

3. *Poor:* Relationship lacks all or most of the qualities rated "good."

III. OCCUPATIONAL FUNCTIONING

1. *Good:* Full-time, stable, and successful homemaking, employment, or school activity.

2. *Fair:* Only part-time involvement with homemaking, work, or

school; or significant occupational problems such as truancy, acting out, underachievement, instability over time.

3. *Poor:* Unable or unwilling to perform occupational tasks on a regular basis.

Assessments of outcome from the three judges on the Peer, Parent, and Occupational Scales were summed to yield a Global Level of Functioning. Interrater reliabilities ranged from .68 to .84; all reliability coefficients were significant ($P < .001$).

Results

Data from Closeness Surveys were divided into three sections: (1) the adolescent's evaluation of their closeness to peers, (2) the adolescents' evaluation of their closeness to staff, and (3) staff rankings of their feelings of closeness to the adolescents. It was hypothesized that data in these three areas would be predictive of postdischarge follow-up level of functioning.

CLOSENESS TO PEERS

Within this area two methods of categorizing the data were developed: mutual relationships and popularity. Mutual relationships were defined as two adolescents' selecting each other as one of the three peers to whom they felt closest. An example would be adolescent A's selecting adolescent B and adolescent B's selecting A as one of three listed on the Closeness Survey. Such an occurrence would be counted as one mutual relationship for each adolescent. The average number of mutual relationships per survey was determined for each member of the sample. It was anticipated that those adolescents most able to engage in mutual relationships would have better long-term outcome.

Popularity was measured by counting the number of times an adolescent was selected by unit peers. An average number of times selected per survey was then computed for each adolescent. It was felt that popularity would be a rough measure of the ability of an adolescent to have an impact on his or her peer group and also would be valuable prognostically.

While the majority of patients with more mutual relationships did attain Good or Fair Global Outcome, these data failed to attain statistical significance (see table 1). However, the ability to attain mutual relationships during hospitalization did significantly predict independent assessment of level of functioning in peer relationships several years after discharge ($\chi^2 = 3.97$). Although the data in table 1 suggest a degree of relationship between popularity with peers during treatment and Global Outcome, this relationship did not attain statistical significance. The data demonstrate that popularity with peers during hospitalization did correlate significantly with Level of Functioning with peers several years after discharge ($\chi^2 = 6.2$).

CLOSENESS TO STAFF

The adolescents' relationships to five categories of staff were evaluated: administrative psychiatrists, individual psychotherapists, nurses,

TABLE 1
OUTCOME AT FOLLOW-UP AND CLOSENESS RATINGS

In-hospital Selections	Outcome*	
	Good or Fair	Poor
	Assessment of Global Functioning	
Average number of mutual choices:		
≥ 1	18	5
< 1	4	5
Popularity with peers:		
Chosen ≥ 2.5 times	14	3
Chosen < 2.5 times	8	7
Continuity of choice of staff:		
Chose same nurse at least two times	13†	1
No consistent choices	9	9
Staff perception of closeness:		
Above median	11	5
Below median	11	5
	Assessment of Peer Relationships	
Average number of mutual choices:		
≥ 1	18†	5
< 1	3	6
Popularity with peers:		
Chosen ≥ 2.5 times	15‡	2
Chosen < 2.5 times	6	9

* $N = 32$.
† Probability $< .01$.
‡ Probability $< .01$.

aides, and others (such as teachers, psychiatric residents, and activities therapists). Within each category an adolescent was judged to have formed a significant relationship with a staff member if the adolescent selected that staff member as one of his or her three choices on two or more consecutive surveys. The adolescents' relationships within one staff category, the nurses, were found to be a significant predictor of future overall functioning ($\chi^2 = 4.89$).

Similar tables constructed for other staff groups demonstrated essentially random distributions, very low χ^2 values, and P values approaching zero.

STAFF CLOSENESS TO PATIENTS

Within each staff category (administrative psychiatrists, teachers, nurses, and aides) an average rank was computed for each adolescent on each survey. The median rank of the adolescent was then determined in each staff group for the entire period of the surveys. Data organized in this manner demonstrated essentially a random relationship to postdischarge level of functioning. As an illustration, staff rankings of feelings of closeness toward patients averaged across all staff categories are included in table 1.

Contrary to expectations, staff's feelings of closeness to, or distance from, adolescent patients during treatment bore no apparent relationship to any measure of the adolescents' level of functioning several years after discharge.

Discussion

The research attempted to differentiate adolescents who had Good or Fair posthospital treatment outcome from those with Poor outcome, based on data concerning their interpersonal relationships during hospitalization. Certain measures of interpersonal relationships during inpatient treatment did appear to have predictive value for future functioning. These were the adolescents' ability to form mutual relationships with peers, their popularity with peers, and their ability to form a meaningful relationship with a member of the unit nursing staff. Patients' feelings of closeness toward other staff members and staff members' feelings of closeness toward patients did not have long-term predictive value. These findings are of particular clinical meaning in view of the implicit assumption of many treatment personnel that their affective reactions to patients contain much greater prognostic power than patients' feelings toward each other. Our findings, however, appear to replicate, in a psychiatric setting, data derived from a large body of longitudinal work summarizing information from a comprehensive review of childhood predictors of adult mental status. Kolhberg et al. (1972) stated, "In a certain sense, this evidence suggests that children are better diagnosticians than are adult clinicians, i.e., that their spontaneous evaluations of each other are more predictive than are the ratings of adults on mental health behavior." No definitive explanation is available for the superior long-term predictive value of adolescent peer-relationship assessments over those made by adult clinicians. However, a partial explanation may derive from the observation that all such studies have been conducted in some form of institutional setting (hospital, school, or other residential or educational program). Within such settings, staff members' affective responses to a patient or student may be influenced by the youngster's apparent conformity to institutionalized goals and procedures. Adolescent peers' sociometric ratings of each other, however, may be sensitive to a broader range of more enduring and more meaningful characterological qualities.

Of related interest is the finding that adolescent patients' feelings of closeness toward unit nurses were predictive of later adult functioning while their feelings toward other staff members did not predict outcome, and that this occurred in a program strongly emphasizing the importance of the youngsters' relationship to their administrative psychiatrist, their individual psychotherapists, teachers, and other members of the treatment team. Within a highly organized, long-term milieu program, it may be the unit nurses who most clearly embody the simultaneous roles of nurturing, supporting, and giving with confrontation, control, and limit setting. In this regard, it is perhaps not surprising that an adolescent's ability to integrate these very different aspects of relationships with adults in a consistent, close relationship has important prognostic significance.

Conclusions

A comprehensive review of adolescent psychiatric hospital follow-up studies identified a number of predictors of later adult functioning: severity of psychopathology on admission, the chronicity of the illness, intelligence, a specialized adolescent treatment program, completion of inpatient treatment goals, and continuation of psychotherapy following hospital discharge (Gossett et al. 1973). Subsequent reports refined these variables and emphasized the importance of family interactional assessment (Gossett et al. 1977; Gossett et al. 1976; Lewis et al. 1976). Results from this study suggest the importance of including an in-hospital evaluation of adolescents' interpersonal relationships as a prognostic variable and indicate a practical survey procedure to facilitate this evaluation. Such surveys could provide a measure of treatment progress during hospitalization, thus yielding valuable clinical as well as prognostic information. The results suggest the prognostic superiority of patients' feelings of closeness toward each other over staff members' perceived relationship to the patients and emphasize the pivotal role of unit nurses within a complex multimodality milieu treatment program. Increased staff sensitivity to adolescent patients' perceptions of each other could promote closer staff-patient collaboration and thereby enrich hospital treatment process and outcome.

REFERENCES

Blos, P. 1962. *On Adolescence: A Psychoanalytic Interpretation.* New York: Macmillan.

Carter, B. 1947. The prognostic factors of adolescent psychosis. *Journal of Mental Science* 88:31–81.

Garber, B. 1972. *Follow-Up Study of Hospitalized Adolescents.* New York: Brunner/Mazel.

Gossett, J. T.; Barnhart, F. D.; Lewis, J. M.; and Phillips, V. A. 1977. Follow-up of adolescents treated in a psychiatric hospital: predictors of outcome. *Archives of General Psychiatry* 34:1037–1042.

Gossett, J. T.; Barnhart, F. D.; Lewis, J. M.; and Phillips, V. A. 1980. Follow-up of adolescents treated in a psychiatric hospital: measurement of outcome. *Southern Medical Journal* 73:459–466.

Gossett, J. T.; Lewis, S. B.; Lewis, J. M.; and Phillips, V. A. 1973. Follow-up of adolescents treated in a psychiatric hospital: a review of studies. *American Journal of Orthopsychiatry* 43:602–610.

Gossett, J. T.; Meeks, J. E.; Barnhart, F. D.; and Phillips, V. A. 1976. Follow-up of adolescents treated in a psychiatric hospital: onset of symptomatology scale. *Adolescence* 11(42): 195–211.

Hartmann, E.; Glasser, B.; Greenblatt, M.; Solomon, M. H.; and Levinson, D. J. 1968. *Adolescents in a Mental Hospital.* New York: Grune & Stratton.

Havighurst, R. J.; Bowman, P. H.; Liddle, G. P.; Matthews, C. V.; and Pierce, J. V. 1962. *Growing Up in River City*. New York: Wiley.

Kohlberg, L.; LaCrosse, J.; and Ricks, D. 1972. The predictability of adult mental health from childhood behavior. In B. B. Wolman, ed. *Manual of Child Psychopathology*. New York: McGraw-Hill.

Lewis, J. M.; Beavers, W. R.; Gossett, J. T.; and Phillips, V. A. 1976. *No Single Thread: Psychological Health in Family Systems*. New York: Brunner/Mazel.

Masterson, F., and Costello, J. L. 1980. *From Borderline Adolescent to Functioning Adult: The Test of Time*. New York: Brunner/Mazel.

Pollack, M.; Levenstein, S.; and Klein, D. 1968. A three-year post-hospital follow-up of adolescent and adult schizophrenics. *American Journal of Orthopsychiatry* 38:94–109.

Robins, L. N. 1966. *Deviant Children Grown Up: A Sociological and Psychiatric Study of Sociopathic Personality*. Baltimore: Williams & Wilkins.

Roff, M. 1961. Childhood social interactions and young adult bad conduct. *Journal of Abnormal Social Psychology* 63:333–337.

Van Alstyne, D., and Hattwick, L. A. 1939. A follow-up study of the behavior of nursery school children. *Child Development* 10:43–70.

34 THE TEST OF TIME: BORDERLINE ADOLESCENT TO FUNCTIONING ADULT

JAMES F. MASTERSON, WILLIAM V. LULOW, AND JACINTA LU COSTELLO

This chapter, a follow-up report of psychoanalytically oriented psychotherapy of hospitalized borderline adolescents and casework treatment of their parents, describes how well the treatment results obtained with thirty-one adolescents, between 1967 and 1974, have stood the test of time. It presents compelling evidence that supports the theory that the borderline syndrome is a stable diagnostic entity owing to a failure in separation-individuation and related to the mother's libidinal unavailability.

It demonstrates that a therapeutic approach based on this theoretical assumption has a wide range of effectiveness, depending on the patient, from relief of symptoms and improvement in functioning to profound and enduring change in intrapsychic structure—that is, in ego development and object relations. Beyond that, it illustrates that the theory not only illuminates the daily clinical vicissitudes of psychotherapy but also serves as a powerful prognostic tool. It brings full cycle twenty-four years of study of what has now come to be labeled the borderline syndrome (Masterson 1967b, 1972).

The Psychiatric Dilemma of Adolescence

The work, begun in 1954, was an effort to distinguish those adolescents whose psychiatric symptomatology was an expression of illness and therefore required treatment from those whose symptomatology was an expression of adolescent turmoil that would subside with further growth and therefore did not require treatment (Masterson 1956, 1958,

1966, 1967a; Masterson, Corrigan, Kofkin, and Wallenstein 1966; Masterson, Tucker, and Berk 1963; Masterson and Washburne 1966).

A five-year follow-up study of seventy-eight adolescent outpatients found that adolescent turmoil was at most an incidental influence, subordinate to that of psychiatric illness in the onset, course, and outcome of the patient's various emotional disorders. The decisive influence of psychiatric illness was clearly seen in the outcome five years later when these patients had not grown out of their illnesses.

Nor did psychotherapy significantly alter this course of events. Approximately one-third of the patients diagnosed as personality disorder received psychotherapy (once a week) for periods of time varying from six months to several years. Although the adolescents improved during their treatment, when seen five years later they were found to be suffering from moderate to severe impairment. The preeminent theme in the treatment was of a patient who ventilated his feelings about current conflicts and complaints. The symptoms subsided, the behavior improved, and treatment ended. However, pathologic character traits such as acting out, avoidance, passivity, dependency, and negativism were dealt with little if at all in the psychotherapy. These sobering findings caused our research interest to move on to an intensive clinical study of the personality disorders in adolescents in an effort to understand better what was wrong and to design a more appropriate and effective treatment (Masterson 1967a).

Treatment of the Borderline Adolescent: A Developmental Approach

This study began in 1968 in an adolescent inpatient unit where personality disorders in adolescents could be observed in microscopic detail and the patients' twenty-four-hour behavior could be monitored and correlated with interviews. At the same time, dramatic strides were being made by researchers in other related areas such as early childhood development (Bowlby 1969, 1973; Mahler 1968, 1975; Spitz 1965) and the borderline syndrome in adolescents and adults (Adler 1973; Frosh 1960, 1964; Giovacchini 1965, 1967; Kernberg 1967, 1968, 1975; Modell 1961, 1963; Rinsley 1968, 1971, 1977).

Integration of all this work with our study of the adolescent inpatient and his family led to a clinical concept of the borderline adolescent as a developmental arrest which was quite specific and resembled in most particulars the concept of the borderline adult elaborated by others through psychoanalytic work with adults.

Beyond this, through a unique vantage point—observing patient and family interactions in joint interviews—a theory evolved that the cause of the developmental arrest of the borderline adolescent was the mother's libidinal unavailability to the child's efforts to separate and individuate, which itself could come from a number of causes. In most of our cases, it was owing to the fact that the mother herself had a borderline syndrome or a more serious emotional disorder that led her to reward regressive behavior and to withdraw from separation-individuation in order to maintain her own intrapsychic equilibrium. There were a number of other possibilities: for example, a long physical separation from the mother; a mother who is psychotic, depressed, or emotionally empty and unable to nurture; or one who dies.

A specific therapeutic design—repair of the faulty separation-individuation through intensive psychoanalytic psychotherapy—emerged and was found to be effective. The therapeutic design, reported in detail elsewhere (Masterson 1972), will be briefly summarized. As the therapists dealt with each clinical issue, the patients presented a sequence of events that occurred with such regular repetition as to form a natural therapeutic design. The first, or testing, phase, where the therapist established a therapeutic alliance by confronting the patient's defenses against his abandonment depression, was worked through via memories, fantasies, dreams, and the transference. The clinical sign that the second phase had been adequately worked through was the patient's having faced and dealt with his feelings of hopelessness and helplessness regarding the frustration of his wish for unconditional love (approval for separation-individuation) and his feeling that if he separates he will die and the mother will die. This led to the third and final separation phase, when the depression markedly decreased, reality perception improved, and adaptation took over from defense with a flowering of individuation.

The thirty-one patients reported in this follow-up were treated in this fashion, and twenty were discharged as improved. Improvement was defined not just as improvement in functioning but as the presence of the capacity to continue to grow, develop, and individuate, while handling separation stress without sacrificing adaptation to defense.

The details of the theory and the treatment are reported extensively elsewhere and will not be reviewed here (Masterson 1975a, 1975b, 1975c, 1976; Masterson and Rinsley 1975). The literature on adolescent follow-up studies was reviewed by Gossett, Lewis, Lewis, and Phillips

496

(1973) and in subsequent studies (Herrera, Lifson, Hartmann, and Solomon 1974; Kalman 1974; Kirowitz, Forgotson, Goldstein, and Gottlieb 1974). The differences in study samples, method of follow-up, and analysis of data make comparisons impossible.

Method

The method was clinical, exploratory, and descriptive, rather than hypothesis testing. The findings reported are based on the clinical approach: a case-by-case review integrating all the data into a comprehensive clinical picture of onset, course, and outcome. Efforts were made by the three clinical researchers to control for individual bias and to define as much as possible the variables studied. The statistical correlations to be reported in detail later will only be mentioned in this report where appropriate.

SELECTION OF CASES

The patients were admitted neither at random nor consecutively but only after careful and thorough evaluation had demonstrated that the diagnosis was most likely a borderline syndrome and that the patient had potential to respond to treatment. In addition, a small group admitted for six-week evaluation and diagnosed as either psychotic or psychopathic have been excluded from this study.

The entire group consisted of fifty-nine adolescent patients hospitalized at the Payne Whitney Clinic between September 1968 and November 1974. This group was divided into two subgroups. A treated sample consisted of thirty-seven patients who were hospitalized for more than twelve months and therefore had an opportunity for a reasonable trial of treatment. The control group consisted of an untreated sample (twenty-two) who were hospitalized for less than twelve months.

THE UNTREATED SAMPLE

The control group is described to complete the clinical picture of the original fifty-nine patients. We contacted nine of the twenty-two patients (40 percent), had personal interviews with three, and interviewed at least one parent of each of the remaining six. Two of these patients had had eighteen months or more of treatment at another hospital, and their impairment rating was mild. One, a girl, age twenty-four, was working

497

and living on her own the life of a homosexual; the other, a sixteen-year-old boy, was a senior in high school. Two of the remaining seven were rated as having mild impairment, but there was strong clinical evidence that the underlying basis for their adjustment was pathological and therefore tenuous. The five remaining patients were rated moderately to severely impaired; their conditions were unchanged since their hospitalization, despite the passage of time. They were unable to continue in school or to hold jobs, suffered from a variety of symptoms, had poor relations with both family and peers, and seemed to drift from crisis to crisis, unable to impose any direction on their lives.

FOLLOW-UP EXAMINATION PROCEDURES

After a series of pilot interviews demonstrated that the observations of the social worker and the two psychiatrists were comparable, each patient was seen by both the social worker and one of the two psychiatrists. The social worker, who had no prior knowledge of the patient, served as a control for any bias the psychiatrist may have had because he had known the patient's past history. The interview technique was similar to that used in a psychiatric consultation. The interviewer began with the interval history, the order of topics was not fixed, and an effort was made to obtain the desired information while preserving the flexibility necessary to pursue clinical leads as they arose. After the examination, each of the interviewers filled in a protocol covering the salient features the interview was designed to elicit.

The parent or parents were seen only by the social worker, who concentrated on attempting to answer with the parents the same questions asked the patients. In addition, changes in each parent's relationship with the other were investigated.

ORGANIZATION AND ANALYSIS OF DATA

At the time of the interview, each of the two interviewers used his or her clinical judgment to rate the patient's impairment, using the following definition: The degree to which the patient's total capacity to function is impaired by his psychiatric illness: minimal, 0–10 percent; mild, 20–30 percent; moderate, up to 50 percent; and severe, over 50 percent. All the material on each patient was reviewed by the two psychiatrists to make a final impairment rating for each patient. Differences between the two were discussed and resolved. Each patient's record was then thoroughly reviewed to specifically assess each of the following: (1) capacity to deal with separation stress; (2) persistence of pathological defenses; (3) change in self- and object representations; (4) degree of autonomy; (5) degree of creativity; (6) capacity for intimacy.

The patient's hospital treatment record was then reviewed to get a clinical impression of the important contributing factors. All of the residents who conducted this treatment were supervised by one of the two psychiatrists or a third colleague. Therefore, it was possible to make some judgment of the therapist's contribution to the treatment process.

The parents' interviews were studied again to answer the questions: How much change were the parents able to make? How much did the parents support or resist the patient's separation-individuation? How did the adolescent's separation-individuation affect the marital relationship? What pathology remained in the family?

Clinical Outcome for Adolescents

The results are presented first in terms of functional impairment. Table 1 presents follow-up functional psychiatric impairment. Sixteen percent of the patients had minimal impairment, 41.9 percent mild, 22.5 percent moderate, and 19.4 percent severe impairment. To summarize, 58 percent were adapting well, whereas 42 percent (moderate and severe) continued to have serious trouble. The six patients rated severe impairment consisted of two who continued to be hospitalized, two others who became psychotic, and two who committed suicide.

To shed more light on these results, we compared them with the rather dismal results of the follow-up study done ten years previously on adolescent outpatients (Masterson 1967a). Although the group cannot

TABLE 1
FOLLOW-UP FUNCTIONAL PSYCHIATRIC IMPAIRMENT

Level of Impairment	No. of Patients	Percent
Minimal	5	16.2
Mild	13	41.9
Moderate	7	22.5
Severe	6	19.4
Total	31	100.0

serve as a control, they can form a useful backdrop against which to contrast the present findings.

Table 2 presents the follow-up functional impairment on those patients diagnosed personality disorder in the earlier study. There is a relatively dramatic shift of patients between tables 1 and 2 from the moderate and severe impairment categories to mild impairment. The 75 percent of the patients who were moderately to severely impaired at follow-up in 1967 has decreased in the present study to 42 percent; the mild from 11.6 to 41.9 percent in the present study. Treatment has doubled the number of patients who are doing well.

From another perspective, the number who maintained their improvement on follow-up four years later was almost the same as the number improved on discharge; that is, eighteen versus twenty. Examining further we found that they were the exact same patients; that is, those who improved, for the most part, maintained their improvement.

Statistical correlations, to be reported in detail elsewhere, found a statistically significant correlation between the degree to which the patient's clinical course followed the optimum therapeutic design and follow-up status—that is, the closer the patient's course came to the design, the better the outcome; the more the patient's course deviated, the worse the outcome. A statistical correlation of prognosis on discharge with later outcome showed the same statistically significant relationship.

An additional, more refined evaluation of the therapeutic process itself was made from those cases where the therapeutic input was optimal. The second-year residents who conducted the psychotherapy lacked knowledge and were prone to massive countertransference re-

TABLE 2
FOLLOW-UP FUNCTIONAL IMPAIRMENT

Level of Impairment	No. of Patients	Percent
Minimal	6	14.0
Mild	5	11.6
Moderate	16	37.2
Severe	16	37.2
Total	43	100.0

SOURCE.—Masterson (1967a).

actions. This single factor caused prolonging and stretching out of the therapy. However, our mission included teaching as well as research. The principal task of supervision was to help the resident to resolve his countertransference. We found if the supervisor could help the resident with his countertransference, the adolescent would teach him what he needed to know about treatment.

To get a purer sample for evaluation of treatment, we teased out a subsample of twelve patients whose treatment was relatively free of contamination by countertransference. Nine (75 percent) of these patients did well (minimally or mildly impaired)—perhaps the truest measure of the effectiveness of the treatment. One can easily imagine how experienced and knowledgeable therapists could have improved on these results.

These findings report a macroscopic level of observation. In order to get closer to the extraordinary variations in detail, with variations so wide as to almost defy efforts at generalization, as well as to go more deeply into some of the changes in ego development and in object relations, each of the four impairment categories is summarized and illustrated with a case example.

This review gives special attention to the degree to which the previous pathologic defense mechanisms had subsided and had been replaced by more adaptive mechanisms: changes in the capacity to manage separation stress; the degree to which the patient had individuated and developed whole self- and object representations and object constancy; and the development of the capacities for autonomy, intimacy, and creativity.

MINIMAL IMPAIRMENT

These five patients showed the most dramatic improvement. They had worked through the rage, depression, and despair of their abandonment depression, separated from the symbiotic relationship with the mother, and received the resultant benefits for ego development and the development of object relations.

Their ego development either achieved or came very close to achieving the stage of ego autonomy with whole self- and object representations that were realistically based and a considerable capacity for object constancy. Splitting and the other pathologic defense mechanisms had been replaced by higher-level mechanisms. Acting out, avoidance, denial, projection, projective identification, clinging, passivity, and regressive behavior gave way to self-assertive attempts to cope with and adapt to reality. Adaptation no longer drastically reduced function and, as they individuated, the self emerged to be consolidated and expressed in a flowering of newly found wishes, interests, creativity, and autonomy. Intimacy still posed some problems, but the patients were dealing with these by experimentation rather than avoidance and denial.

Case illustration 1. Carl, eighteen, a senior at boarding school, was admitted with a one-year history of change in personality, truancy, running away from school, and a suicidal attempt by scratching his wrists. Carl had had a long history of school difficulty, despite the fact that he had a relatively high IQ. At the beginning of the year his schoolwork had begun to improve, but he underwent a drastic change from being quiet, compliant, and conservative to rebellious, hippie-like behavior. He developed sudden obsessive interests in the Beatles and in Russia and communism.

Carl had a domineering mother who tried to oversee and control his every action and a distant, compulsive, overworking, but successful father. Carl responded with passive-aggressive behavior. He did poorly throughout childhood, and when he first went to camp had to be returned because of separation anxiety. This was followed shortly by a transient period of fear of the dark.

On admission examination, he denied the existence of any feelings whatsoever, including depression. He also denied any content to his suicidal attempt. When razor blades were found in his luggage, he admitted placing them there to use in case his hospital treatment did not work. Carl's pathological defense mechanisms consisted of avoidance and denial of feelings, a facade of over-compliance which made a caricature of expectations, passive-aggressiveness, marked avoidance of any aspect of individuation or self-expression, intellectualization, and emotional withdrawal.

Psychotherapy lasted eighteen months. When the therapist confronted Carl with the destructiveness of his behavior, the patient would deny any affect and, as a resistance, comply with what he perceived as instructions. The resident therapist, who had similar defenses of intellectualization and passive-aggressiveness, developed an intense countertransference, and patient and resident colluded to present an illusion of psychotherapy based on instructions and compliance, devoid of affect.

This impasse lasted eight months, until the supervisor helped the resident to become aware of and contain his countertransference and therefore to stop resonating with the patient's transference acting out. The therapist was then able to confront the patient. Integration of the confrontation led the patient back to his terror of individuation, which related to his fear that if he expressed any anger toward his mother she would abandon him. From time to time, when his transference acting out was blocked, in order to manage his depression and rage, he would resort to the splitting defense by turning to the nursing staff. When this was confronted, he would resume working through his depression and anger. He managed family conferences extremely well. Despite the fact that he was savagely and bitterly attacked by his mother for self-assertion, he continued to improve and was discharged to attend college.

Carl was seen at age twenty-five, five and one-half years later. He had continued psychotherapy with the same therapist for four years throughout college and had stopped about eight months before. He graduated cum laude and has been an executive in his father's business for several years. He lives in his own apartment, supporting himself. In the intervening years he had coped with the breakup of two love relationships and his father's illness without an abandonment depression. He reported no symptomatology. He was dating but not seeking a close relationship at the moment.

He had many interests: camping, tennis, bicycling, arts, music, ballet, and creative writing. He hoped to publish some short stories. He had a close relationship with his father, who had continued in treatment, and with his brother, but felt that he had to avoid his mother who was still trying to run his life. Carl had taken charge of his life and was able to assert himself to activate his thoughts and wishes in reality, work, and recreation and to regulate his self-esteem and pursue his objectives.

There was no evidence of the former, predominant, pathological defense mechanisms of intellectualization, suppression and denial of affect, overcompliance, passive-aggressiveness, and various forms of acting out of his dependency. He seems to have achieved whole object relations with adequate self- and object representation. There is much clear evidence of creativity and autonomy, but he still may have problems moving toward intimacy. At the moment he is playing the field and may be avoiding involvement by keeping himself busy.

The parents viewed their involvement in treatment as ancillary. The major purpose of their sessions was for them to provide information to the social worker who in turn would keep them up-to-date on Carl's progress. The father was particularly affected by the parent's group, viewing the other parents as poor excuses for adults and feeling that it was no wonder that they had children with problems. He would often leave feeling that he was healthier than he thought—especially after seeing how "crazy everyone else was." Though he viewed Carl as a competent adult, he felt it had nothing to do with his own involvement in treatment: "Carl grew up; that's the only difference." He was indebted to the hospital for Carl's improvement.

The mother did believe that she had changed since treatment in relation to Carl. She described herself as "flying off the handle" with Carl at the slightest provocation before treatment. Now she felt in more control of her own anger. Both parents view Carl as exaggeratedly touchy about his independence, to which they grudgingly acquiesce.

Carl saw no change in his mother and described her as rigid, controlling, and intolerant of his independence. He had for the most part avoided being in her company. He felt that he had changed as a result of treatment but that his parents had not. However, he felt quite relaxed now with his father and enjoyed working and discussing business with him: "His strength doesn't scare me anymore."

MILD IMPAIRMENT

The minimal and mild groups differ little in impairment of functioning, but there is a chasm of difference from the perspective of ego development and object relations. The patients in the mild group have not achieved whole object relations and require pathologic defenses against separation, anxiety, and abandonment depression to maintain an adequate level of functioning. Beyond that, we were able to subdivide the mild into two subgroups based on the intensity of the need for pathologic defenses as well as on the degree to which there had been consolidation of the self; that is, the degree to which the patients had increased their capacity to assert themselves, to regulate self-esteem, and to activate their wishes in reality.

SUBGROUP A (SIX PATIENTS)

All have shown an improvement in self-representation; a feeling of the self being worthwhile that is more realistically based. They are more open to their own feelings, have a greater capacity to identify their own individuated wishes and thoughts and express them in reality, to regulate their own self-esteem as well as to assert themselves, and to take charge of the direction of their lives.

However, they have not fully separated and do not have whole self- and object representations. Although their self-representation is better and their adaptation is improved, they have made one or another environmental arrangement, usually a relationship, which acts out the rewarding object relations unit to defend against further separation anxiety and abandonment depression. There is a mild to moderate persistence of one or more of the original pathological defense mechanisms. As a result, they remain vulnerable to separation stress and further experiences of depression. There is not the flowering of individuation or self-expression seen in the minimal group.

Case illustration 2. Bill, age fifteen, a model student at school, had begun at about age nine to have outbursts of anger and aggressiveness at home. These usually occurred when his father, a successful theatrical producer, was away and he was left with his permissive, indulgent mother, on whom he made excessive demands. In the beginning, his tantrums were mild, occurred about once every several months, and did not involve destructive behavior. By age eleven or twelve, however, he began to smash his own possessions, for example, a telescope that he valued highly. These would later be replaced by the parents. On occasion, if Bill had an outburst when the father was at home, the father would expel him from the house for the night, forcing him to sleep in the garage or at a friend's house.

The conflict with the mother and father, exemplified by the outbursts, gradually escalated. Then six months before Bill's admission to the hospital, the father left home for a period of a month. The patient's anger increased to a point where he began to threaten his young brother and talk about killing his mother. In one of these outbursts of anger, he accidentally fractured his mother's finger. The poignant thing about this story is that this patient's behavior was clearly a plea for help. The mother's lack of firmness and the father's inconsistency forced the patient to escalate his pleas. Having received no help, he finally turned from destroying his own property to destroying the property of others.

Despite this history of acting out, the patient's basic defenses were obsessive, schizoid, and paranoid. For example, on examination, his facial expression had the quality of a mask—a superficial smile with almost no emotion underneath. The defense of intellectualization was manifested by his obsessive interest in spending large amounts of time on science projects, at which his performance was excellent, although his meticulous attention to detail consumed endless hours. The schizoid quality of his character was illustrated by the fact that, although he was a good student and had no behavior problems in school, he either became the class clown to get attention or had no friends at all. He had fantasies of retreating to the North Pole, where he would have no contact with humans and could become like a machine—a task at which he seemed to have almost succeeded. He idolized Mr. Spock, of the television show "Star Trek," because Spock was devoid of human feelings.

His clinging and paranoid defenses became apparent soon after admission to the hospital. He adopted the same clinging, demanding relationship with a nurse that he had had with his mother. Socially, he could not relate to his peers because he was constantly preoccupied with fear that they might attack him. The minimal role of acting out as a defense was confirmed by the fact that his aggressive behavior never became a problem during his entire hospital stay.

In his fifteen months of hospitalization, the patient projected the rewarding unit on the nursing staff, picking out specific nurses who would permit him to cling and from whom he would angrily demand attention. He projected the withdrawing unit on his therapist, whom he would constantly attack for not taking responsibility for interviews, asking questions, directing interviews, and not giving him enough attention. In addition, his rage was handled through a projection that his peers would attack him. There was also isolation and almost detachment of affect. He had fantasies of becoming the commandant of his own concentration camp and torturing inmates, while he had dreams of the Holocaust and his own death. In addition, there was much intellectualization and social withdrawal. It was necessary to have interviews increased to four times a week, instead of the customary three, in order to help him to get in touch with his anger and depressive affect.

Bill was seen at age twenty-four, seven years after discharge. In his second year of professional school, he was functioning well but was undergoing an abandonment depression of a much milder degree, with feelings of loneliness, depression, and anger since graduation from college and leaving his prior therapist.

Bill was discharged in order to finish his junior year in high school. He lived at the local YMCA, went to a private school, and was in treatment three times a week for eighteen months, until his graduation. He then attended college for four years, graduating cum laude. At college he was seen by another therapist who, rather than confront Bill to enable him to continue to work through the rest of his abandonment depression, behaved more as a father: "We worked on everyday issues; he became a father to me; he was fulfilling my fantasies of being taken care of."

As might be expected, Bill seemed to flourish under this therapeutic approach, with many outside interests and several short-term relationships with girls. However, when he left college to enter professional school, he had an abandonment depression which he defended against by projecting and acting out against the school. At this point in his first year of school, his father died, which deepened his depression. He then reentered treatment and was being seen three times a week, again tending to split, project, and act out the anger at his old therapist on his new therapist; that is, he described his new therapist as cold, stone-faced, withdrawn, and quiet. He reported, "The anger, depression, and wish to be cared for are still there, although I cope with them much better."

There have been two serious separation stresses: leaving his therapist and the death of his father. Mastery and coping are much improved. He still uses avoidance, denial, splitting, projection, and acting out. However, the paranoid phenomenon, the intellectualization, and detachment of affect have not returned. His self-image is dramatically improved. He reported, "Before, I felt blind about myself; blind, angry, scared, grasping at anything to avoid feeling, and would have killed myself without treatment." Now he can identify feelings, likes many parts of himself, thinks he has great potential, and is able to do more and to cope better. In addition, he has a more realistic perception of his parents and does not project as much on his peers. Although not "one of the boys," he has close friends and does socialize.

Relationships with girls are still difficult. He has had sexual intercourse with quite a number, but two long-term relationships were terminated because of his demanding and possessive behavior. As far as independence and autonomy, Bill has been more or less living on his own and managing his own life since his senior year in high school. He is much better in coping with the external world but still lacks intrapsychic autonomy. He has intense abandonment fears about intimacy, with demanding and possessive behavior as a defense. Bill has always been creative, and since discharge pursues many interests avidly, such as marine biology and classical music.

Bill is presently and temporarily suffering from an abandonment depression at leaving his prior therapist. However, like the other patients in this particular category, Bill's adaptation throughout college was based on transference acting out of the rewarding unit with his therapist. This led to seeming dramatic improvement, but it was based heavily on this transference relationship. There was marked improvement of his self-image, improved self-representation, increased capacity to be assertive, along with a more realistic image of both parents. A good deal of the passive-aggressive compliance, isolation, intellectualization, and paranoid defenses are gone and have not returned.

There remains a reliance on splitting, with the rewarding unit projected on the old therapist and the withdrawing unit on the new therapist. However, if the treatment is successful, it could go far toward resolving this intrapsychic problem. It is important to note that Bill's defenses against the abandonment depression are much less intense and more adaptive. He does not retreat into detachment, paranoid projections, isolation, or withdrawal. Although he has always been a person of many interests, his ability to pursue them remains impaired also by his lack of full individuation and whole self-representation. Despite the fact that impairment persists, this is no small improvement for a boy who at age fourteen was diagnosed as paranoid schizophrenic.

Two years after the study was completed, Bill suddenly dropped in to see me. He was in his senior year of professional school, had changed his interest from clinical to industrial psychology, and had been going with a girl for a year and a half. His depression and acting out had resolved, and his perspective had improved with treatment. For example, he was now aware of the regressive effect of his college therapist's treatment and of how he had acted out to defend against the depression on leaving for professional school. He felt more "grown up" and had a "better sense of reality." He still became depressed on occasion but felt he would be able to conclude his treatment in the near future.

SUBGROUP B (SEVEN PATIENTS)

These patients were rated mild impairment because their surface functioning was adequate. However, when one looked beneath that surface at the psychodynamic basis responsible for that functioning, it became apparent that these patients warranted a separate subcategory. There was less improvement in self-representation than in the subgroup A patients and a more intense need for defense against separation anxiety and abandonment depression. Although they felt better about themselves and were somewhat better able to assert themselves, this change was mild compared to the subgroup A patients: they could not take charge of their lives; they could not identify what they wanted and activate and pursue their interest in reality; and there was moderate pathology in the self-representations as well as in object relations.

Case illustration 3. Ruth is a sixteen-year-old girl whose present illness began at age fourteen. Two years prior to admission, she was sent to a Catholic girls' high school which required two hours of commuting. She was unable to manage and failed all subjects. The next year she repeated the grade and began to come into increasing conflict with her mother over rules and restrictions. She sought out rebellious peers, fought with her mother, became depressed and withdrawn, spent more time alone, and began to have difficulty relating to peers. Mother finally gave up efforts to discipline and control her. Ruth became more depressed, hated the rules of the school, began to take drugs, slashed her wrists, and was referred for private therapy. She developed a fear of leaving the house and cut her wrists again, at which time she was hospitalized. The patient denied the need for the hospital, and her mother was torn over the recommendation to hospitalize Ruth. Pathological defenses consisted of avoidance, denial, acting out through clinging, splitting, and projective identification.

Father deserted mother when the patient was an infant and mother had to go to work. The patient was cared for by a series of substitute figures, but the mother remained tied to the patient.

From ages two to five she lived, during the day, with a foster mother so that her mother could work. She clung to her mother on the long walk home each evening after work. At age five mother was hospitalized for a hysterectomy. At age nine father died, at age twelve mother was hospitalized for a thyroidectomy, and at age fifteen the neighbor taking care of the patient died.

Hospital treatment lasted twelve months. Ruth's behavior was characterized by splitting of staff and doctor, intense clinging and demanding, transference acting out with denial of affect, projection, projective identification, and avoidance of individuation. Confrontation eventually led to the depression. Ruth's main difficulty was in getting in touch with her rage at her mother, followed by her extreme anxiety about autonomy.

Ruth was seen again at age twenty-two, four years after discharge. The first year following discharge, the patient stopped treatment, "I wanted another fling with babyhood; I didn't want to grow up." She had great difficulty adjusting, was caught up in a constant round of promiscuity, pot smoking, and was unable to hold a job. Feeling lost, she did not know what to do with all her freedom.

Approximately one year after discharge, Ruth moved back with her mother, gave up drinking and promiscuity, and became generally anxious. At this point, she met a boy whom she fell in love with "because he did not push sex." She got married but became increasingly dependent on him as well as resentful. She found him having an affair with another woman, walked out on him, but then was reunited with him. She is now living with her husband and her mother, is not on drugs or promiscuous, and is supporting herself.

Ruth continues to idealize her prior therapist, her mother, and her husband. She complies with both mother and husband, subjecting herself to abuse. She uses splitting and projects anger on others so that there is less acting out but a persistence of avoidance of individuation, denial, splitting, clinging, and projection. Though she says, "I don't feel helpless anymore; I can protect and assert myself," there is evidently much denial in this. Object representations are split, idealized, or devalued as in the rewarding or withdrawing unit. She still seems unable to tolerate the separation stress as evidenced by her reaction on discharge from the hospital and her continuing to live with her mother, though married. There is little autonomy; she seems to vacillate in dependency between mother and husband. However, she no longer acts out destructively. She still describes herself as not feeling very worthwhile much of the time. The relationship with her husband is based on clinging rather than real intimacy. There are few interests and little creativity.

Mother felt she gained a lot for herself from her treatment. She noted that when Ruth was hospitalized, she had come to the end of her rope. She understands now that she had difficulty in facilitating Ruth's becoming independent, "The social worker helped me to see . . . you not only have to rear them, you have to release them too. . . . She also helped me to see I wasn't just a mother, I was a person."

Following Ruth's discharge, mother felt Ruth went "crazy with freedom." At one point she was so distraught she called the doctor for help and "the doctor told me it was up to Ruth now." The mother provided partial support, but beyond that let Ruth alone, "I didn't intrude, I waited for an invitation, even though I worried. I knew she had to get through it." Ruth returned to live with her mother at nineteen. She realized she had "to get away from drugs and promiscuity or it would kill me." She remained home until her marriage, kept a steady job, and helped to defray expenses. Ruth returned to live with mother following the separation from her husband. She had been with her for six months at the time of the follow-up.

This patient has clearly some better self-representation, seeing herself as not being helpless, being able to assert herself, being able to hold a job, and to be married. The fact that there is a fair amount of denial in this self-observation is also true.

Through acted-out environmental arrangements and clinging to mother and to her husband, Ruth is able to deal with her failure to individuate and thereby perpetuates her problem. Though there is some improvement in the self-representation, it is minimal. Object representations remain the same, there is the same vulnerability to separation stress, and persistence of the same pathological defense mechanisms: denial, avoidance, splitting, and acting out. There is very little independence, intimacy, or creativity. At best one can say that the destructiveness of the acting out has decreased and the self-representation has improved somewhat. One wonders how long this will hold up under stress.

MODERATE IMPAIRMENT

These patients were not substantially helped by treatment. They continued to suffer from severe symptomatology and impairment of functioning. Their clinical pictures were dominated by the need to defend against the abandonment depression at the cost of adaptation to reality. There was little or no autonomy, intimacy, or creativity and no change in intrapsychic structure.

However, even within this gloomy picture there were some positive aspects which may have been related to treatment. For example, one patient finished the second year of college, another graduated from high school, and a third was able to graduate from college. The destructiveness of the acting out of three patients was markedly decreased, and one patient, after living the life of a junkie for five years, was able to overcome his drug habit through the help of Odyssey House. It is entirely possible that without hospital treatment, none of these achievements would have taken place. Consequently, although the treatment made very little change on their defenses against abandonment depression, it did evidently increase to some extent their capacity to cope with reality.

Case illustration 4. The present illness of Jill, age thirteen, began around age ten when her sister, age seventeen, began acting out and her stepbrother attempted to molest her sexually. Stepmother had became preoccupied with sister's problems, at which time Jill began to cut classes, take and sell drugs, steal, and sexually act out. Jill became involved with a nineteen-year-old criminal who sold drugs and often took the punishment for him because they felt that she would be spared because of her young age. Jill was first placed in a reform school and then hospitalized. On admission she denied any difficulties, "All I want to do is drink, take drugs, and have a good time."

Jill was adopted at age two and one-half; her adoptive mother died when she was four. From age four to six she was taken care of by a grandmother and several housekeepers. At age six, her father remarried and Jill was described at first as a model child. At age seven her older sister became involved with drugs and had Jill hold the tourniquet for injections. School and social history were good until age ten, when the patient matured physically before her peers, felt embarrassed about it, and began manifesting behavioral difficulties.

Once hospitalized, Jill's acting out was readily controlled. She began to deal with her anger, which was associated with much regression and acting out, and to work through some of her abandonment depression. She finally started family sessions, where there was revealed equal resistance on the part of both the patient

and the family to separation. The discharge planning was complicated by the patient's reluctance to give up her reunion fantasy
and the parents' resistance to supporting Jill's individuation. This
resistance on both parts was reinforced by a former family psychiatrist. Nevertheless, Jill was discharged to a local boarding school
near home to continue in treatment with her doctor.

Jill did well her first semester after discharge, continuing with her
therapist. She then dropped out of therapy and returned home, and her
clinical condition has deteriorated ever since. She has chronic and
recurrent acute depressions, intense mood swings, temper outbursts,
overeating, and increased drug use, smoking marijuana every day. She
occasionally steals from her mother and, when confronted, says that
she is entitled. She became reinvolved with the same criminal as before
hospitalization, an involvement which became sadomasochistic with
intermittent beatings. She finally terminated the relationship a few
months before the interview, after she had had a pregnancy and an
abortion.

At age seventeen, four years later, Jill has returned to work again,
but now she is beginning to think about college. Part of her present
status is due to a relationship with a new boyfriend whom she idealizes
"because he doesn't want to have sex." She continues to handle separation stress poorly, with the need for destructive acting out as a
defense against abandonment depression. Her original pathological
mechanisms of defense continue more or less unchanged. Her self-
representation, although a little better, is quite infantile and unrealistic.

SEVERE IMPAIRMENT

Two patients failed to respond to treatment and have had to remain
in the hospital. These patients were on our unit in the last year of its
existence when there was extreme separation stress for everyone, and
it is doubtful that they received adequate treatment. One patient who
became psychotic had what seemed to be a good course of inpatient
treatment but broke with his therapist after discharge and later became
psychotic. Either we misdiagnosed this patient or his psychosis
emerged only later. The second patient who became psychotic refused
treatment after discharge. In this case, it is clear that we were wrong in
attributing his temporary psychotic symptoms as being due to drugs
and separation stress, rather than underlying psychosis.

One suicide was a patient whose hospital treatment was thoroughly defeated by her resident's countertransference, and she was discharged unimproved. The second suicide had a seemingly effective course of hospital treatment, but we were unable to find a place for him to live and had to relinquish our therapeutic control to place him with an agency. Shortly afterward he stopped therapy and returned home.

Clinical Outcome for Parents

Both parents received casework treatment, once weekly, throughout the adolescents' hospital stay, usually individually but sometimes jointly. In addition, they participated in weekly group psychotherapy along with a period of family interviews with their adolescent. We were interested in changes in the parents' attitudes toward themselves, toward the spouse, toward the adolescent, toward their role as a parent, and toward the communication patterns with the adolescent and with each other. Did they support or resist the adolescent's individuation? What mechanisms of adaptation compensated for the adolescent's emancipation from the family?

Fourteen of the thirty-one sets of parents improved, sixteen showed no change, and one became worse. Three clusters emerged among the fourteen who improved: both the mother and father (three cases) improved; only one parent (usually the mother) improved (ten cases); one mother improved in treatment but relapsed.

The three families where both parents improved were a marked exception in that all continued individual psychotherapy after the hospital therapy. Usually the parents refused suggestions for continued treatment after the hospitalization. One pair of parents from this group were the only parents of the entire sample who were able to provide sustained positive parental support for their adolescent's individuation.

The most common theme was the mother's (in one case the father's) responding to treatment almost exclusively in terms of herself and her own problems. This enabled her to pull back from the intense involvement with the adolescent, contain her negative projections, invest more affect in herself, and achieve greater self-autonomy. These mothers' behavior became self-directed, often for the first time, with new or better jobs and interests and activities outside the family. However, the mothers were not able to go beyond this and provide maternal nurturing and support for their adolescent's individuation. Nevertheless, the withdrawal of the projection itself was an assist.

Six of the ten mothers (and one father) paid a price for this change in their relationship with their spouses, who did not change. Three mothers divorced and three other marriages are in severe conflict that may lead to divorce. Only 15 percent of the fathers improved.

PARENTS OF MARY

Mother became aware of the ways in which her deep attachment to her daughter compensated for her dissatisfaction with herself and her relationship with her husband. Prior to hospitalization she never admitted the existence of marital problems. Since she has continued in treatment and "became more of an individual," she has returned to work, no longer defines herself only in terms of her role as a mother, feels she has more control of her own destiny, is able to control her urge to reengulf her daughter, and has been able to establish a relationship with her own mother, who is dying. The price that she paid is a greater awareness of her conflict with her husband, who has continued to deny emotional problems in himself and to project upon his wife and daughter.

PARENTS OF DAVID

David's mother, despite her negativism about her treatment, seemed to benefit a good deal. She obtained a substitute teaching job, became interested in and finished a masters' degree in special education, and is now working full time. This has increased her self-confidence and ability to assert herself. Father was more negative about his experience and remains quite uncommunicative with his son. Both parents are tired and frustrated with David and, in essence, wish he would leave them alone.

PARENTS OF HELEN

Helen's mother and father have divorced. Mother continued in treatment and "has gained strength to leave her husband and become an individual." She has pursued her education and is presently completing a degree program in college and hopes to pursue a career in labor law. She describes herself as being unable to be involved with her daughter, since she needs all her energy to stay integrated herself. Father seems to have gained nothing from his treatment.

Discussion

Eighteen out of twenty, or 90 percent, of the patients discharged as improved have passed a test of time by maintaining that improvement four years later. This represents 58 percent of the total sample. The 16 percent minimally impaired improved not just in symptomatology and functioning but also in ego development and in object relations. They developed close to the stage of ego autonomy, with whole self- and object representations, the disappearance of splitting, substantial object constancy with improved capacity to handle separation stress, and with the flowering of individuation—creativity, independence, and beginning capacity for intimacy.

Those mildly impaired (42 percent) showed not only dramatic improvement in symptomatology and functioning but also in self-image development and the capacity for self-assertion. However, they had not achieved full separation and required pathologic defense mechanisms against separation anxiety and abandonment depression, including a clinging relationship, to maintain a high level of functioning. Nevertheless, the improved self-assertive capacity markedly lessened the need to sacrifice adaptation to defense.

The improvement with hospital therapy was closely related to the degree to which the patient's clinical course followed the therapeutic design; that improvement was maintained four years later and could be predicted with a high degree of accuracy at discharge. These findings are compelling evidence that support both the accuracy of the theory and the effectiveness of the therapeutic approach. The method was observational and exploratory rather than hypothesis testing, and, therefore, in the scientific sense, the findings cannot be considered final proof; but short of that their weight and consistency are more than persuasive.

The salient clinical features of the patients who improved were the continuation of outpatient psychotherapy for many years, not returning to live at home again, and the constant support of their own individuation against the parents' regressive projections and other pressures. The parents were not able usually to give positive support for separation-individuation. For example, three of the five patients minimally impaired had to actually cut off all contact with their parents for long periods of time to combat the parents' regressive influence.

The patients who were mildly impaired, although they did not achieve full separation with whole self- and object representations, nevertheless showed substantial clinical change in adaptive capacity through the gradual transfer of emotional investment from object representation to self-representation, with gradual improvement of self-image and self-assertive capacity. This finding, by demonstrating the mechanism of change, offers a strong argument for long-term supportive or confrontive psychotherapy of the borderline.

The salient clinical features of those who did not improve included: overt symptomatology and environmental separation trauma in childhood; clinical illness having its onset around prepuberty (eight to ten years); greater difficulty in the hospital psychotherapy with parents' and patient's resistance to separation; and more intense countertransference problems with the resident. These difficulties crystallized during the family interviews and later during discharge planning, when the joint resistance would result in continued seemingly inseparable obstacles to appropriate plans. Soon after discharge, the patient stopped his outpatient psychotherapy and returned home to live.

A word is in order here about a problem that dogged our footsteps from the beginning to the end. Despite our intense attempts, we were unable to provide a halfway house. This led us to sometimes heroic efforts to find places for the adolescent to live, intensified the adolescent's abandonment depression on discharge, placed a pressure on his capacity to adapt at a time when his new ego structure was most fragile, and may well have been the particular or specific defeat for some of these patients who were moderately impaired. Although a few patients may have received inadequate treatment, a more likely explanation for the majority was the patient's not having the ability to internalize the self- and object representations in order to achieve separation-individuation. They were able to manage throughout childhood with the support available for their dependency, but the approach of adolescence, with the task of becoming independent, interrupted their defenses. Their inability to internalize representations made it impossible to function autonomously, and they were thus exposed to an abandonment depression. This sequence was repeated in the hospital, where they were able to manage as long as the hospital reproduced the childhood environment. But when patients had to leave, not having internalized the object, they again had an abandonment depression against which their only defense was to return to the childhood environment of the family, giving up the struggle for individuation and thus sealing their fate. A halfway house could have provided some of them with a longer period of treatment and more opportunity to internalize.

The relatively poor results with the parents reflect the severity of their pathology, which limited the therapeutic goal. More mothers improved than fathers. One of the keys to the mothers' intrapsychic system for relieving anxiety was change; that compelled them to find other means of adaptation. The tie with the fathers was less intense, and, therefore, they did not feel compelled in the same way. Let me emphasize that we did not neglect the fathers, and they did attend the sessions regularly. In one case, the father was more attached to his daughter; he improved and later divorced the mother, who had not improved at all.

Although the decrease and/or the removal of the intensity of the regressive parental projections is no small achievement, nevertheless, the goal of therapy with the parents—their support of the adolescent's individuation—was not always achieved. This raises questions about the role parents should play in the adolescent's treatment. The dilemma springs from the fact that the borderline adolescent is usually a central cog in the family's communication system and removal of the adolescent creates a change in the rest of the system that must be managed. However, a relatively large amount of therapeutic input achieved a minimal goal for the mothers, less for the fathers, and helped the adolescent indirectly. Should we accept this as a reasonable goal in view of the severity of the parents' psychopathology? Should the parents be advised to also receive psychotherapy on their own, rather than as part of the treatment plan? Would they be motivated enough to accept it? Should the therapeutic approach with mother play down confrontation of the destructiveness of maternal behavior, in favor of emphasizing the need for mother to invest her emotion in her own autonomy?

Some perspective is gained by comparing these findings with those of Offer (Offer 1969; Offer and Offer 1975), who studied the development of healthy adolescents. He divided normal adolescents into three groups (continuous growth; surgent growth; and tumultuous growth) and observed that only the parents in the continuous growth group (25 percent) took pleasure in and were able to give unqualified support to their adolescents' independence. The parents in the other two groups had some difficulty letting go, with those in the tumultuous group having the most resistance. If parents of healthy adolescents can support emancipation and independence only ambivalently, it may be too much to expect seriously ill parents, even with psychotherapy, to support the earlier, more fateful task of separation-individuation.

518

The average age on follow-up was twenty-one, too young to provide more than beginning evidence of the patient's eventual capacity for intimacy. The patients who married seemed to do so as a defense against abandonment depression and not to fulfill mature genital desire for intimacy. The rest of the patients are still experimenting with their capacities for intimacy. Who is not at twenty-one? It would be useful to follow a selected sample through the adult years to trace out the evidence for the capacity for intimacy and finally, and most ultimately important for the assessment of development, to follow this sample into parenthood to evaluate whether, unlike their parents, these patients, particularly the women, had sufficiently overcome their separation-individuation and resultant need for parenting enough to be able to offer appropriate parenting, particularly during the separation-individuation phases of their own offspring.

The stability of the diagnosis of the borderline syndrome is indicated by the fact that it was sustained throughout the follow-up period in all but two cases. These disorders began in early childhood and were constantly reinforced throughout childhood and adolescence. All these patients were ill enough to have to be hospitalized for suicide attempts which expressed desperate pleas for help. Without treatment, many of them would no doubt be dead, in hospitals, or prisons. From this perspective, the results for many reflect a true triumph over tragedy.

Conclusions

The inpatient hospital part of the long course of therapy these patients received was crucial in that it changed a regressive spiral to an adaptive pathway. It changed the balance from defense to adaptation, enabling the patient to participate in later inpatient psychotherapy. These patients then found new capacities to direct their own lives, to perceive realistically, to cope with challenges in work and relationships in a constructive, self-motivated manner, and to contain separation stress without sacrificing adaptation. These were building blocks with which to build a new life whose structure would sustain and support them rather than drag them down. In the 16 percent most clearly, but also to a lesser extent in the others, the work of the psychotherapy had been internalized and became a part of the patient. They had made it their own.

These results go far toward laying to rest, it seems to us, the notion that borderline patients cannot benefit from psychoanalytic psychotherapy. The therapy is arduous, time-consuming, filled with seductive and deceptive obstacles, but is far from impossible. When it is pursued faithfully, it more than justifies the effort by providing a beacon to guide them to overcome their developmental trauma, reconstruct their psyche, and rejoin the mainstream of life. These objectives, a fulfillment of both the therapist's and patient's deepest wishes, enhance the mutual struggle and endow it with a vitality and nobility that gives the work its enduring satisfaction and significance.

REFERENCES

Adler, G. 1973. Hospital treatment of borderline patients. *Journal of Psychiatry* 130:32–36.

Bowlby, J. 1969. *Attachment and Loss*. Vol. 1. *Attachment*. New York: Basic.

Bowlby, J. 1973. *Attachment and Loss*. Vol. 2. *Separation: Anxiety and Anger*. New York: Basic.

Frosch, J. 1960. Psychoanalytic considerations of the psychotic character. *Journal of the American Psychoanalytic Association* 8:544–548.

Frosch, J. 1964. The psychotic character: clinical psychiatric consideration. *Psychiatric Quarterly* 38:81–96.

Giovacchini, P. L. 1965. Maternal introjection and ego defect. *Journal of the American Academy of Child Psychiatry* 4:279–292.

Giovacchini, P. L. 1967. The frozen introject. *International Journal of Psycho-Analysis* 48:61–67.

Gossett, J.; Lewis, S.; Lewis, J.; and Phillips, V. 1973. Follow-up of adolescents treated in a psychiatric hospital: a review of studies. *American Journal of Orthopsychiatry* 43:602–610.

Herrera, E.; Lifson, B.; Hartmann, E.; and Solomon, M. 1974. A 10-year follow-up of 55 hospitalized adolescents. *American Journal of Psychiatry* 131(7): 769–774.

Kalman, F. 1974. Outcome of treatment for adolescents. *Adolescence* 9:57–66.

Kernberg, O. 1967. Borderline personality organization. *Journal of the American Psychoanalytic Association* 15:641–685.

Kernberg, O. 1968. The treatment of patients with borderline personality organization. *International Journal of Psycho-Analysis* 49:600–619.

Kernberg, O. 1975. *Borderline Conditions and Pathological Narcissism*. New York: Science House.

Kirowitz, J.; Forgotson, J.; Goldstein, G.; and Gottlieb, F. 1974. A follow-up study of hospitalized adolescents. *Comprehensive Psychiatry* 15(1): 35–42.

Mahler, M. S. 1968. *On Human Symbiosis and the Vicissitudes of Individuation*. New York: International Universities Press.

Mahler, M. S. 1975. *The Psychological Birth of the Human Infant*. New York: Basic.

Masterson, J. F. 1956. Prognosis in adolescent disorders—schizophrenia. *Journal of Nervous and Mental Diseases* 124:219–232.

Masterson, J. F. 1958. Prognosis in adolescent disorders. *American Journal of Psychiatry* 114:1097–1103.

Masterson, J. F. 1966. Delineation of psychiatric syndromes. *Comprehensive Psychiatry* 7:166–174.

Masterson, J. F. 1967a. The symptomatic adolescent five years later: he didn't grow out of it. *American Journal of Psychiatry* 123(11): 1338–1345.

Masterson, J. F. 1967b. *The Psychiatric Dilemma of Adolescence*. Boston: Little, Brown.

Masterson, J. F. 1972. *Treatment of the Borderline Adolescent: A Developmental Approach*. New York: Wiley-Interscience.

Masterson, J. F. 1975a. Intensive psychotherapy of the adolescent with a borderline syndrome. In G. Kaplan, ed. *American Handbook of Psychiatry* (Special Edition on Adolescence). New York: Basic.

Masterson, J. F. 1975b. Intensive psychotherapy of the borderline adolescent. *Adolescent Psychiatry* 2:240–268.

Masterson, J. F. 1975c. The splitting defense mechanism of the borderline adolescent: developmental and clinical aspects. In J. Mack, ed. *Borderline States*. New York: Grune & Stratton.

Masterson, J. F. 1976. *Psychotherapy of the Borderline Adult: A Developmental Approach*. New York: Brunner/Mazel.

Masterson, J. F.; Corrigan, E. M.; Kofkin, M. I.; and Wallenstein, H. G. 1966. The symptomatic adolescent: comparing patients with controls. Presented to the American Orthopsychiatry Association, March, San Francisco.

Masterson, J. F., and Rinsley, D. B. 1975. The borderline syndrome: the role of the mother in the genesis and psychic structure of the borderline personality. *International Journal of Psycho-Analysis* 56:163–178.

Masterson, J. F.; Tucker, K.; and Berk, G. 1963. Psychopathology in adolescence: clinical and dynamic characteristics. *American Journal of Psychiatry* 120:357–365.

Masterson, J. F., and Washburne, A. 1966. The symptomatic adolescent: psychiatric illness or adolescent turmoil. *American Journal of Psychiatry* 122:1240–1247.

Modell, A. H. 1961. Denial and the sense of separateness. *Journal of the American Psychoanalytic Association* 9:533–547.

Modell, A. H. 1963. Primitive object relationships and the predisposition to schizophrenia. *International Journal of Psycho-Analysis* 44:282–292.

Offer, D. 1969. *The Psychological World of the Teenager*. New York: Basic.

Offer, D., and Offer, J. 1975. *From Teenage to Young Manhood*. New York: Basic.

Rinsley, D. B. 1965. Intensive psychiatric hospital treatment of adolescents: an object relations view. *Psychiatric Quarterly* 39:405–429.

Rinsley, D. B. 1968. Economic aspects of the object relations. *International Journal of Psycho-Analysis* 49:38–48.

Rinsley, D. B. 1971. The adolescent inpatient: patterns of depersonification. *Psychiatric Quarterly* 45:1–20.

Rinsley, D. B. 1977. An object relations view of borderline personality. In P. Hartocallis, ed. *Borderline Personality Disorder: The Concept, the Syndrome, the Patient*. New York: International Universities Press.

Slavin, M., and Slavin, N. 1976. Two patterns of adaptation in late adolescent borderline personalities. *Psychiatry* 13(9): 41–50.

Spitz, R. A. 1965. *The First Year of Life*. New York: International Universities Press.

35 KORO IN AN ADOLESCENT: HYPOCHRONDRIASIS AS A STRESS RESPONSE

STUART ROSENTHAL AND PERIHAN A. ROSENTHAL

Koro, first described by Brero (1897), is a rare syndrome found predominantly among the south Chinese, characterized by acute, severe anxiety associated with a patient's conviction that his penis is shrinking and will eventually disappear, leading to death. A psychogenic etiology is consistently postulated (Devereaux 1954; Gwee 1968; Lapierre 1972; Lehmann 1975; Rin 1963; Veith 1975; Yap 1965a), with cultural expectations about virility and the expression of genital impulses a major predisposing factor.

Veith (1975) refers to a belief in the loss or shrinkage of the primary sex organ among some who thought themselves bewitched; Veith labeled it a sexual delusion. Kraepelin (1921) mentioned shrinkage of the penis among the hypochondriacal delusions in the depressive state of manic-depressive psychosis. Schilder (1950) described two cases of concerns about penile shrinking which he ascribed to pathological distortion of body image. In the most comprehensive literature survey to date, Yap (1965a) collected nineteen cases over a fifteen-year-period and concluded that koro was a depersonalization syndrome that should be classified as an "atypical culture-bound psychogenic psychosis." He and others reported some cases of koro as a symptom of a schizophrenic syndrome (Edwards 1970; Gittleson and Levine 1966; Yap 1965b).

Lapierre (1972), reporting a case of koro in a French Canadian with a frontotemporal brain tumor, acknowledged the importance of cultural factors in the development of the syndrome but suggested "the possibility of a psychogenic localized depersonalization, such as a postoperative stress phenomenon." Yap (1965a) emphasized that his series of patients were not precipitated into illness by acute stress, which he thought often produced depersonalization, but that the partial depersonalization in koro was "specially structured and brought into being by particular cultural beliefs and expectations." Moreover, he did not consider the conviction of penile retraction itself evidence of a loss of touch with reality or a delusion because he thought the conviction is based only on partial depersonalization—a perceptual distortion of proprioceptive penile impulses—and is reinforced by "a folk belief in the reality of a possibly dangerous koro illness." To Yap, the limited insight of koro patients into their condition and the absence of a general disturbance of affective responsiveness differentiate this syndrome from ordinary states of depersonalization. In general, the literature recognizes the interaction of cultural, social, and psychodynamic factors in predisposed personalities.

Case Report

K, a thirteen-year-old, white Roman Catholic eighth grader, was referred by a pediatrician because of psychotic-like episodes over the previous six months. These episodes were characterized by extreme anxiety and agitation, nightmares with frequent nocturnal awakenings, a fear of dying, and an inability to fall asleep because of a dread that his penis was shrinking and disappearing. He touched his penis repeatedly to assure himself of its integrity, making several trips, each two to three hours long, to the toilet for an added visual check and to hold his penis. In the last month K complained of a choking sensation associated with a difficulty in swallowing and threatened his mother with jumping from a window of their second-story apartment, an attempt he tried a year earlier. A neurological evaluation just prior to psychiatric referral, including the EEG and CAT scan, was negative.

K's thirty-year-old beautician mother had an uncomplicated pregnancy and birth. Six months later she divorced K's father, a heavy drinker. Except for a bilateral herniorrhaphy at one year, K's early development was unremarkable. Mother remarried when K was four, and from the age of five K was bothered nightly by sleep awakenings, also a childhood problem of mother. School

behavior and relationships were as tempestuous as his relationships with his older brother and stepfather, and K fought
frequently with other children, his anger escalating to the point of
smashing windows, swearing at teachers, and, once, throwing a
chair.

K got along fairly well with his younger eight-year-old stepbrother, with whom he shared a room. The heavy-drinking, wife-
abusing stepfather—an admitted victim of child abuse—rejected
K. This contrasted with stepfather's extremely friendly relationship with K's older brother, who began two years earlier to constantly bait K with accusations of "fag," "gay," "homosexual,"
and "crazy," inciting K to verbal and physical retaliation and a
feeling of wanting to "kill or hurt people."

K confided to his mother that often when he was scared his
penis became numb and he thought it would disappear. During the
psychiatric evaluation he told a story of being hit in the genital area
in a fight with another boy while playing football. On returning
home he told the incident to his brother who said, "Why don't you
go and kill him?" A few days later K experienced numbness of his
penis, felt that it was shrinking, and went to the toilet to see if it
was still there. He also confided to the evaluator (P. A. R.) that at
school, a few hours earlier, he became very anxious that the insect
the class was studying might die, a subject that disturbed him.
Moreover, on several occasions, he told his mother he was afraid
of dying, saying it was because they were discussing the subject in
school. His tremulous awakenings from nightmares evoked
brother's hostile teasing that he risked dying if he fell out of bed, a
prospect K took seriously. Similarly, his mother frightened him
into believing he risked being drawn into the mirror that he used to
inspect his penis. K's year earlier attempt to jump from the apartment window was precipitated by his mother's threat to throw him
out of the window after finding him fondling his younger brother's
penis.

K's biological father remarried and has two young children. K
reported that one of his legs was injured in war. The father phones
occasionally, making unkept promises to visit his children. His
prolonged absence has aroused intense yearning in K, who as-
cribes his absence to his father's irregular working hours at a bar.
Notwithstanding his fear of his stepfather's alcohol-precipitated assaults on his mother, and despite his feelings of being rejected by

him, K wishes his stepfather would give him his surname, expressing dislike for his own.

Though initially hesitant, wringing his hands, fidgeting throughout the diagnostic interview, and speaking with a tremulous voice, K willingly described his feelings and the family environment. He repeatedly assured the interviewer that he was not homosexual and enthusiastically welcomed the opportunity to discuss his problems further in individual sessions.

Failing to enlist the stepfather's involvement, the therapist saw the mother alone. She was told of K's identification with and concern about his stepfather's aggressive behavior and that she would have to help her spouse set limits for the eldest boy and for himself.

In the next individual session K said his brother had ceased baiting him. K's nightmares had abated and his sleep had improved, though his fear of dying or becoming ill and his concern that his penis was shrinking remained. Though unable to explain it, he said his anxiety had diminished since talking with the therapist. Moreover, he felt better about himself since his brother stopped picking on him. At a brief meeting with the mother at the end of this session, the therapist expressed concern for mother's safety and the need to control her spouse's assaults if her children were going to be helped. In the individual sessions that followed, K expressed guilt about masturbating and fear that he would die or go crazy because of it. The therapist's assurances that masturbation was normal and innocuous and that he did not risk death from falling out of bed or looking into a mirror greatly relieved his anxiety.

Following some canceled appointments, the mother and three children were seen jointly over several sporadic sessions. In the first family session the children, including the youngest, described sadistic teasing among themselves. The therapist acknowledged to them that although sibling rivalry was commonplace, their behavior toward one another was destructive and was a cause of nightmares in K and the youngest. She confronted the mother about her passive, helpless attitude and urged her to enlist her husband's support in jointly controlling the children. Toward the session's end the children spoke about the assaults on their mother and began to cry as they expressed feelings of helplessness and anger toward the stepfather. In the second family session, after several

cancellations, the therapist suggested that the mother acknowledge the children's age differences by setting differential limits
around bedtimes and allowances. In an aside to the mother, she
reiterated the need to get the spouse into marital counseling and
emphasized that both parents' absences, due to long working
hours, gave the eldest boy leeway to express sadistic behavior as
an outgrowth of his identification with the stepfather. In the third
family conference the children fidgeted less, fought less, and mod-
erated their name-calling language. K appeared calmer and said he
was less fearful and no longer having nightmares.

During the subsequent two-month hiatus created by cancellations, the mother related by phone that the children were better. In
the fourth conjoint session the children appeared much calmer and
fought less. However, the eldest boy was breaking into cars and
his case was pending in court. The final family session demonstrated marked progress. Cessation of the stepfather's and
brother's attacks on K was associated with normal sleep, disappearance of fear, marked reduction in violent behavior, and the
disappearance of K's concern about his penis. Improvement was
stable on one-year follow-up.

Discussion

To our knowledge, this is the youngest case of koro response described in the literature. The case illustrates an interaction encompassing social beliefs, sexual myths, major family-induced stressors,
and a critical developmental life stage. Early adolescent concerns with
self-differentiation, sexuality, and controlling aggressive impulses
reached crisis level in K. Identity confusion was exacerbated by sibling
taunts of homosexuality and by ambivalent identifications with his
father and stepfather.

Given the level of verbal and physical aggression pervading the
household and his anger toward his ambivalently regarded father,
stepfather, and older brother, we infer that K experienced guilt from
the unacceptable aggressive impulses engendered. Probably he was
unconsciously angry at his mother, who was helpless to protect him but
did threaten and punish him. Much of his anger was displaced onto
peers and authority figures at school. K felt guilty about his sexual
impulses and behavior; he admitted as much about his masturbation
and tried to jump from the apartment window when shamed and

threatened by his mother for fondling his younger brother's penis. During treatment K acknowledged feeling bad about himself, and he experienced a marked rise in self-esteem when the therapist was able to induce the family to ameliorate their attacks on him and each other. In fact, that outcome and the therapist's assurances that his masturbatory concern and concern about dissolution into the mirror were unfounded brought a rapid and stable cessation of symptoms.

Immature mechanisms of defense are common in adolescence. Vaillant (1977) concluded from his analysis of the data from the Grant Study members at thirty-year follow-up that most showed immature mechanisms during adolescence. He found these immature mechanisms to be "dynamic modes of adaptation and not simply a rigid armor that deforms the personality." In our judgment, this case of koro response demonstrates in larval form the immature mechanism of hypochondriasis, not depersonalization. Unlike depersonalization, K was not keenly aware of the disturbance in his reality sense, evidenced by his conviction of penile shrinkage and disappearance. Yap (1965a) observed lack of insight in his series but explained it as due to reinforcement from a folk belief, a factor not present in our case. Notwithstanding an outbreak of epidemic koro in Singapore (Mun 1968), the typical syndrome is rather rare (Lehmann 1975). This rarity indicates that this folk belief (with a castration anxiety theme) is neither a predisposing nor a precipitating factor in koro, but a socially acceptable mode for expressing deep, individual castration anxiety in a larval form of hypochondriasis. K's symptoms and the absence of psychotic thought processes or major affective illness militate against labeling his conviction a delusion. Nemiah (1975), discussing hypochondriacal neurosis, notes that the fixity and intensity of somatic preoccupation often make the "line between anxious concern and delusional conviction seem very thin indeed, and one often finds it difficult to determine the degree to which their reality testing remains intact."

This case showed some of the behavioral characteristics of hypochondriasis, with some significant departures (Nemiah 1975; Yap 1965a). Though K presented his complaints in detail and with some pressure of speech, the clinical encounter was not a monologue; he listened and responded to the interviewer. K showed the characteristic worry, anxiety, and concern about his symptoms, but, unlike the typical hypochondriacal patient, he spontaneously spoke of his painful human relationships, activities, and feelings unconnected with his somatic preoccupations. His penile numbness, which occurred with intense fear, fits observations of hypochondriacal concern arising from physiological sensations overlooked or unobserved by the normal person. A variety of psychological stresses have been noted to precede the onset of such symptoms (Yap 1965a). Contrasted with the typical patient, K did not use medical jargon, complain on the smallest pretext, insist on endless examinations, or arouse feelings of frustration and resentment. K's response to therapy also contrasted with the refractoriness to treatment of such patients.

This case illustrates symptoms beyond the experience of penile shrinkage: K dreaded that his penis would disappear. Although K did not mention penile retraction into the abdomen or a fatal consequence of penile disappearance, he was preoccupied with a fear of dying. Some would consider this a case of koro pattern, reserving the term "koro" only for cases showing a belief in penile disappearance into the abdomen with a fatal outcome. The folk belief of so-called classical koro has heuristic value in that it facilitates an overt expression of castration anxiety, which in occidental cultures is covert, expressed in neurotic symptoms, or acted out. We think more would be gained from viewing this syndrome from a psychodynamic perspective than from a phenomenological one. We think this case is in the borderland between koro pattern and true koro.

Conclusions

This adolescent demonstrates many of the elements implicated in current theoretical formulations of the psychodynamics of hypochondriasis. This symptom can be used to deal with anger, unmet dependency needs, and guilt over aggressive and sexual impulses, and to protect against low self-esteem by substituting an image of self as ill or physically defective in place of one as a worthless person. Moreover, K's ambivalent relationship with both male adults allows one to postulate an identification with his father's injured leg that produced penile symptoms, or that he introjected the anticipated castrating aspects of his stepfather's violent behavior.

We think that the massive family-induced stressors of rejection, verbal and physical attack, and the absence of maternal succor produced surging emotions of fear, anger, and depressive affect. The physiological penile sensations produced by fear (and possibly other dysphoric emotions) triggered the patient's conviction of penile shrinkage, abetted by castration anxiety from the overt violence in the household and

K's unconscious anticipation of retaliation by the stepfather for K's aggressive fantasies. Elucidation of the actual dynamics of this case would require extensive exploration in a prolonged therapeutic intervention. However, the outcome of this case adds a note of optimism to the treatment of a larval form of hypochondriasis.

REFERENCES

Brero, P. C. J. van. 1897. Koro, eine eigenthumliche Zwangsvorstellung. *Allgemeine Zeitschrift fur Psychiatrie und Psychisch-Gerichliche Medicin* 53:569–573.

Devereaux, G. 1954. Primitive genital mutilations in a neurotic's dream. *Journal of the American Psychoanalytic Association* 2:484–492.

Edwards, J. G. 1970. The koro pattern of depersonalization in an American schizophrenic patient. *American Journal of Psychiatry* 126:1171–1173.

Gittleson, N. L., and Levine, S. 1966. Subjective ideas of sexual changes in male schizophrenics. *British Journal of Psychiatry* 112:779–782.

Gwee, A. L. 1968. Koro—its origin and nature as a disease entity. *Singapore Medical Journal* 9(1):3–5.

Kenyon, F. E. 1964. Hypochondriasis: a clinical study. *British Journal of Psychiatry* 110:478–488.

Kraepelin, E. 1921. *Manic-Depressive Insanity and Paranoia.* Edinburgh: Livingston.

Lapierre, Y. D. 1972. Koro in a French Canadian. *Journal of the Canadian Psychiatric Association* 17:333–334.

Lehmann, H. E. 1975. Unusual psychiatric disorders and atypical psychoses. In A. M. Freedman, H. I. Kaplan, and B. J. Sadock, eds. *Comprehensive Textbook of Psychiatry/II.* Baltimore: Williams & Wilkins.

Mun, C. T. 1968. Epidemic koro in Singapore. *British Medical Journal* 1:640–641.

Nemiah, J. C. 1975. Hypochondriacal neurosis. In A. M. Freedman, H. I. Kaplan, and B. J. Sadock, eds. *Comprehensive Textbook of Psychiatry/II.* Baltimore: Williams & Wilkins.

Rin, H. 1963. Koro: a consideration on Chinese concepts of illness and case illustrations. *Transcultural Psychiatry Research* 15:23–30.

Schilder, P. 1950. *The Image and Appearance of the Human Body*. New York: International Universities Press.

Vaillant, G. E. 1977. *Adaptation to Life*. Boston: Little, Brown.

Veith, I. 1975. The Far East, reflections on the psychological foundations. In J. G. Howells, ed. *World History of Psychiatry*. New York: Brunner/Mazel.

Yap, P. M. 1965a. Koro—a culture-bound depersonalization syndrome. *British Journal of Psychiatry* 111:43–50.

Yap, P. M. 1965b. Koro in a Briton. *British Journal of Psychiatry* 111:774–775.

THE AUTHORS

ALAN APTER is Assistant Professor of Psychiatry, Tel-Aviv University, Israel.

NANCY AUGER is Clinical Nursing Supervisor, McLean Hospital, Belmont, Massachusetts.

F. DAVID BARNHART is Research Sociologist, Timberlawn Psychiatric Research Foundation, Dallas.

THOMAS BOND is Instructor in Psychiatry, Harvard Medical School, and Associate Psychiatrist, McLean Hospital, Belmont, Massachusetts.

GABRIELLE CARLSON is Assistant Professor of Child Psychiatry, University of California at Los Angeles Center for the Health Sciences.

REGINA C. CASPER is Associate Professor of Psychiatry, Abraham Lincoln Medical School, University of Illinois, and Associate Director of Research, Illinois State Psychiatric Institute, Chicago.

PETER T. CHORAS is Instructor in Psychiatry, Harvard Medical School, and Associate Psychiatrist, McLean Hospital, Belmont, Massachusetts.

JACINTA LU COSTELLO is Research Assistant, The Masterson Group, New York.

GLENN CURTISS is Research Scientist, Adolescent Program and Tri-Agency Adolescent Services, Illinois State Psychiatric Institute, Chicago.

LEON CYTRYN is Clinical Professor of Psychiatry, George Washington School of Medicine, and Staff Psychiatrist, Unit on Childhood Mental Illness of the Biological Psychiatry Branch and the Laboratory of Developmental Psychology, National Institute of Mental Health.

PAOLO DECINA is Director, Lithium Clinic, New York State Psychiatric Institute.

AARON A. ESMAN is Professor of Clinical Psychiatry, Cornell University Medical College, and Faculty Member, New York Psychoanalytic Institute.

SUSAN FARBER is Assistant Professor of Clinical Psychology, New York University.

SHERMAN C. FEINSTEIN is Clinical Professor of Child Psychiatry, Pritzker School of Medicine, University of Chicago, and Director, Child Psychiatry Research, Michael Reese Hospital and Medical Center. He is Coordinating Editor of this volume.

RONALD FIEVE is Professor of Psychiatry, Columbia University College of Physicians and Surgeons, New York.

LOIS T. FLAHERTY is Assistant Professor and Director of Training, Division of Child and Adolescent Psychiatry, University of Maryland, Instructor in Child Psychiatry and Pediatrics, Johns Hopkins University School of Medicine, and Director, Child and Adolescent Services, Walter P. Carter Community Mental Health and Retardation Center of the State of Maryland, Baltimore.

SELMA FRAIBERG (deceased) was Professor of Child Psychoanalysis and Director of Infant-Parent Program, University of California, San Francisco. She was the 1981 recipient of the William A. Schonfeld Distinguished Service Award.

JUDITH A. FREEDMAN is Staff Social Worker, Institute of Contemporary Psychotherapy, New York.

MARGARET GARGAN is a graduate student in clinical psychology, New York University.

534

JOHN T. GOSSETT is Associate Director of Timberlawn Psychiatric Research Foundation, and Director, Department of Psychology, Timberlawn Psychiatric Hospital, Dallas.

HELENE COOPER JACKSON is a Doctoral Fellow, Smith College School for Social Work, and Staff Clinical Social Worker, Veterans Administration Mental Hygiene Unit, Boston.

EUGENE H. KAPLAN is Associate Professor of Clinical Psychiatry, State University of New York at Stony Brook, and Adjunct Associate Professor of Clinical Psychiatry, Cornell University Medical College, New York.

CLARICE J. KESTENBAUM is Clinical Professor of Psychiatry, Columbia University, and Director, Child and Adolescent Psychiatry Division, St. Luke's–Roosevelt Hospital Center, New York.

JONATHAN KOLB is Lecturer on Psychiatry, Harvard Medical School, and Associate Psychiatrist, McLean Hospital, Belmont, Massachusetts.

LEON KRON is Assistant Director, Child and Adolescent Psychiatry Division, St. Luke's–Roosevelt Hospital Center, New York.

MARY C. LAMIA is Clinical Supervisor, Department of Psychiatry, Children's Hospital of San Francisco.

MARTINE LAMOUR is a Fellow, Biological Psychiatry Branch and the Laboratory of Developmental Psychology, National Institute of Mental Health.

SAUL V. LEVINE is Professor of Psychiatry, University of Toronto, and Head, Department of Psychiatry, Sunnybrook Hospital, Toronto.

MELVIN LEWIS is Professor of Pediatrics and Psychiatry, Yale Child Study Center, Yale University School of Medicine, New Haven, Connecticut.

JOSEPH D. LICHTENBERG is on the Faculty, Washington Psychoanalytic Institute and the Baltimore–District of Columbia Institute for Psychoanalysis.

ELLEN LOCKE is Social Worker, Adolescent Program and Tri-Agency Adolescent Services, Illinois State Psychiatric Institute, Chicago.

WILLIAM S. LOGAN is Psychiatry Medical Officer, United States Medical Center for Federal Prisons, Springfield, Missouri.

WILLIAM V. LULOW (deceased) was Assistant Clinical Professor of Psychology, Cornell Medical College, and Assistant Director, The Masterson Group, New York.

DONALD H. MC KNEW, JR., is Clinical Associate Professor of Psychiatry, George Washington School of Medicine, and Staff Psychiatrist, Unit on Childhood Mental Illness of the Biological Psychiatry Branch and the Laboratory of Developmental Psychology, National Institute of Mental Health.

SIDNEY MALITZ is Professor of Clinical Psychiatry and Acting Chairman, Department of Psychiatry, College of Physicians and Surgeons, Columbia University, and Acting Director, New York State Psychiatric Institute.

RICHARD C. MAROHN is Associate Professor of Psychiatry, Rush Medical College, and Director, Adolescent Program and Tri-Agency Adolescent Services, Illinois State Psychiatric Institute, Chicago.

A. DAMIEN MARTIN is Associate Professor, New York University, and Founding Member of the Institute for the Protection of Lesbian and Gay Youth.

JAMES F. MASTERSON is Director, The Masterson Group, and Director, The Character Disorder Foundation, New York.

HYMAN MUSLIN is Professor of Psychiatry, University of Illinois School of Medicine, Chicago.

SOL NICHTERN is Assistant Clinical Professor of Psychiatry, New York Medical College, and Director of Psychiatric Services, Jewish Child Care Association.

JACQUELINE OLDS is Instructor in Clinical Psychiatry, Harvard Medical School, and Assistant Attending Psychiatrist, McLean Hospital, Belmont, Massachusetts.

MICHELLE RODEN is a student at Rice University, Houston, Texas.

RUDOLPH G. RODEN is Associate Professor of Psychiatry and Behavioral Sciences, the University of Texas Medical Branch, Galveston, and Lecturer, Houston-Galveston Psychoanalytic Institute.

PERIHAN A. ROSENTHAL is Associate Professor of Psychiatry and Pediatrics, University of Massachusetts School of Medicine, Worcester.

RONALD ROSENTHAL is Director, Research and Evaluation Section, Adolescent Program and Tri-Agency Adolescent Services, Illinois State Psychiatric Institute, Chicago.

STUART ROSENTHAL is Associate Clinical Professor of Psychiatry, Tufts University School of Medicine, and Clinical Instructor of Psychiatry, Harvard Medical School, Boston.

PAUL G. ROSSMAN is Assistant Professor of Psychiatry, University of New Mexico Medical School, and Medical Director, New Mexico Children's Psychiatric Center.

HAROLD A. SACKEIM is Associate Profess or Psychology, New York University, Research Scientist, Department of Biological Psychiatry, New York State Psychiatric Institute, and Lecturer in Psychiatry, College of Physicians and Surgeons, Columbia University.

EDWARD R. SHAPIRO is Assistant Clinical Professor of Psychiatry, Harvard Medical School, and Associate Psychiatrist, McLean Hospital, Belmont, Massachusetts.

JON A. SHAW is Professor of Psychiatry and Vice-Chairman, Department of Psychiatry, Uniformed Services University of the Health Sciences, Clinical Associate Professor, Georgetown University, and Chief, Department of Psychiatry, Walter Reed Army Medical Center, Washington, D.C.

JOYCE D. SHIELDS is Assistant Clinical Professor of Psychiatric Nursing, Boston University, and Clinical Specialist in Psychiatric Nursing, McLean Hospital, Belmont, Massachusetts.

ADRIAN SONDHEIMER is Clinical Assistant Professor of Psychiatry and Coordinator of Child Psychiatry Training, University of Medicine and Dentistry of New Jersey, New Jersey Medical School, Newark.

MICHAEL STROBER is Assistant Professor of Medical Psychology, School of Medicine, University of California at Los Angeles.

LEVON D. TASHJIAN is Assistant Professor of Clinical Psychiatry, University of Pennsylvania, and Director, Adult Program and University Services, Horsham Clinic, Ambler, Pennsylvania.

ERNEST S. WOLF is Assistant Professor of Psychiatry, Northwestern University, and Training and Supervising Analyst, Chicago Institute for Psychoanalysis.

538

CONTENTS OF VOLUMES I–IX

NAME INDEX

557

SUBJECT INDEX